Autism Spectrum Disorders in Adults

Bernardo Barahona Corrêa
Rutger-Jan van der Gaag
Editors

Autism Spectrum Disorders in Adults

Springer

Editors
Bernardo Barahona Corrêa
Department of Psychiatry and Mental Health
NOVA Medical School
Lisbon
Portugal

Rutger-Jan van der Gaag
Child and Adolescent Psychiatry
University Medical Centre Nijmegen
St. Radboud
Nijmegen
The Netherlands

ISBN 978-3-319-82642-4 ISBN 978-3-319-42713-3 (eBook)
DOI 10.1007/978-3-319-42713-3

Softcover reprint of the hardcover 1st edition 2017

Printed on acid-free paper

This Springer imprint is published by Springer Nature
The registered company is Springer International Publishing AG
The registered company address is: Gewerbestrasse 11, 6330 Cham, Switzerland

Foreword

When I was invited to write the introduction for this book, my son was 15. The invitation made me think about what my life would be when my son reached his adulthood. It made me speculate about the differences in the lives of adults with autism.

Children with autism grow into adults with autism. There is no other way. It is up to us to make the transition as easy as possible, to prepare these children for their lives as adults to the best of our abilities. Just like any parent or relative of any child or teenager would do.

I intend to write about my personal experience, my road, my understanding, and my view of the future. And at this point, I can say that my experience has been amazing. No doubt, it has been difficult and demanding, requiring hard work every single day, not short of occasional emotional trials. Nevertheless, all in all, it has been truly amazing.

In the initial stage, the primary focus of the parents of children with autism is on teaching particular skills – to speak, to read and write, and to understand the social norms and behavioral models and must "dos" and "don'ts." Our task is not to change our children in the hope to make them become "ordinary citizens," but to try to explain the model of the society they live in and facilitate the child's adaptation to it. It is our task to teach the child to follow certain social norms, thus becoming a part of the society. This, of course, also requires society's understanding and readiness to interact and cooperate.

We have to deal with numerous challenges, such as how to prevent the aggression fits, how to best explain the planned events, and how to give adequate warnings on unforeseen circumstances. As years go by, we find appropriate solutions. We teach our children, and we learn and grow ourselves in the process. Later on, we focus on issues such as further education, employment, and establishing family. Yet, the main driving force of our actions is our desire to ensure that our children are happy, as simple as that. And autism is not an obstacle either to this desire or to its fulfillment. As for any parent, my child's happiness is the main goal of my life.

Happiness can mean many different things for different people. A good job, or a job in general, or certain opportunities in life are certainly not the most important preconditions for happiness. It may not be even good health. I will not try to find the answer to the philosophical question "What is happiness?" I will simply tell the story of my amazing life experience with my son Jānis.

We can assume that parents know when their child is happy: when he is joyful, satisfied, interested, calm, and cooperative. Even in the case I could receive a verbal response from my son, I doubt if he was able to reply to the question "Are you happy?" Thus, it makes no difference if the child can or cannot speak or whether or not he is autistic.

Autism opens up many new opportunities that we might miss if we did not have a child with autism. Of course, there are many rules we should follow regarding an autistic member of a family, but do we not do the same with any other person, child, or a choice that we make? I want to emphasize that while autism imposes some limitations, it simultaneously offers a variety of opportunities. What is important is the ability to see and seize the opportunities. It is both my experience and my conviction. I regard my son's autism as the big opportunity of my life to make new discoveries, to learn, and to gain new knowledge and new experience.

Thanks to my son, I have learned much not only about autism but the world in general. In the beginning of the 2000s, the information on autism was scarce in Latvia; I had to look for it beyond the borders of my country, in other countries, other languages, books, and in the Internet. I realized that my son is not the only child with autism and that there are many other people in a similar situation. The difference lies in the fact that in a number of countries, there are good support systems in place and people with autism who live in those countries lead dignified lives as full-fledged members of society. As this was not the case in Latvia at the time, this information and knowledge served as an impetus to work toward a better future for people with autism in Latvia, in cooperation with teachers, medical specialists, psychologists, speech therapists, and, most of all, parents.

In 2006, we founded the *Latvian Autism Society* and started working on establishing contacts with similar organizations abroad, later becoming also a member of the *Autism Europe* organization. We also collected information on Latvian specialists in various fields providing assistance to people with autism and their families.

My son has helped me to discover many new opportunities just because of his autism. Despite the fact that he is incapable of performing many activities and functions, such as staying home alone, getting to school by himself, or using public transportation autonomously, he has a number of talents that need to be recognized and developed. I have discovered many of them, but, I am sure, there are more.

Many of my own achievements in life I attribute to my son. For 17 years, I have established a successful career as a diplomat, having become also Ambassador Extraordinary and Plenipotentiary of Latvia. Thanks to my son, I have developed stronger self-discipline, planning skills, ability to foresee extraordinary situations, and quick reaction skills. Being in a management position, I can make good use of my ability to focus on the "big picture," not wasting time on minor and insignificant details, to overcome obstacles and advance toward the goal, and to make crucial decisions. It was early in my life that I came to realize that there is no use crying over the things I lack in life; instead, I should appreciate and be grateful for the things I do have. And there are so many of those.

There is a stereotypical opinion that it is extremely difficult for people with autism to change the environment and adapt to new people, customs, and rhythms of everyday life. It was because of this opinion that I could not make a decision in favor of taking up a diplomatic posting abroad, which is an integral part of a diplomat's life. After my very first posting in Germany, I spent the following 13 years working at the Ministry of Foreign Affairs in Riga. Now I know that there are no accidents in life, as the long years spent in Riga finally resulted in the wonderful opportunity to have a posting in Lisbon, as the Ambassador of Latvia to Portugal.

It was no coincidence either that in 2010, at the European IX Autism Conference in Catania, I met *Mrs. Isabel Cottinelli Telmo*, the President of the Portuguese Autism Federation. We talked about the various opportunities and challenges that my moving to Portugal might entail. I took the decision, relying on my intuition that has usually proved to be the best advisor in similar situations.

Looking back, I can say in full confidence that the four years spent in Portugal have had a very favorable impact on my son's development. The agreeable climate and positive atmosphere and, most importantly, the people we met – Portuguese teachers, medical specialists, sports coaches, friends, and acquaintances – have all contributed to the development of my son's artistic talent. Sometimes it was even difficult to meet the high demand for the ceramic pieces of art that my son and his classmates were making. The awards received in several drawing competitions and two very successful photo and drawing exhibitions in the Portuguese Parliament and at *Champalimaud Foundation Centre for the Unknown* are just a few other testimonies of the artistic talents of people with autism.

In Portugal, as in most European countries, there is still room for improvement in many areas regarding the quality of life of people with autism. Nevertheless, our stay in Portugal offered an amazing experience for my son, especially, in acquiring new skills, such as to read and write, understand and articulate in Portuguese, and even horse-riding. Jānis had done equine therapy before in Latvia, but in Portugal, the land of horse-riders, he learned to manage a horse by himself. It brought my son a lot of joy and unforgettable emotions.

But Jānis' greatest attraction is water. For three years, he regularly attended swimming lessons within the framework of the program offered by an ONG that specializes in adapting a variety of sport activities and modalities to individuals with a motor deficiency or any other form of special need (*Associação de Actividade Motora Adaptada, A.A.M.A.*). During this time, he learned various swimming styles and also made new friends. The young and enthusiastic swimming teachers became good friends of Jānis, and it was difficult to part with them upon leaving Portugal.

Since his childhood, Jānis has enjoyed music, dance, and rhythm. In Portugal, he became a member of a jazz band supported by the country's national autism association (*Associação Portuguesa para as Perturbações do Desenvolvimento e Autismo*), trying out various instruments and finally settling for the drums. While in Lisbon, we had the opportunity to enjoy a lot of unforgettable concerts by the band. Now, back in Latvia, the CD of the band's songs is one of the favorites in Jānis' CD collection.

Our weekly long walks on the shore of the Atlantic Ocean, with a view to Cabo de Roca, the westernmost promontory of the European continent, was another source of energy not only for the body but also for the soul.

Indeed, Portugal and the Portuguese people we were lucky to meet and cooperate with did their utmost for Janis to return to Latvia with new invaluable experience, knowledge, skills, and goals in life.

I touched upon just a few of the many opportunities we had and made use of while in Lisbon. There are many others, and they may differ for everybody. The most powerful point in Janis' story is that it shows how the often repeated, stereotypical belief that people with autism are unable to benefit from profound environmental changes such as migrating to a whole new and different country is simply wrong. Moving abroad offered Janis a host of enriching opportunities which he was able to take advantage of, despite his autistic disorder. Now, back in Latvia, we will continue working on gaining new experiences, brought about by new activities, hobbies, traditions, and, most importantly, new people – teachers, speech therapists, medical specialists, and others – all working toward the common goal of improving the life for people with autism in Latvia, Europe, and in the world.

The Autism Society of Latvia, Riga, Latvia Ambassador Alda Vanaga

Contents

Autism Spectrum Disorders: Developmental History of a Concept

1

Rutger-Jan van der Gaag

The term autism was first introduced in 1908. The famous Swiss psychiatrist Eugen Bleuler used the term autism to describe the very aloof and withdrawn condition of some patients with what he called schizophrenia. Leo Kanner (1943), when describing eleven children with "an autistic disturbance of affective contact", clearly had Bleuler's thoughts in mind. Likewise Hans Asperger (1944) called the atypical boys in his study "autistic psychopaths", hereby also alluding to some resemblance with schizophrenia. Despite the fact that "autistic aloofness" does not by far cover the complexity of the pervasive developmental disorder described nowadays as "autism spectrum disorder", the term has become the common way to describe the large range of individuals with a syndrome characterized by impairments of the development of social and communicative reciprocity and a rigid and restricted repertoire of interests and behaviours. In this chapter a historical overview of the development of a concept in psychopathology will be presented.

It may be interesting to note, before entering into the matter, that Bleuler believed that there was a continuum between psychiatric disorders and normality. This is very much in line with the current concept of a broad autism spectrum ranging from severe cases to well-adapted individuals with autistic features bordering what Simon Baron-Cohen would call an *autistic condition* including 5 % of the population.

This chapter aims at giving the reader a stepwise overview of the development of the concept of the condition/disorder currently labelled as "autism spectrum disorder" (ASD) to get a better understanding of what is understood by ASD, what the current issues are both in terms of clinical problems and integration of individuals with ASD in our complex societies and what is at stack in terms of

R.-J. van der Gaag
Radboud University Nijmegen Medical Centre, Nijmegen, The Netherlands
e-mail: r.vandergaag@radboudumc.nl

B. Barahona Corrêa, R.-J. van der Gaag (eds.), *Autism Spectrum Disorders in Adults*, DOI 10.1007/978-3-319-42713-3_1

research. This chapter has no pretention of being exhaustive, and readers interested in more details will find references to solid overviews at the end of this chapter.

1.1 Autism Has Always Been Around as an Evolutionary Trait

Johan Cruyff, a brilliant Dutch soccer player and coach who recently passed away, was well known for his very down to earth pragmatic sayings: one sounded like, "You can only see it when you know about it". This holds true for the condition that we have been calling autism for the past seven decades since the seminal reports in the 1940s of the past century. But that does not mean that the condition since then called autism had not been not around for ages already. Simon Baron-Cohen (2002) refers to autism as the "extreme male brain". If so there must have been good evolutionary reasons why the male brain developed in a different way compared to the female brain. Before going further on the pathway of evolutionary speculation, it is good to note that apart from clear bodily distinctions between males and females, the distribution of psychological and behavioural characteristics is by no means clearly split between sexes but shows a huge overlap.

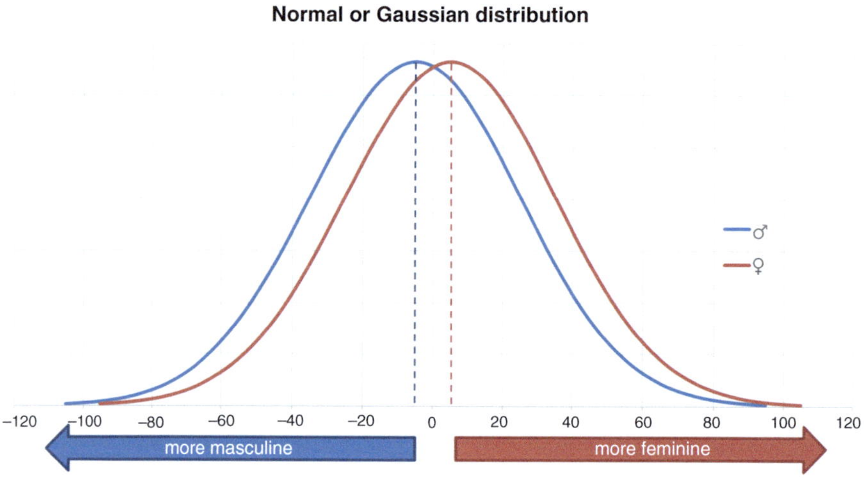

But when it comes to the gross differentiation of the evolution of the male and female brain, the speculation is (Skuse et al. 1997) that the differences are linked to adaptive behaviour. In primitive societies, male and female roles were clearly distinct: females were sedentary and occupied with raising children, preparing food and socializing with other families to ensure a peaceful co-existence. The faculties required for such tasks are empathy (understanding what others mean and intend and feel) and a global way of perceiving situations in order to understand its dynamics and act in consequence. In that sense the pattern of thinking in those women was mostly "analogue", in other words open to different interpretations in the context. In those primitive societies, men were the hunters who went out to gather food and make sure the community was not under threat from other groups or tribes, eager to steel their goods and eventually wives and children. This asked for quite a different set of skills: perseverance, detailed observation (in order to find the trails of their prey and signs of the presence of potential enemies) and a rather digital way of thinking as they had to make quick and clear decisions such as take a left or a right and inhibit all kinds of interferences to be completely focused on their task. As we know, in evolution neither the brightest ones nor the strongest survive but those that can adapt best to the circumstances under which they live. Thus, in those societies warm and socially oriented females and detail-geared perseverant males were favoured and often chosen as mating partners to ensure the survival of the species. This differentiation was of course by no means absolute. As societies evolved, men differentiated to become responsible for law and order, and those "poli(=city)ticians" obviously needed all kinds of qualities earlier more attributed to women, such as awareness of what is happening and a certain social shrewdness to "manipulate" others to reach one's goals. But the earlier described "male traits" of detail-focused and digital thinking were popular in another area, namely, scientific development of tools, agriculture and later culture altogether and science. It goes beyond the scope of this chapter, but it is obvious that from monks to great scientists, men (and women) with autistic traits/"extreme male brains" have contributed enormously to scientific progress and innovation in technology. We are all acutely aware of the fact that no progress in the seminal computer science would have been achieved without the contribution of binary thinking, single-minded (wo)men that invented and still help promote our rapidly expanding digital world. So in many cases "the extreme male brain" seems to (have been) be a definitive asset. Yet we all realize that many of these geniuses were cognitively brilliant but oftentimes socially odd, or strange, call it eccentric, and in many ways different. Some of them were so absorbed by their research and activities that they did not take time to wonder if they were happy. The ones, who did, often felt isolated and miserable.

We are currently able to better understand this evolutionary trait, much better thanks to the tremendous progress that we have made from studying extreme clinical cases.

Those clinical cases raised interest in different parts of the world, and the tribute should be given to Leo Kanner (1943) and Hans Asperger (1944) who nearly simultaneously, without being aware of each other's publications, drew attention to what they both called a clinical syndrome. A clinical syndrome means the co-occurrence of a similar set of symptoms in different individuals. So let us see how they defined their syndromes, which they called "autistic disturbances of affective contact" and "autistic psychopathy", respectively (the word psychopathy should not be read here as the summon of the callous antisocial personality but merely as "psychopathology").

PATHOLOGY

To understand and measure emotional qualities is very difficult. Psychologists and educators have been struggling with that problem for years but we are still unable to measure emotional and personality traits with the exactness with which we can measure intelligence.

—Rose Zeligs in *Glimpses into Child Life**

AUTISTIC DISTURBANCES OF AFFECTIVE CONTACT

By Leo Kanner

SINCE 1938, there have come to our attention a number of children whose condition differs so markedly and uniquely from anything reported so far, that each case merits—and, I hope, will eventually receive—a detailed consideration of its fascinating peculiarities. In this place, the limitations necessarily imposed by space call for a condensed presentation of the case material. For the same reason, photographs have also been omitted. Since none of the children of this group has as yet attained an age beyond 11 years, this must be considered a preliminary report, to be enlarged upon as the patients grow older and further observation of their development is made.

1.2 Autistic Disturbances of Affective Contact (Kanner 1943)

Leo Kanner (1894–1981) was an Austrian psychiatrist who trained in Berlin and Vienna. He immigrated to the USA in the 1920s and was selected to set up the first child psychiatry department at John Hopkins in Baltimore. There he and his team devoted themselves to very scrupulous case histories and trying to discern similarities between different cases to be able to classify them as syndromes. The first case, Donald T, was followed by ten other cases (together eight boys and three girls) that Kanner wrote up for his seminal publication in 1943. What struck him and his team in the first instance was that they were all *good-looking children*, presenting with the same kind of *inability to relate themselves in the ordinary way to people and situations from the beginning of their life*. They seemed completely secluded from the outside in a state of *extreme autistic aloofness*. Another similarity he described was their *failure to assume an anticipatory posture*. Three of them never developed spoken language, whilst the others spoke late and in various peculiar ways: echoing both directly and as so-called delayed echolalia (repeating long sentences by heart but completely out of the context), speaking nonsense words (neologisms), knowing whole chains of related words and nursery rimes and mostly *naming* instead of using language to communicate. Kanner also observed that when they understood what was being said, these children tended to take everything literally. They all had *excellent rote memory*. Intrusions like *loud noises* and *moving objects* terrified them, each one with specific hypersensitivities. They definitely showed *limitations in the variety of spontaneous activities*, time and again engaging in *monotonous repetitious* movements and habits. And these children all seemed governed by *an anxious obsessive desire for the maintenance of sameness*. They had a good *relation with objects*, with which they would engage in exciting activities, such as spinning, leading in many cases to a seemingly *ecstatic fervour* that eyed as "*masturbatory orgastic gratification*". Though they seemed to have *good cognitive potentials* and all had *strikingly intelligent physiognomies* and came from *highly intelligent families*, their outcome was poor, and they seemed to function at a far lower level of intelligence than one would have expected. Kanner thought the condition could have an *innate disturbance*, pointing to an inborn organic cause (both *physical and intellectual*), although in the last paragraph of his article, he also alluded to "coldness in the parents" and the fact that several marriages of the parents were painful failures. Though Kanner did not specify that he thought these parental conditions were the cause of the disturbance in the children, he never really opposed to those who overread the "organic cause" Kanner suggested and strongly pointed to the parents as bearing responsibility for the condition of their kids.

This is the sad part of an incredibly accurate description that still characterizes autism spectrum disorders in their current definitions.

1.3 Boys with Autistic Psychopathy

Nearly at the very same time, Hans Asperger (1906–1980), an Austrian paediatrician from Vienna, published a very similar paper describing the features of four boys (representative of a group of 200 over whom he published later). The paper is less accessible than Kanner's writings for two reasons, the first being that it was written in German and not translated before the 1980s and the second that it starts with a long and interesting but tough reflection on psychopathology and how to classify syndromes. But strikingly, Asperger seems to describe the other side of the same coin. He uses the same term "autistic" for the lack of "social reciprocity" and the boys' "autistic intelligence". To a certain extent, the resemblance is striking: social aloofness, restricted patterns of interest and hyper-focalisation on specific preoccupations of stereotypies and extraordinary skills on a limited scope.

(Aus der Wiener Universitäts-Kinderklinik [Vorstand: Prof. *Franz Hamburger*].)

Die „Autistischen Psychopathen" im Kindesalter[1].

Von

Doz. Dr. Hans Asperger,

Leiter der Heilpädagogischen Abteilung der Klinik.

(Eingegangen am 8. Oktober 1943.)

Problemstellung.

Ordnung und Erkenntnis des Aufbaues der Dinge ist eines der letzten Ziele der Wissenschaft. In der Fülle der Erscheinungen des Lebens, die voller Gegensätze sind, die mit verschwimmenden Grenzen in einander übergehen, sucht der denkende Mensch dadurch einen festen Standpunkt zu finden, daß er den einzelnen Erscheinungen einen Namen gibt, sie abgrenzt gegen die anderen Erscheinungen, Zusammenhänge, Ähnlichkeiten und Gegensätze feststellt, kurz, die Dinge in eine Ordnung, in ein System bringt. Diese Arbeit ist eine wesentliche Voraussetzung des Erkennens.

Die Wissenschaft vom Menschen mußte ähnliche Wege gehen. Nirgendwo aber sind die Schwierigkeiten größer als hier:

Jeder Mensch ist ein einmaliges, unwiederholbares, unteilbares Wesen („In-dividuum"), darum auch letztlich unvergleichbar mit anderen. In jedem Charakter finden sich einander scheinbar widersprechende Züge — gerade aus Gegensätzen und Spannungen lebt ja das Leben.

On the other hand, there are definitive differences: a high, though disharmonic and oddly focussed intelligence, motor clumsiness and high verbal skills lacking pragmatism (yet again not used for communication). But Asperger described other areas that Kanner did not mention or mentioned only briefly. First he pointed at the extremes in emotions (panic and anger) and the terrorizing behaviours these boys showed vis-à-vis their parents in order to have it always their way (a behaviour that parallels the need for sameness in Kanner's autistic children); secondly he was far more explicit in his causal thoughts: he refers to the "erbbiologisches" aspects, meaning that he was strongly convinced that this condition was hereditary as the sons (he only described boys) looked very much like their fathers. However, he was intrigued by the fact that the fathers seemed rather successful in their careers as scientists and engineers and seemed to be just less subject to strong emotional swings and single minded than their offspring. This is despite the fact that what Asperger referred to as "autistische intelligenz" (digital – strictly and extremely logical – rigid in its reasoning) seemed to apply both to the fathers and the sons. Finally, Asperger was far more optimistic about the outcome. Where Kanner complained that most of the patients he described where *dumbed in schools for feeble-minded*, Asperger saw that many of his patients grew over their ill tempers and dictatorial behaviour towards their parents, did well in science and were able to pursue a career in that field.

But as stated earlier, Asperger had hardly any impact abroad until Lorna Wing (1981) (through Uta Frith, who could read German) rediscovered Asperger's work, where she found an adequate description of those patients with autistic features who, in her studies, did not meet Kanner's diagnostic criteria by far.

1.4 Dark Times of Blaming Parents for the Autism in Their Children

Meanwhile, as an unintended consequence of Kanner's allusions to the typology of the parents of his patients as cold and distant, blaming the parents for the autistic condition of their child had been taken up by the dominant stream within psychiatry in those days and especially by psychoanalysts, with a great deal of tragic, unnecessary suffering as a consequence. For nearly two decades, it was strongly put forward that these "refrigerator" mothers should be blamed for the autistic condition of their children. The culmination of this movement was the publication of the book *The Empty Fortress* by Bruno Bettelheim (as late as 1967). For parents these were extremely painful years, not only did they suffer from the dramatic condition of their children, moreover they were overloaded with accusations by those treating their children and felt utterly guilty. Though this ceased in the 1970s in most of the Anglo-Saxon world and the Nordic countries in Europe, the influence of psychoanalysis remain(ed)s very strong in Latin countries in Europe and South America. It is painful because the evidence that the parents are not to blame in causal terms is extremely strong. Firstly, most of the parents with an autistic child also have healthy children, which makes it even more intriguing as to why one should be affected! Secondly, it has become evident that the despair of the parents, perceived as coldness, is not the cause of the autism in their children but, on the contrary, is a consequence of having, and being burdened by, a child who does not at all respond as one should expect, hardly relates, and is extremely difficult to sooth.

1.5 Emergence of a Pragmatic Empirical Approach

The psychoanalytical approach had a great impact and lasted worldwide for nearly two decades. But slowly changes started to occur. Parents united in users-group associations and expressed their discontent with the unfair blaming. A nice illustration was formed by a button in the USA stating "*Madness is hereditary, you get it from your kids*". This was a heartbreaking appeal. It illustrates the immense burden of having a child with autism. On the other hand, it indirectly calls for a different, more scientific approach. And that is what emerged in different ways in the 1960s and 1970s of the twentieth century. Different approaches were favoured, including epidemiology, neurophysiology and genetics. Emerging attention was given also to treatment and guidance approaches, as the intensive psychoanalytical approaches did not seem to bring cure or, at best, produce an improvement that was so slim, which without any intervention development might have had the same result.

Yet in order to study a condition/disease/disorder, it is of great importance to have consensus on how to identify those cases who are targeted in those studies. This was the start of the movement aiming at defining autism as a distinct clinical entity by offering a set of diagnostic criteria. In the UK Mildred Creak's working party (1961) came up with a list of nine criteria to be used as when diagnosing autism or when doing research into this condition. These criteria enabled systematic research such as the first prevalence study on autism by Victor Lotter (1966). This study yielded an estimated prevalence for this condition of 4.5/10.000. Subsequent replications of this study showed that the prevalence worldwide was practically the same, rendering it rather unlikely that autism might be caused by parents' way of bringing up their child, as child-rearing styles vary greatly from one culture to the other.

Tentatively some psychoanalysts started studies into the hypersensitivity of children with autism such as Ritvo and Freeman (see Ritvo and Freeman 1984) at Yale Child Study Centre, where Sally Provence favoured a dual approach to developmental psychopathology.

But in those days, parents who were also health professionals and scientists made the difference. To illustrate this point, let us look into the contributions of Bernard Rimland and Lorna Wing.

Rimland (see Rimland 1968) was triggered by his son's behaviours. Marc Rimland, in later life a talented artist, had a most atypical development. His father attributed this to autism and perceived it as a neurodevelopmental disorder. Leo Kanner himself acknowledged this when he wrote the foreword in Rimland's book *Infantile Autism: The Syndrome and Its Implications for a Neural Theory of Behavior* (1964) that paved the way to more research into the neurological correlates of this intriguing disorder.

Lorna Wing, mother of a daughter with autism and intellectual disability and spouse to John Wing, a well-known expert in the field of schizophrenia, took a very different approach. Together with her Maudsley colleague Judy Gould, she undertook a comprehensive epidemiological study in the London Borough of Camberwell (Wing and Gould 1979). This was an absolutely seminal tipping point in the developmental history of the concept of autism.

The Camberwell Study The initial goal was to replicate the Lotter study by a comprehensive and systematic study of the prevalence of autism in a defined area with approximately 150.000 inhabitants. The results were of great interest especially because of the way Wing and Gould analysed the huge data set in a population of 155.000, including 35.000 children and adolescents, but even more so by the very clear manner in which they reported their results:

- Firstly, they discovered that the prevalence of "autism" as defined by Kanner was in line with Lotter's findings: 4.9 in 10.000. But they found a much larger group adding up to nearly 0.21 % of the population that displayed a number, but not all, of the symptoms described by Kanner. Amongst these they identified cases very similar to those that Asperger had discovered. Thanks to her collaborator Uta Frith, Wing was able to introduce Hans Asperger work to the Anglo-Saxon community: a welcome finding as many clinicians knew these individuals but failed to diagnose them correctly because they were not familiar with Asperger's work.

- Secondly, Wing and Gould clustered the symptoms in different dimensions. The three first, known as the Triad of Wing, still form the basis of the international classification systems to date:
  - Impairment of the quality of social interaction
  - Impairment of the development of reciprocal communication
  - Restricted and repetitive stereotypies and preoccupations
  - (Impaired development of imagination)
- Thirdly, they point to the variety of expression on the different dimensions. For example, on the impairment of the social interaction, the expression ranged from aloof, via passive to what they named "active but odd". And likewise for all the other dimensions, they could show that in individuals with autism, or autism in a broader sense, the presenting symptoms varied greatly both in the way they expressed themselves but also in the way they would change as development progressed.

Thus, Wing and Gould changed our perception of autism profoundly, from a very rare disorder with dramatic impairments to a developmental syndrome with a core group and lesser variants and an evolving clinical picture from early childhood into adulthood with variations both for the better as for the worse as time progresses. Wing (1997) was the first one to take an even broader view, stating that autism was not only a spectrum disorder but that the autistic features were on a continuum ranging from profoundly impaired with mental retardation via bright eccentricity into normality.

This concept of autism as a developmental disorder was strongly supported by reports from the group at Yale Child Study Centre (Cohen, Volkmar, Klin) who in a comprehensive study of cases from 1947 onwards (Dahl et al. 1986) could identify four distinct groups of children with developmental disorders: (1) those with a global retardation; (2) those with classic Kanner autism (with and without learning disability); (3) the autism-related group including the more rigid Asperger group and the group with severe problems in behaviour, emotion and thought regulation multiple complex developmental disorders (McDD); and finally (4) children with specific isolated developmental disorders (motor coordination, language, reading, calculating, etc.).

Lorna Wing's triad, as mentioned above, has from 1980 formed the core triad of impairment criteria for diagnosing autism and related disorders. This recognition of autism as a disorder in its own right led to an explosion of research in autism… but also to a fivefold increase in the prevalence of autism!

In the following paragraphs, we will look into these developments step by step.

1.6 Inclusion of Autism and Pervasive Developmental Disorders in DSM III (1980)

Though the Camberwell study made it clear that "autism" is a very heterogeneous condition, the international classification systems (DSM III and ICD 9) opted for a strictly categorical approach. In 1980 the committee of the American *Diagnostic and Statistical Manual of Mental Disorders* proposed to include "autism" within a broader category they named "pervasive developmental disorder (PDD)" (in contrast with general and specific developmental disorders). The DSM III subdivided the PDD category into five disorders: (1) infantile autism, (2) residual infantile autism, (3) child-onset PDD, (4) residual child-onset PDD, and (5) PDD – not otherwise specified.

This induced a major change in the approach to autism. Well-defined behavioural criteria were very welcome and helped shape sound and broad research. In the following paragraphs, we will review the progress of research along very different pathways to end up with the current situation.

Splitting or Lumping? The greatly regretted Donald Cohen (1940–2001), from Yale Child Study Centre, emphasized that classification systems should, in principle, be heuristic. That is, they should incite research to make them even better and, in the case of pervasive developmental disorders, lead to further exploration of areas that are still unclear. As the approach was mainly categorical, the search was for distinct subgroups that would help to specify the fuzzy areas called "Childhood onset Developmental Disorders" and even more the ill-defined "PDD-NOS" area. Some even at that time, in the late 1980s/early 1990s, preferred the idea of a continuum ranging from infantile autism to normality via subgroups where the symptoms appeared less severe and finally would fade away into normality (Wing 1997). Others focussed more on describing distinct groups. On the one hand were those who mainly addressed the "aloof" side of the autistic triad as described by Wing and Gould. Obviously, Wing herself favoured Asperger's description to define this group. Asperger's was the term used by Christopher Gillberg and his Swedish group. They published a great number of impressive population-based studies to underscore the face validity of Asperger's concept… with emphasis on the social and motor awkwardness that they eventually also coined as DAMP syndrome (Deficits in Attention, Motor control and Perception). They thus broadened the scope by putting more emphasis on the developmental aspect of the condition than on a static disease category. Interestingly, very similar children and adolescents were well described by Sula Wolff from Edinburgh under the name schizoid children, summarized in a beautiful book as *Loners*. Moving more to the "active but odd" part of the continuum were those who tried to categorize those children with autistic features who were not aloof but eager and boundless in approaching others and also characterized by mood swings, strong affects and thought problems. This group had been described by Scandinavian authors as from 1968 under the label "borderline syndrome in children" (Aarkrog 1981 – Wergeland 1979), but after the apparition of DSM III and the Dahl study on subtyping of developmental disorders, this group received scrupulous scientific attention under different names: Peter Szatmari from Canada published several studies in which the term schizotypal was used, whilst others embraced the concept of multiplex developmental disorders (later multiple complex developmental disorders (McDD)) proposed by Donald Cohen, based on the Dahl et al. study, to describe this group. Different groups studied these patients in depth: Kenneth Towbin et al. (1993) in the USA and Rutger Jan van der Gaag in the Netherlands (1993) and Jonathan Green (1998) in his seminal book on in-patient treatment in childpsychiatry. These studies, though clinically very relevant, were not taken on board in the revisions of DSM and ICD for two possible reasons: they appeared too late (DSM III was already revised by 1987), and they were not in line with the, at that time, generally favoured view that autism and schizophrenia were entirely distinct conditions.

Now why was DSM III revised so quickly? In general one can say that this happened because DSM III was an armchair consensus document that needed empirical evidence. But when it comes to the autism section, more was at hand: It appeared quite rapidly that the proposed categories were not fit for clinical nor for scientific use. Infantile autism had such strict criteria with regard to age of onset and severity of symptoms that many children clinically diagnosed with autism did not meet the criteria. Childhood-onset PDD could only be classified if the onset was after 30 months of age, and atypical autism and PDD-NOS appeared to be indistinct. The DSM-III-R revision into autistic disorder and PDD-NOS dropping of the age of onset criteria and stretching out of the criteria for autistic disorder to a less stringent interpretation of the Wing triad did not help much either. It was rightly criticized for being overinclusive. Yet another move would follow quickly as DSM IV appeared as soon as 1994. Within those 7 years, whilst research was going on to test the validity of the PDD subgroups, the DSM committee took on board three rather randomly chosen subgroups and based the face validity on armchair field trials. Two new subgroups – Rett syndrome (in girls) and disintegrative disorders (formerly Heller's syndrome) – were in fact more neurological than psychiatric. Both had severe regressive characteristics in children who, after a seemingly sound development of 9 months to 3 years, lost speech and motor skills and who, during their regression, could display "autistic" features. But no real reasons existed to assume they had anything in common with autism in essence. The last inclusion was neither a happy one either. Asperger's disorder was introduced in DSM IV as "autism with a normal language development". Quite unfortunate as Asperger had described children with apparently good speech but no language skills in terms of reciprocal communication. Thus, the DSM IV criteria for Asperger were not fit for Asperger's original cases, who in DSM terms would either be diagnosed as autistic disorder or merely PDD-NOS.

But empirical research made it clear that a categorical approach to autism and PDD was the right way to go. So what have these studies revealed thus far?

1.7 Scientific Progress from Different Angles

The movement that led to the publication of DSM III with its theoretical criteria along with an explosion of new techniques in neuroimaging and genetics fostered an incredible amount of empirical research in autism, in various domains.

1.7.1 Findings from Electrophysiology

In the 1970s of the past century, it became possible to measure the arousal levels in experimental conditions through combined measures of skin conductance and heart rate. In the 1980s computer technology enabled filtering out all the noise in the electroencephalogram to analyse the brain's response to external stimuli (evoked response potentials). These studies showed that individuals meeting the criteria for pervasive developmental disorders (from autism to PDD-NOS) have aberrant neurophysiological patterns. Their levels of arousal are either too high or too low to process (social) information correctly. They also appear to process incoming (social) information in a different way; where typical individuals show high responses to novel information and a pattern of habituation when the same information is repeated or encountered, individuals with autism in the broad sense tend to either ignore novelty or respond very intensely. As they do not show normal habituation patterns, the world for them seems new over and over again, making life fraught with anxiety.

These conclusions seem solid, as they were independently reproduced worldwide. At the same time, they raised a fundamental question, namely, if people with autism do in fact perceive the information that is offered to them. This is a pertinent interrogation, since, from the first descriptions by Leo Kanner, gaze aversion has been described as a prominent feature in individuals with autism. Further technical developments led to studies in which gaze patterns of individuals could be monitored by linking eye movements to eye tracking of images perceived on a screen. This lead to a series of seminal studies by Ami Klin (2002) and his team that showed that where typical individuals look at the eyes to appraise the other person's emotions and intentions, people with autism are more inclined to look at moving parts, thus missing essential social information.

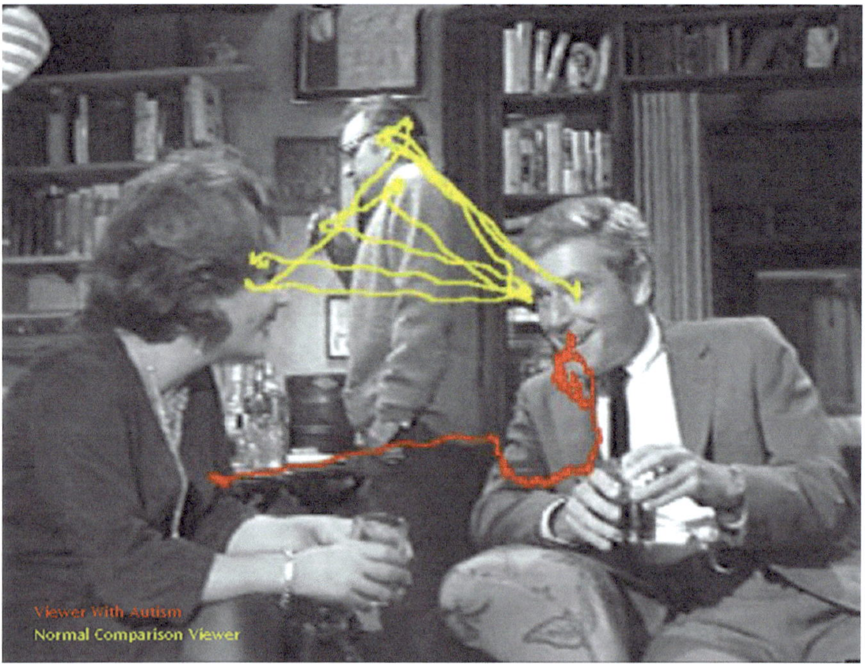

This picture (Klin et al. 2002) clearly illustrates this point: typical individuals (yellow) scan the scene in such a fashion that they look at the interaction between the two individuals on the foreground but also include the third person, clearly showing that they understand that the conversation relates to that third person. Individuals with autism (in this study high functioning college students) clearly miss the point by paying too much attention to mouth movements and clothing.

These information processing findings matched well with the great leap forward made in neuropsychology by groups in the UK and USA, helping greatly to understand why people with autism are so different when it comes to their appraisal of, and reactions to, social situations.

1.7.2 Findings in Neuropsychology

Neuropsychology yielded two important contributions to our understanding of autism. The first is the fact that individuals with autism appear in general to have very disharmonic profiles when it comes to their IQ as measured, for instance, on the classic Wechsler scales. But here again it is more the disharmonic pattern that emerges rather than "one" and the same disharmonic pattern common to all individuals with autism. Roughly speaking individuals with "Kanner-like" autism seem to have higher scores on their performance IQ than on their verbal IQ, whereas individuals with Asperger's tend to have the reverse pattern, namely, high verbal IQ versus low performance IQ (a pattern extensively studied by Rourke (1989) and his team as "nonverbal learning disabilities" but that appears by no means to be specific for autism nor for a subgroup within autism spectrum).

The second contribution refers to more complex information processing related to understanding other individuals and appraising their emotions and intentions. The first series of studies referred to what is commonly called the *theory of mind* (Uta Frith and Francesca Happé 1994). This relates to the development, at an early age, of the child's ability to understand that other people have other perspectives, intentions and motives than oneself. It refers to the individual's capacity to take the other's perspective in order to understand what he/she thinks and why he/she should think this. In a series of well-conducted experiments, it appeared that the development of the theory of mind in individuals with autism is most often delayed and in many cases different. This insight has greatly helped outsiders to better understand why people with autism can so grossly misunderstand others and react so awkwardly in social situations.

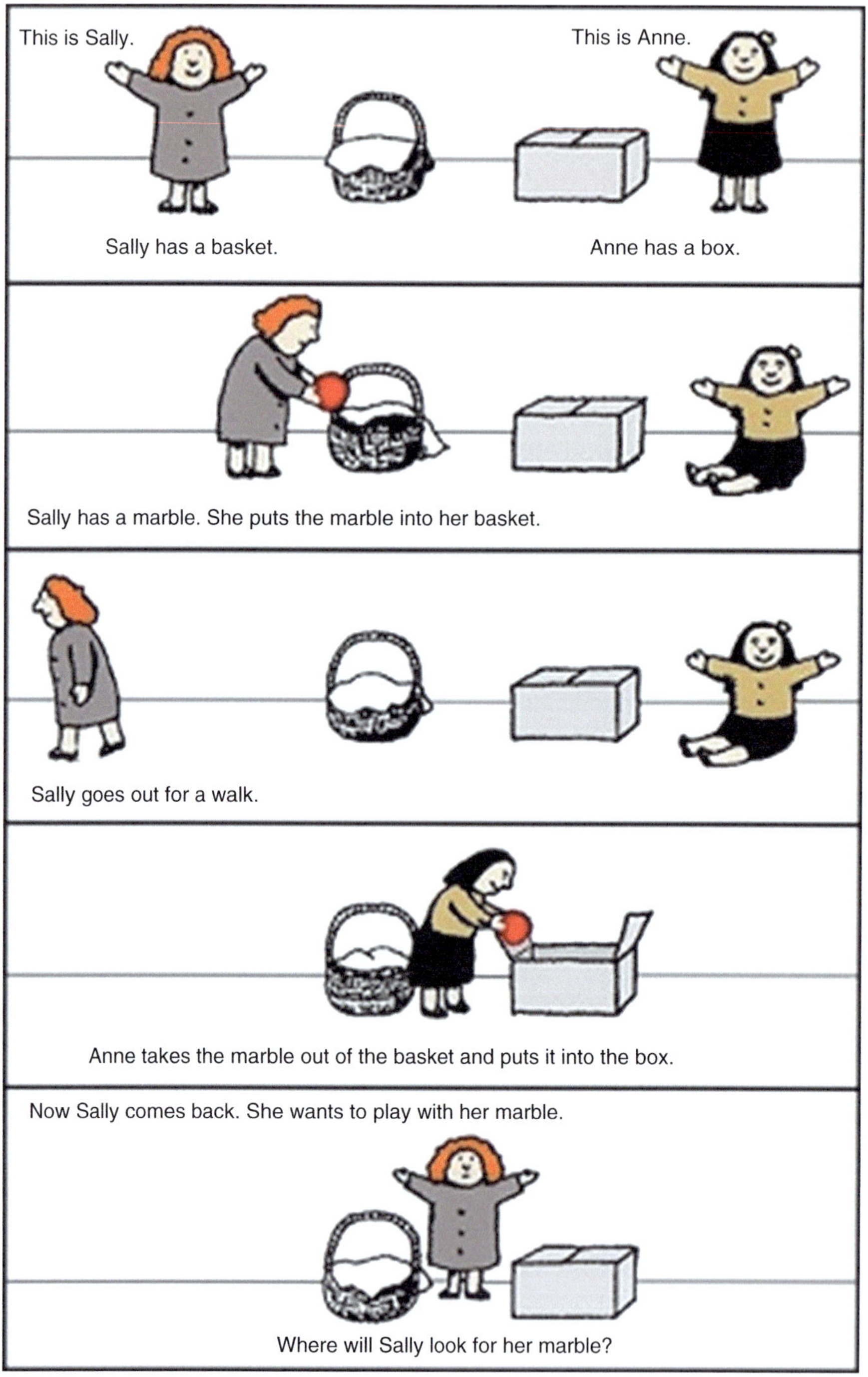
This is Sally.
This is Anne.
Sally has a basket.
Anne has a box.
Sally has a marble. She puts the marble into her basket.
Sally goes out for a walk.
Anne takes the marble out of the basket and puts it into the box.
Now Sally comes back. She wants to play with her marble.
Where will Sally look for her marble?

Along with these studies, it became obvious that individuals with autism lacked a sense of *central coherence.* This relates to one's capacity to focus on relevant clues and ignore irrelevant details. The focus on details was described both by Kanner and Asperger, and neurophysiological studies made it clear that the impaired information processing in individuals with autism implies that they are not able to process well-known information automatically, leading them to focus again and again on details to understand the whole, whereas in typically developing individuals as from the seventh year of life, a global appraisal of a (new) situation makes it possible to orient oneself quickly, details being only processed, if relevant, later. Thus, the finding that a different development of *theory of mind* and *central coherence skills* hampers individuals with autism in their understanding of others, as summarized by Simon Baron-Cohen (1995) as "*mind-blindness*", helps us to understand how people with autism are handicapped by their defective understanding of social situations. The third finding in the field of neuropsychological research was on the complex topic of *executive functioning* (Happé et al. 2006). This refers to the activities within the frontal areas of our brain that help us to choose how to act and then plan and execute our actions in consequence. Here again it appeared that individuals with autism have greater difficulties when it comes to smoothly and flexibly acting and reacting in social circumstances.

Thus, empirically based neuropsychological theories elaborated in the 1980s and 1990s of the past century have greatly contributed to our understanding of why individuals with autism are "different". But it soon appeared both in neurophysiology and in neuropsychology that the findings for autism were by no means specific. Very similar findings of aberrant arousal, deviant theory of mind and difficulties with executive functioning were found in clinical conditions as diverging as schizophrenia and depression, amongst others. This poses a fundamental question when it comes to the construct validity of clinical syndromes such as they were conceived in the twentieth century and that form the backbone of our classifications in psychopathology.

1.7.3 Findings on Neurotransmitters

A beginning of an explanation or augmentation of our confusion was given by studies combining (dis)functional pathways in the brain linked to certain neurotransmitters, e.g. dopamine. In an extensive review of animal and human studies on fronto-cortico-striatal pathways related to patterns of rigidity, Langen et al. (2011) were able to discern three different loops and relate them, if dysfunctional, and with regard to abnormal dopamine release in the striatum and prefrontal cortex, to conditions as different as "addiction" (in the case of limbic dysfunctioning, leading to rigid skewedness on substances and habits), Parkinson's (in the case of sensomotor dysfunctioning, leading to rigid patterns of motor functioning) or on the contrary disinhibition in the case of attention deficit disorder when the cognitive fronto-cortico-striatal pathway is functionally impaired. This explains the behavioural overlaps between these disorders and autism that can exhibit more or less all of these different expressions of dysfunction:

"addiction" like obsessions and preoccupations, the "active but odd" behavioural disinhibitions and emotional swings in, e.g. Asperger's and Multiple Complex Developmental Disorders (McDD), whereas many individuals with autism also show motor rigidity and stereotypies, as illustrated in the figures here below.

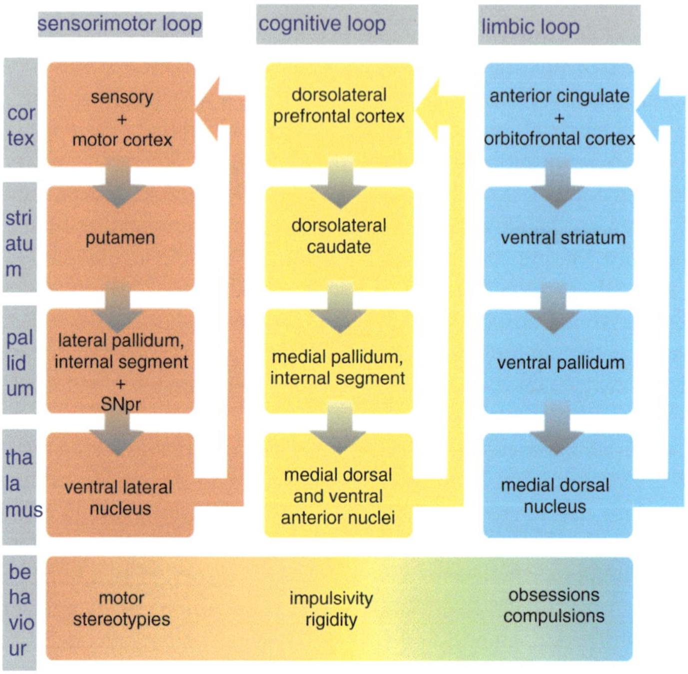

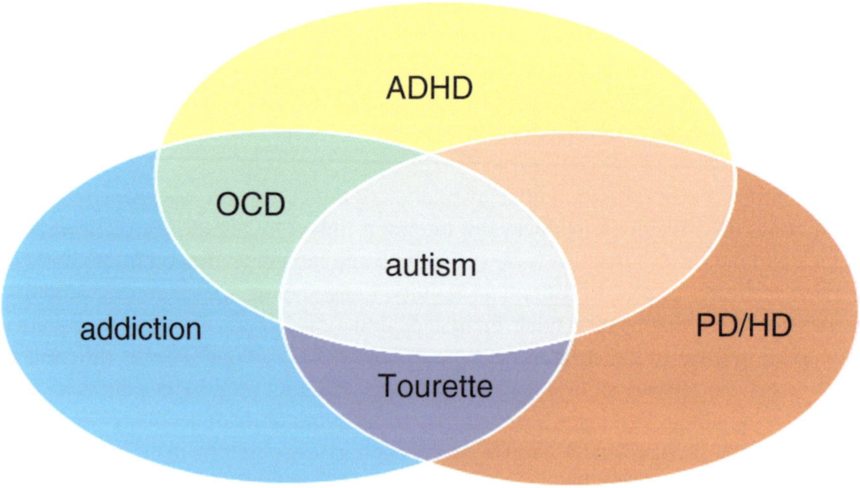

OCD=Obsessive Compulsive Disorder – PD= Parkinson's disease – HD= Huntington's disease (Langen et al. 2010)

How far have we moved from the very accurate clinical pictures by Kanner, wrongly attributed to bad parenting and autism, as underlying brain dysfunctioning becomes more evident, and from a condition very distinct to other forms of psychopathology and normality? What about heredity, which Asperger supposed to be in play?

1.7.4 Findings from Genetics

The first study relating to genetics and autism (Folstein and Rutter 1977) was on concordance of the condition in monozygotic twins. Monozygotic twins are by definition genetically identical. Thus, if a condition has "a" genetic cause, the concordance in identical offsprings should be 100 %. In first instance, focussing only on very strict Kanner criteria, Folstein and Rutter found only a concordance in infancy of 30 %. From their clinical point of view, they interpreted it as proof that genetic factors played a limited role in the aetiology of autism. Geneticists perceived this very differently: if a condition only occurs, at the most, in 0.3 % of the general population, and if 30 % of the cases in monozygotic twins are concordant for the disorder (i.e. a hundredfold increase in incidence), then there must be a high degree of heritability! Rutter later admitted his mistake, when 10 years later, the twins were reassessed, taking into account the broader phenotype, and the concordance raised to 90 %, by far the highest in psychopathology (far higher than in cancer, diabetes, cardiovascular diseases, depression, schizophrenia, etc.). But the fact that concordance never reaches 100 % means that it is not the disease that is inherited but the vulnerability to develop the disease! And where on the human genome would that vulnerability to developing autism be located? Admitting that it is only a vulnerability to develop the condition that is indeed inherited, which external factors then could be in play and which can trigger that predisposition?

The answer to the second question is yet to be resolved, but there are clear indications for prenatal adversity in the form of infections (e.g. rubella), toxins (medication, alcohol, etc.) and stress. Whereas no clear evidence has been found for a relation between perinatal hazards and autism, the postnatal environmental factors that could contribute to developing autism still have to be identified.

With respect to the specific genetics of autism, much was expected from the mapping of the human genome. Unfortunately here again the heterogeneity of autism is huge. Correlations between functional defects (e.g. polymorphism, deletions, inversions) on all chromosomes and autism have to date been established, with a higher number of positive findings involving chromosomes 7, 15, and 22 and the X chromosome (Staal et al. 2015). Moreover, there is evidence that parental inheritance may only account for part of the genetic risk, with a higher frequency of de novo mutations than previously thought.

So for the time being, there are clear-cut indications for genetic involvement in the aetiology of autism, but here again there appears to be not one cause but a huge variety of genetic vulnerabilities leading to heterogeneous phenotypic (clinical) expressions within the autism spectrum. Do they lead to clinical expression through anatomical and functional brain abnormalities? If this is the case, the tremendous technical advances in neuroimaging could provide us with some answers.

1.7.5 Findings from Neuropathology and Neuroimaging

There is in fact one abnormal feature that seems to characterize autism as a whole and that is the fact that, statistically, individuals with autism have bigger brains (macrocephaly) than not only typically developing individuals but also individuals with other developmental disorders such as schizophrenia or ADHD. It has been hypothesized that this could be due to deficient pruning of irrelevant brain connections, a process that normally takes place in the second year of life. This in turn could explain the information processing difficulties that we have described previously. Post-mortem studies of brains of individuals who had autism confirm this finding. Moreover, Kemper and Bauman (2005) found evidence of developmental brain immaturity in autistic brains, such as aberrant patterns of cell density, with increased cell packing density and reduced numbers of axons, as well as reduced cell sizes in regions that are crucial for information processing, namely, the hippocampus, the amygdalae and the cerebellum. Specifically in the latter, Kemper and Bauman found fewer Purkinje cells, pointing at reduced efficiency of the normal relaying, by the cerebellum, of primary sensory information to the frontal cortex for further processing. These findings point at vulnerabilities in those brain networks that enable humans to rapid and flexible adaptation to varying (social) circumstances. In the absence of any global indications for anatomical differences between typical brains and those of individuals with autism (Verhoeven et al. 2010), the (preliminary) neuroanatomical findings tend to point at functional deficits or abnormal functional patterns of information processing. This hypothesis (functional differences in individuals with autism) gained support from neuroimaging studies using newer techniques. Chris Frith (2003), for instance, using PET and functional MRI, showed that individuals with autism involve far more brain regions when solving theory of mind problems than neurotypical individuals. The latter tend to show increased BOLD signal in regions such as the fusiform cortex when appraising social situations, which they do much faster than individuals with autism. These findings were confirmed using the even newer DTI (diffuse tension imaging) technique that makes it possible to visualize interconnected brain networks involved in specific tasks. Just et al. (2004) found – and this has been extensively replicated – that individuals with autism have different connectivity patterns when compared to typical individuals: where typical individuals develop so-called “long range” connectivity networks, people with autism tend to stick to the far less mature “short range” local connectivity patterns as seen in very young children. This is an appealing theory because it helps to explain a great number of peculiarities in autism that Kanner and Asperger had already signalled from a clinical point of view, such as excessive focus on details, excellent rote memory and hypersensitivity to "noise" that they cannot inhibit in order to focus on the signal. The following figure illustrates these connectivity differences between individuals with autism and neurotypical individuals.

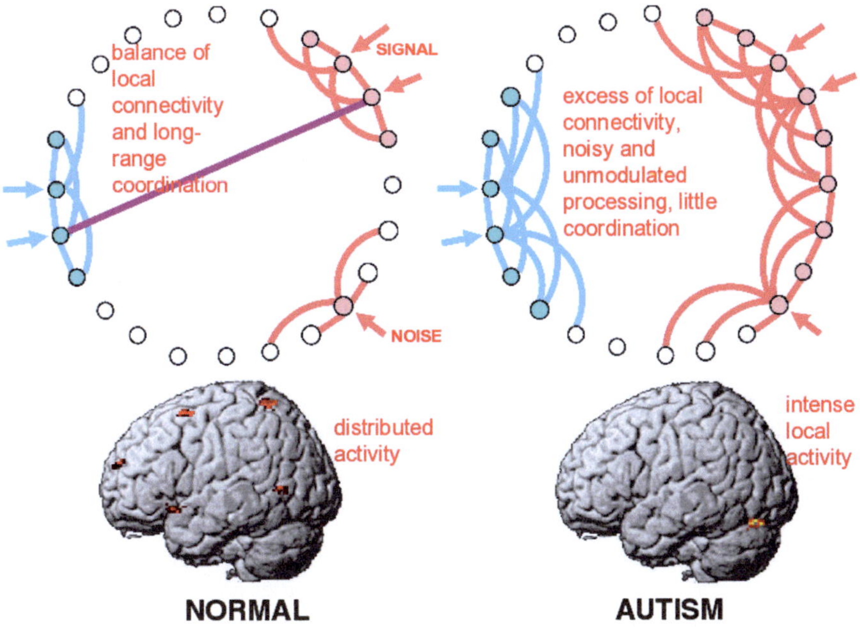

But here again the connectivity differences are not "the biological marker" for autism, as there is not such a marker yet. The question is will we ever find one? Not really and that is because we still tend to perceive autism as a distinct category, whereas Wing (1988) already pointed at autism as a continuum.

At this point we need to open a small parenthesis. DSM III proposed to rename autism into "pervasive developmental disorder". Yet as you noticed, the authors tended to revert to the "inadequate" terms autism and autistic, inadequate as individuals with "autism" are far from all being aloof and autonomous, whilst the term autism tends to reflect a condition rather than a developmental disorder. The reason seems to be twofold: the first one is of a linguistic nature. In English the adjective "pervasive" has the connotation of "existing in all parts" of "spreading to affect all parts", which differentiates poorly from a "general" developmental disorder, which would refer to intellectual backwardness such as in "learning disability". Secondly, parents and users preferred the term autism, because they had grown used to it over the years. Thus, "pervasive developmental disorder" was gradually changed into the currently common denomination of "autism spectrum" (disorder).

So what has changed over the years?

1.8 In Conclusion: From Autism to PDD to Autism Spectrum Disorder (DSM V), Where Are We Currently?

Quite a lot has changed, frankly speaking, since the seminal papers in the 1940s and the DSM revolution in the 1980s. In sum and to conclude, let us look at the current situation and hypothesize on what may happen in the (near) future:

1. Epidemiology:
   - "Autism" has evolved from a very rare condition with a high overlap with learning disability towards a quite common condition. The current estimated prevalence (Baird et al. 2006) of autism spectrum disorder is 1 % of the population worldwide. This figure refers to the prevalence of individuals presenting symptoms on the autism spectrum and impairments in functioning as a result.
   - There could be different reasons why the prevalence of autism has increased to such a degree:
     - One of the obvious reasons why ASD prevalence is on the rise is that more is known about it and thus it is better acknowledged in clinical practice.
     - Another one is that ASD is diagnosed far more often in "high functioning" individuals. Subsequently, the core group of 30 years ago – those with a co-occurring learning disability – is now a minority.
     - Another reason could be that individuals with lesser forms of ASD that could maintain themselves pretty well in predictable well-structured societies are at loss in the current culture that requires great flexibility and fast information processing from many sources.
     - A final reason could be the benefits that come along with a diagnostic label in terms of access to services, special education and social security. Somehow, "medical classifications" serve nowadays as a passport to gain access to these services in most countries worldwide.
2. A changing view on ASD as the ill part of a form of intelligence to be seen as a societal asset:
   - "Autism spectrum disorder" points at the group of individuals with autistic features who are impaired by them, in contrast with a larger group of individuals who have a so-called autistic condition but do not suffer and even sometimes benefit from being so.
   - Simon Baron-Cohen (2012) estimates that the prevalence of an "autistic condition" amounts to 5 % of the population. Not everyone who has "an autistic intelligence" – i.e. a skewed, systematic, strictly logical way of thinking, with a strong perseverance – suffers as a result. It has become clear that much of the scientific and technical progress of mankind has come from highly gifted individuals with this kind of intelligence (from middle age monks through Newton and Einstein to all those involved in the development of computer technology). Thus, many of the scientists and engineers (male and female) have more than a touch of autism. In other words, next to a lot of impairment and consequent difficulties and suffering, autism over the years has undoubtedly been an evolutionary asset.

- This new perspective on autism has surely been of great advantage for the self-awareness and pride of individuals with ASD.

3. Autism as a developmental condition:
   - There is consensus on the fact that ASD is a developmental condition that evolves as age progresses.
   - In other words it is sometimes difficult, in clinical practice, to differentiate between developmental effects and progress that results from treatment interventions.
4. Gender:
   - "Autism" is not merely a "male" condition though it appears to be more common amongst boys and men than in girls/women, but there are clear indications that this could be caused by a "criterion" bias, as the defining criteria for ASD are still very much focussed on male characteristics.
5. Diagnosis, treatment and guidance:
   - Where autism was, historically, more or less synonymous with a poor outcome and lifelong (institutional) dependency, nowadays an educational approach to treatment and guidance can help to foster meaningful societal participation and high degrees of independence.
   - Unfortunately, oftentimes the classification ASD is equated with the individual diagnosis.
   - As we have seen, autism is a highly heterogeneous condition at very different levels. A comprehensive assessment of the individual case should take all these different levels, aspects and interactions into account (see figure by van Wijngaarden-Cremers et al. (van Wijngaarden-Cremers et al. 2014) below) in order to tailor an individualized treatment/guidance plan.

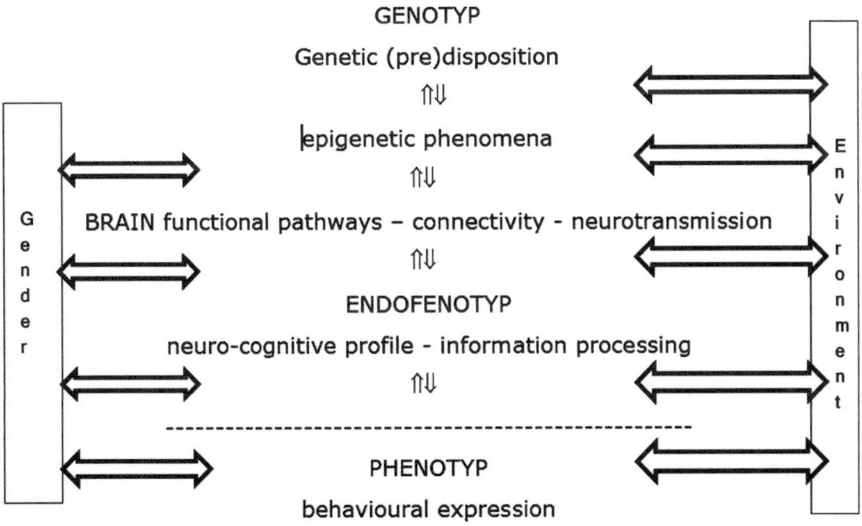

- When it comes to treatment, it must be noted that to date no "cure" for autism has been found, despite claims in that direction. Schopler et al. (Schopler et al. 1982) elaborated the TEACCH program (*Treatment and Education of Autistic and Related Communication Handicapped Children* www.teacch.com) to date the most effective and best validated approach to educate individuals with autism and those most near to them both personally and professionally to learn and cope with the difficulties that autism presents to the person himself and those in his near environment. In that sense Schopler and his team set the pace to a modern concept of dealing with chronic diseases and handicaps, that is, not to seek to cure them but far more to help handicapped individuals develop skills that will help them to live a most independent and worthwhile life in the community.

- Though TEACCH is a structured program based mainly on working with visual cues and prompts, the program also taught users that it should be tailored to the individual's profile of strengths and weaknesses and thus adapted to individual needs. This augmented the tension between individual assessment (in English "diagnosis" knowing thoroughly) and classification (in American diagnosis). The illusion created by the classification DSM was and is that autism is a distinct disorder and that "one size fits all" when it comes to treatment and guidance. So how has DSM coped with this dilemma in the long years that lead from DSM IV to DSM 5?
- DSM 5 (2015) has opted for a "lumping" approach to the category "autism spectrum disorders", with dimensional aspects as indicators of severity of the symptoms and impairment. Interestingly, the two first characteristics from the triad of Wing – social and communicative impairment – have been merged into one, whereas some of the characteristics signalled by Kanner and Asperger, for instance, hypersensitivity, have been "reintroduced".
- The "classification" ICD 10 criteria are

Autism Spectrum Disorder 299.00 (F84.0)

Diagnostic Criteria

A. Persistent deficits in social communication and social interaction across multiple contexts, as manifested by the following, currently or by history (examples are illustrative, not exhaustive; see text):
   1. Deficits in social-emotional reciprocity, ranging, for example, from abnormal social approach and failure of normal back-and-forth conversation to reduced sharing of interests, emotions or affect and to failure to initiate or respond to social interactions
   2. Deficits in nonverbal communicative behaviours used for social interaction, ranging, for example, from poorly integrated verbal and nonverbal communication to abnormalities in eye contact and body language or deficits in understanding and use of gestures and to a total lack of facial expressions and nonverbal communication
   3. Deficits in developing, maintaining and understanding relationships, ranging, for example, from difficulties in adjusting behaviour to suit various social contexts to difficulties in sharing imaginative play or in making friends and to the absence of interest in peers

Specify current severity:
Severity is based on social communication impairments and restricted repetitive patterns of behaviour.

B. Restricted, repetitive patterns of behaviour, interests or activities, as manifested by at least two of the following, currently or by history (examples are illustrative, not exhaustive; see text):
   1. Stereotyped or repetitive motor movements, use of objects or speech (e.g. simple motor stereotypies, lining up toys or flipping objects, echolalia, idiosyncratic phrases).
   2. Insistence on sameness, inflexible adherence to routines or ritualized patterns or verbal nonverbal behaviour (e.g. extreme distress at small changes, difficulties with transitions, rigid thinking patterns, greeting rituals, need to take same route or eat food every day).
   3. Highly restricted, fixated interests that are abnormal in intensity or focus (e.g. strong attachment to or preoccupation with unusual objects, excessively circumscribed or perseverative interest).
   4. Hyper- or hyporeactivity to sensory input or unusual interests in sensory aspects of the environment (e.g. apparent indifference to pain/temperature, adverse response to specific sounds or textures, excessive smelling or touching of objects, visual fascination with lights or movement).

Specify current severity:
Severity is based on social communication impairments and restricted, repetitive patterns of behaviour (see Table 1.1).

C. Symptoms must be present in the early developmental period (but may not become fully manifested until social demands exceed limited capacities or may be masked by learned strategies in later life).
D. Symptoms cause clinically significant impairment in social, occupational or other important areas of current functioning.
E. These disturbances are not better explained by intellectual disability (intellectual developmental disorder) or global developmental delay. Intellectual disability and autism spectrum disorder frequently co-occur; to make comorbid diagnoses of autism spectrum disorder and intellectual disability, social communication should be below that expected for general developmental level.

Note: Individuals with a well-established DSM IV diagnosis of autistic disorder, Asperger's disorder or pervasive developmental disorder not otherwise specified should be given the diagnosis of autism spectrum disorder.

Individuals who have marked deficits in social communication, but whose symptoms do not otherwise meet criteria for autism spectrum disorder, should be evaluated for social (pragmatic) communication disorder.

Table 1.1 Severity levels for autism spectrum disorder

Severity level	Social communication	Restricted, repetitive behaviours
Level 3 "requiring very substantial support"	Severe deficits in verbal and nonverbal social communication skills cause severe impairments in functioning, very limited initiation of social interactions and minimal response to social overtures from others. For example, a person with few words of intelligible speech who rarely initiates interaction and, when he or she does, makes unusual approaches to meet needs only and responds to only very direct social approaches	Inflexibility of behaviour, extreme difficulty coping with change or other restricted/repetitive behaviours markedly interfere with functioning in all spheres. Great distress/ difficulty changing focus or action
Level 2 "requiring substantial support"	Marked deficits in verbal and nonverbal social communication skills, social impairments apparent even with supports in place, limited initiation of social interactions and reduced or abnormal responses to social overtures from others. For example: a person who speaks simple sentences, whose interaction is limited to narrow special interests, and how has markedly odd nonverbal communication	Inflexibility of behaviour, difficulty coping with change or other restricted/repetitive behaviours appear frequently enough to be obvious to the casual observer and interfere with functioning in a variety of contexts. Distress and/or difficulty changing focus or action
Level 1 "requiring support"	Without supports in place, deficits in social communication cause noticeable impairments. Difficulty initiating social interactions and clear examples of atypical or unsuccessful response to social overtures of others may appear to have decreased interest in social interactions. For example, a person who is able to speak in full sentences and engages in communication but whose to-and-fro conversation with others fails and whose attempts to make friends are odd and typically unsuccessful	Inflexibility of behaviour causes significant interference with functioning in one or more contexts. Difficulty switching between activities. Problems of organization and planning hamper independence

Specify if:

With or without accompanying intellectual impairment.
With or without accompanying language impairment.
Associated with a known medical or genetic condition or environmental factor.
(Coding note: Use additional code to identify the associated medical or genetic condition.)
Associated with another neurodevelopmental, mental or behavioural disorder.
(Coding note: Use additional code[s] to identify the associated neurodevelopmental, mental or behavioural disorder[s].)

With catatonia (refer to the criteria for catatonia associated with another mental disorder, pp. 119–120, for definition). (Coding note: Use additional code 293.89 [F06.1] catatonia associated with autism spectrum disorder to indicate the presence of the comorbid catatonia.)

6. Outcome and stigma:
   - Understandably with the broadening of the definition, the outcome has changed too. Nevertheless ASD remains a very chronic condition that requires a lot of guidance and lifelong support, especially in periods of transition: adolescence, moving from school to work and, in old age, coping with retirement.
   - Many individuals with ASD suffer unnecessarily from the stigma that results from widespread stereotyped ideas about what ASD is like (e.g. being like "Rain man") and from the fact that most people do not understand the immense difficulties "good-looking" individuals with ASD encounter in everyday life.

Future Directions

The concept of autism has greatly evolved since the first descriptions, under this name, of a clinical syndrome characterized by social and communicative developmental impairments and rigid and restricted patterns of behaviour and interest. Yet it has become evident that there is not one cause for this heterogeneous syndrome. There is certainly a genetic vulnerability in play, but the external triggers and causal pathways are certainly different and remain yet to be elucidated. Despite the causal and clinical heterogeneity, there is enough in common to speak of a spectrum of disorders. But for treatment and guidance, despite the fact that an educational approach shows the best evidence in terms of developmental outcome, a thorough individual assessment is of the uttermost importance in order to tailor treatment and guidance at the individual's and his environment's needs. In this respect, too often the diagnostic classification "ASD" leads to a "one-size-fits-all" therapeutic approach based on the wrong supposition that all individuals with autism would benefit, for example, from visual cues to prompt their behaviour.

For research it is likewise a relevant question whether the category ASD is useful when trying to unravel the underlying causal pathways that lead to the clinical impairments. At this stage of our knowledge, it seems more appropriate to take endophenotypes within the autistic spectrum at a neuropsychological, neurophysiological or connectivity level to understand why in those individuals (e.g. in contrast with their healthy siblings) the interaction of genetic vulnerability and environmental factors has led to a certain clinical profile. These more individually skewed approaches may contribute greatly to the amelioration of individual profile-oriented assessment and diagnostics in order to provide well-adapted treatment and guidance.

Finally as we have seen all along this chapter, most of the research in autism has been performed in children and mostly boys. Too little is known about autism in adults. And that is what this book is about.

References

Recommended Further Readings

Silberman S (2015) *NeuroTribes:* The legacy of Autism and how to think smarter about people who think differently. Allan and Unwin, London

Volkmar FR (2013) Encyclopedia of autism spectrum disorders. Springer, New York (Five Volumes)

Historical References

Aarkrog T (1981) The borderline concept in childhood, adolescence and adulthood. Borderline adolescents in psychiatric treatment and 5 years later. Acta Psychiatr Scand Suppl 293:1–300

Asperger H (1944) Die autistischen psychopathen im kindersalter. Archly für Psychiatrie und Nervenkrankheiten 117:76–136

Baird G, Simonoff E, Pickles A, Chandler S, Loucas T, Meldrum D, Charman T (2006) Prevalence of disorders of the autism spectrum in a population cohort of childrenin South Thames: the Special Needs and Autism Project (SNAP). Lancet 368(9531):7–136

Baron-Cohen S (1995) Mindblindness: an essay on autism and theory of mind. In: A Bradford Book. The MIT Press, Cambridge, MA/London

Baron-Cohen S, Hammer J (1997) Parents of children with asperger syndrome: what is the cognitive phenotype? J Cogn Neurosci 9(4):548–554

Baron-Cohen S (2002) The extreme male brain theory of autism. Trends Cogn Sci 6(6):248–254

Baron-Cohen S (2012) Autism and the technical mind: children of scientists and engineers may inherit genes that not only confer intellectual talents but also predispose them to autism. Sci Am 307(5):72–75

Bauman ML, Kemper TL (2005) Neuroanatomic observations of the brain in autism: a review and future directions. Int J Dev Neurosci 23(2–3):183–187

Bruno B (1967) The empty fortress: infantile autism and the birth of the self. The Free Press, New York

Cohen DJ, Paul R, Volkmar F (1987) Issues in the classification of pervasive developmental disorders and associated conditions. In: Cohen DJ, Donnellan AM, Rhea P (eds) Handbook of autism and pervasive developmental disorders. Wiley, New York, pp 20–39

Dahl EK, Cohen DJ, Provence S (1986) Cinical and multivariate approaches to the nosology of pervasive developmental disorders. J Am Acad Child Psychiatry 25:170–180

Folstein S, Rutter M (1977) Genetic influences and infantile autism. Nature 265(5596):726–728

Frith C (2004) Is autism a disconnection disorder? Lancet Neurol 2004(10):577

Frith C (2003) What do imaging studies tell us about the neural basis of autism? Novartis Found Symp 251:149–166 discussion 166-76, 281-297

Frith U, Happé F (1994) Autism: beyond "theory of mind". Cognition 50(1–3):115–132

Frith U (1997) The neurocognitive basis of autism. Trends Cogn Sci 1(2):73–77

Gillberg C (2003) Deficits in attention, motor control, and perception: a brief review. Arch Dis Child 88(10):904–910

Green J. & Jones B. (Eds) (1998) In-patient Child Psychiatry - Modern Practice, Research and the Future. Routeledge London

Kanner L (1943) Autistic disturbances of affective contact. Nerv Child 2:217–250

Klin A, Jones W, Schultz R, Volkmar F, Cohen D (2002) Defining and quantifying the social phenotype in autism. Am J Psychiatry 159(6):895–908

Lotter V (1966) Epidemiology of autistic conditions in young children. I. Prevalence. Social Psychiatry 1:124–137

Lotter V (1967) Epidemiology of autistic conditions in young children. II. Some characteristics of the parents and children. Soc Psychiatry 1:163–173

Nagy J, Szatmari P (1986 Sep) A chart review of schizotypal personality disorders in children. J Autism Dev Disord 16(3):351–367

Rimland B (1968) On the objective diagnosis of infantile autism. Acta Paedopsychiatr 35(4): 146–161

Ritvo ER, Freeman BJ (1984) A medical model of autism: etiology, pathology and treatment. Pediatr Ann 13(4):298–305

Rourke BP (1989) Nonverbal learning disabilities: the syndrome and the model. Guilford Press, New York

Schopler E, Mesibov G, Baker A (1982) Evaluation of treatment for autistic children and their parents. J Am Acad Child Psychiatry 21(3):262–267

Skuse DH, James RS, Bishop DV, Coppin B, Dalton P, Aamodt-Leeper G, Bacarese-Hamilton M, Creswell C, McGurk R, Jacobs PA (1997) Evidence from Turner's syndrome of an imprinted X-linked locus affecting cognitive function. Nature 387(6634):705–708

Towbin KE, Dykens EM, Pearson GS, Cohen DJ (1993) Conceptualizing "borderline syndrome of childhood" and "childhood schizophrenia" as a developmental disorder. J Am Acad Child Adolesc Psychiatry 32(4):775–782

Van der Gaag RJ, Buitelaar J, Van den Ban E, Bezemer M, Njio L, Van Engeland H (1995) A controlled multivariate chart review of multiple complex developmental disorder. J Am Acad Child Adolesc Psychiatry 34(8):1096–1106

Volkmar FR, Cohen DJ (1986) Current concepts: infantile autism and the pervasive developmental disorders. J Dev Behav Pediatr 7(5):324–329

Wergeland H (1979) A follow-up study of 29 borderline psychotic children 5 to 20 years after discharge. Acta Psychiatr Scand 60(5):465–476

Wing L, Gould J (1979) Severe impairments of social interaction and associated abnormalities in children: epidemiology and classification. J Autism Dev Disord 9(1):11–29

Wing L (1981) Asperger's syndrome: a clinical account. Psychol Med 11:115–129

Wing L (1997) The autistic spectrum. Lancet 350(9093):1761–1766

Wolff S, Barlow A (1979) Schizoid personality in childhood: a comparative study of schizoid, autistic and normal children. J Child Psychol Psychiatry 20:29–46

Quoted Articles

Just MA, Cherkassky VL, Keller TA, Minshew NJ (2004) Cortical activation and synchronization during sentence comprehension in high-functioning autism: evidence of underconnectivity. Brain 127(Pt 8):1811–1821

Langen M, Durston S, Kas MJ, van Engeland H, Staal WG (2011) The neurobiology of repetitive behavior: in mice …and men. Neurosci Biobehav Rev 35(3):356–365

Staal WG, Langen M, van Dijk S, Mensen VT, Durston S (2015) DRD3 gene and striatum in autism spectrum disorder. Br J Psychiatry 206(5):431–432

Verhoeven JS, De Cock P, Lagae L, Sunaert S (2010) Neuroimaging of autism. Neuroradiology 52(1):3–14

van Wijngaarden-Cremers PJ, van Deurzen P, Oosterling I, Groen W, Langen M, Lagro-Janssen AL, van der Gaag RJ (2014) A fresh look at psychiatric disorders. Tijdschr Psychiatr 56(10):670–679 English translation available p.vanwijngaarden@dimence.nl

Neurobiology of Autism Spectrum Disorders

2

Gabriela J. Martins

2.1 Introduction

Autism spectrum disorders (ASDs) are a highly prevalent class of neurodevelopmental disorders characterized by impairments in social behavior, atypical communication, and restricted interests and repetitive behaviors. ASDs vary significantly in characteristics and severity, and at present, there is no cure for autism. Currently, there are no effective pharmacological treatments for ASD; instead treatments focus on therapies and behavioral interventions designed to ameliorate specific symptoms. For better treatments to be available and effective, much research is necessary to understand the neurobiological underpinnings of ASDs.

ASDs are not static or simple disorders with fixed effects and characteristics. Instead, both symptoms and causes of ASDs are highly variable and change across development and to different degrees. Co-occurring medical conditions (sleep problems, epilepsy, and gastrointestinal symptoms) and psychiatric disturbances (anxiety, obsessive–compulsive disorder (OCD), and aggression) are common and can appear at different ages in children on the spectrum. Furthermore, children with genetically diverse neurodevelopmental syndromic disorders, including fragile X syndrome, Rett syndrome, tuberous sclerosis, neurofibromatosis, and Angelman syndrome (see Table 2.1), have been reported to have a higher penetrance of ASD diagnosis. However, very few studies closely compare the phenotypic characteristics between single-gene (syndromic) and multigenic (idiopathic) ASDs (Levitt and Campbell 2009).

There is a general consensus regarding a developmental onset of ASDs, but the underlying causes of the disorders and their heterogeneous symptoms remain elusive. Contemporary hypotheses of the causes of ASDs often include

G.J. Martins
Champalimaud Neuroscience Program, Lisbon, Portugal
e-mail: gabriela.martins@neuro.fchampalimaud.org

B. Barahona Corrêa, R.-J. van der Gaag (eds.), *Autism Spectrum Disorders in Adults*, DOI 10.1007/978-3-319-42713-3_2

Table 2.1 Monogenic syndromes associated with ASD

SYNDROME	GENE	LOCUS	PHENOTYPE	PROTEIN FUNCTION
Fragile X syndrome	*FMR1*	Xq27.3	Large, protruding ears, long face, hyperextensible joint, macroorchidism, hypotonia, learning problem, intellectual disability, language impairment, developmental delay, attention problem, impaired cognition, anxiety, hyperactivity, social phobia, and repetitive behaviors, 45–70% co-diagnosis with ASD representing 1–3% of ASD patients	RNA binding
Rett syndrome	*MeCP2*	Xq28	Developmental regression, microcephaly, cognitive and motor impairment, epilepsy, stereotyped hand movement, severe repetitive behavior, represent about 0.5–1% of ASD patients	Methyl-DNA binding
Tuberous sclerosis	*TSC1, TSC2*	9q34, 16p13	Brain tumors, multi-organ involvement, learning difficulties, intellectual disability, self-injurious behavior, obsessive-compulsive disorder, attention deficit hyperactivity disorder, aggression, epilepsy, 40–50% present with ASD; represent about 1% of patients with ASD	Cell cycle
Neurofibromatosis 1	*NF1*	17q11.2	Café au lait spots, neurofibromas, scoliosis, iris tumor, cognitive dysfunction, epilepsy, > 4% co-diagnosed with ASD	PI3K signaling activity
Cohen syndrome	*COH1*	8q22	Ocular abnormalities, obesity, thin arms and legs, micrognathia, deafness, intellectual disability, epilepsy, ASD	Function unclear, may be involved in sorting and transporting proteins inside the cell
Timothy syndrome	*CACNA1C*	12p13.3	Congenital heart disease, cardiac arrhythmias (QT prolongation), syndactyly, dysmorphic faces, developmental delays, immune deficiency, cognitive abnormalities, 60–80% present with ASD	Calcium channel voltage-dependent L type alpha 1C subunit; calcium signaling
Smith-Lemli-Opitz syndrome	*DHCR7*	DHCR7	Facial abnormalities, micrognathia, finger and feet abnormalities, microcephaly, developmental delay, learning disability, behavioral abnormalities, hand mannerism, 50–86% of patients present with ASD	(7-dehydrocholesterol reductase) Cholesterol biosynthesis; Ras-mediated ERK signaling; PI3K signaling

Williams-Beuren syndrome	>25 genes including *ELN*	7q11.23 deletion	Cardiac and gastrointestinal problems, hyperacusis, phonophobia, strabismus, esotropia, problems with visual processing, hypertonia, motor delay, intellectual disability, strong interest in people, lack of social inhibition, ASD	Loss of the *ELN* gene, which codes for the protein elastin, is associated with the connective-tissue abnormalities and cardiovascular disease
Dup15q syndromes	*GABRB3; UBE3A*	15q11–q13 duplication	Hypotonia, facial dysmorphism, small stature, gross and fine motor delays, cognitive delays, speech/language delays, behavior problems, sensory processing problem, epilepsy, present in up to 5% of ASD cases	Gamma-aminobutyric acid (GABA)A receptor beta 3; ubiquitin protein ligase which participates in protein degradation in proteasomes via the ubiquitin pathway
Prader-Willi syndrome	*GABRB3; UBE3A*	Del 15q11–q13 (paternal allele)	Specific face, hypogonadism, small hands and feet, hypopigmentation, hyperphagia, severe obesity, obsessive compulsive disorder, mood and behavior problem, ASD	
Angelman syndrome	*GABRB3; UBE3A*	Del 15q11–q13 maternal deletion	Strabismus, unique facial dysmorphism, prominent mandible, wide mouth, sleep disturbance, severe developmental delay, speech impairment, ataxia, attention problem, frequent laughter, easily excitable personality, epilepsy, >40% of patients present with ASD; account for 1–2% of patients with ASD	
16p11.2 Deletion syndrome	26-29 genes	16p11 deletion	Minor unusual facial and physical features, hypotonia, obesity developmental delay, intellectual disability, language delay, learning difficulty, epilepsy, high prevalence of ASD representing ~1% of ASD patients	Roles in synaptic function, chromatin modification, transcriptional regulation, neuronal development
Smith-Magenis syndrome	*RAI1*	17p11.2 deletion	Facial dysmorphism, short stature, scoliosis, eye abnormalities, reduced sensitivity to pain and temperature, sleep disturbances, behavioral problem, self-injurious behavior, stereotyped behavior, ASD	(*retinoic acid inducible 1*) Transcription factor regulates the expression of multiple genes, including CLOCK
Potocki-Lupski syndrome	*RAI1*	17p11.2 duplication	Mental retardation, infantile hypotonia, sleep apnea, structural cardiovascular anomalies, cognitive deficits, abnormal social behaviors, learning disabilities, attention-deficit disorder, obsessive compulsive disorder, malocclusions, short stature and failure to thrive, 80% co-diagnosed with ASD	Retinoic acid inducible 1 (RAI1)

(continued)

Table 2.1 (continued)

SYNDROME	GENE	LOCUS	PHENOTYPE	PROTEIN FUNCTION
22q11 Duplication syndrome	30-40 genes	22q11.2 duplication	Growth retardation, hypotonia, delayed psychomotor development, learning difficulty, intellectual disability, ASD	Genes and their functions unknown
DiGeorge syndrome (velocardiofacial syndrome)	*TBX1/COMT*	22q11.2 deletion	Multi-organ abnormalities, thymic aplasia, cleft palate, facial dysmorphism, immune system abnormality, low calcium levels, hearing loss, developmental delay, learning difficulty, schizophrenia, anxiety, mood disorders, attention deficit hyperactivity disorder, ASD	(T-box transcription factor) Important role in tissue and organ formation, regulation of differentiation neural crest cells; (catechol-O-methyltransferase) one of several enzymes that degrade catecholamines
Phelan-McDermid syndrome	*SHANK3*	22q13.3 deletion	Dolichocephaly, hand and facial dysmorphism, ptosis, kidney problems, neonatal hypotonia, global developmental delay, intellectual disability, reduced sensitivity to pain, absent or severely delayed speech, pervasive developmental disorder – not otherwise specified with 90% co-diagnosis of ASD representing 1% of ASD patients	Organizes post synaptic density and binds neuroligins; mediates synapse formation and dendritic spine maturation, connects neurotransmitter receptors
PTEN-macrocephaly	*PTEN*	10q23	Macrocephaly, mental retardation, seizures, and 1–17% co-diagnosed with ASD	Protein phosphatase; tumor suppressor gene, regulating the cell cycle; important in neuronal survival and synaptic plasticity; possibly represses PI 3-kinase pathway
Cortical dysplasia-focal epilepsy syndrome	*CNTNAP2*	7q35-36	Congenital disorder characterized by seizures, intellectual disability, and language regression; 2/3 present with ASD	Synaptic binding protein for contactin molecules, clustering potassium channels along myelinated axons

Buxbaum and Hof (2013), Abrahams and Geschwind (2008), Levitt and Campbell (2009), Miles (2011), Yoo (2015) experience-dependent processes through which atypical gene–environment interactions yield pathophysiology in later emerging systems that underlie social, motor, and communication competencies (Levitt and Campbell 2009). Impairments in initial basic processes become expressed in ever more complex systems, with the population heterogeneity of the clinical features of ASD expected to increase from infancy to childhood and through adolescence (Levitt and Campbell 2009). Some hypotheses focus on synaptic function (Polleux and Lauder 2004; Won et al. 2013; Uchino and Waga 2013) while others on neurotransmitter systems including glutamate, GABA, and serotonin (Bear et al. 2004; Polleux and Lauder 2004; Rubenstein and Merzenich 2003; Belmonte et al. 2004b; Chugani 2004; Rose'Meyer 2013; Ismail et al. 2016), most arguing toward a balance between excitation and inhibition (Gogolla et al. 2009). However, with each of these hypotheses, an important question remains: how are cognitive and behavioral profiles attained? The broad functional categories of genes indentified suggest that no single molecular explanation will suffice. However, the advancement of research performed in several fields, including epidemiology, brain imaging, genetics, and neuroscience, has led to new hypotheses regarding possible etiologies.

Genetic studies have provided great advancement to our understanding of ASDs and are the core to the development of appropriate animal models. Human studies are inherently limited due to scarcity of material, high diversity in individual and family histories, variability and uncontrollability of genetic background, inability to isolate genetic and environmental factors, indirect inference of brain operation within the limitations of current noninvasive methods to investigate the brain, and difficulty with which experimental results replicate (Bernardet and Crusio 2006). While no single animal model is likely to encompass all the human traits common in ASDs, they will be crucial to our understanding of the neurobiological mechanisms. Running animal model and human studies in parallel looking at genetic links and neuroanatomical markers will provide great validity to the animal models and begin to elucidate the mechanistic pathways and neural substrates involved in ASDs. This chapter will give an overview of the current areas of ASD research on animal models in the context of data from human studies and discuss our current understanding of the neurobiology of ASDs.

2.2 Neuroanatomical Changes

In recent years, the fields of neuropathology and brain imaging have developed several new technological innovations, such as functional MRI (fMRI), diffusion tensor imaging (DTI), and proton magnetic resonance spectroscopy (^{1}H-MRS) imaging, revealing promising breakthroughs in exploring subtle morphological and neurochemical changes in the autistic brain and their impact on function (Polsek et al. 2011; Ismail et al. 2016). Alterations in brain connectivity and morphology may be a potential endophenotype of ASD. Data suggest that ASD is a dynamic disorder and that the time course of brain development rather than the final product is most disturbed in autism (Amaral et al. 2008; Ismail et al. 2016).

A commonly tested hypothesis is altered structural and functional brain connectivity (Belmonte et al. 2004a; Geschwind and Levitt 2007; Vissers et al. 2012; Hulbert and Jiang 2016). Structural connectivity is the physical connections between different brain regions, while functional connectivity refers to the integrated relationship between spatially separated brain regions. It is believed that structural connections within the brain give rise to functional network activity as measured by coherence or information flow. Neuroimaging investigations indicate that ASDs are associated with perturbed connectivity at both structural and functional levels (Minshew and Keller 2010; Kana et al. 2014; Hulbert and Jiang 2016); however, the exact nature and pattern of this aberrant neural connectivity remains uncertain due to inconsistent findings from neuroimaging studies in patients (Uddin et al. 2013; Kana et al. 2014; Hulbert and Jiang 2016). It is likely that discrepancies between findings of autism-related hypo-connectivity and hyper-connectivity might be reconciled by taking developmental changes into account. The consistent pattern emerging across several studies is that while intrinsic functional connectivity in adolescents and adults with autism is generally reduced compared with age-matched controls, functional connectivity in younger children with the disorder appears to be increased (Uddin et al. 2013). In addition to methodological and conceptual controversy, this uncertainty likely reflects the substantial molecular and genetic heterogeneity of human patients.

Initial observations of children with ASD and studies of head circumference reveal an early abnormal head enlargement followed by an abnormally reduced rate of brain growth, suggesting a dynamic process of age-dependent brain growth abnormalities (Courchesne and Pierce 2005). Studies of young children with autism have consistently found increased total brain volume, particularly in frontal lobes (Redcay and Courchesne 2005; Courchesne et al. 2011). In fact, children with ASD exhibited rapid brain overgrowth during early childhood and then experienced a plateau in brain growth such that brain size was within the normal range by adolescence and adulthood suggesting an atypical trajectory of brain development (Redcay and Courchesne 2005; Courchesne et al. 2011; Stigler et al. 2011). In fact, Courchesne (2005) hypothesizes that cortical systems (e.g., frontal cortex) with a more protracted developmental timetable for synaptogenesis, dendritic growth, circuit formation, and myelination may be more adversely impacted by the growth dysregulation than those that mature rapidly and early (e.g., primary visual cortex). Thus, growth dysregulation will most strongly affect regions mediating higher-order social communication, emotional processing, language, and cognition. Large integrative and projecting pyramidal neurons that normally require several years to fully develop, such as those in frontal cortex, would develop improperly, resulting in a reduction in long-distance connectivity and top-down control signaling, while abnormal increases may occur in local and short-distance connectivity and processing (Courchesne and Pierce 2005). These findings appear to be related to changes in both gray and white matter volumes; however, these structural MRI studies have been inconsistent (Chen et al. 2011; Amaral et al. 2008).

Postmortem and magnetic resonance imaging studies have highlighted abnormalities in brain neuroanatomy including in the corpus callosum, cortex (frontal and temporal lobes), hippocampus, amygdala, thalamus, cerebellum, and the brainstem (Palmen et al. 2004; Amaral et al. 2008; Chen et al. 2015; Ismail et al. 2016). There is also evidence showing abnormal cortical thickness (Hardan et al. 2010; Casanova et al. 2003; Blatt 2012) and cortical minicolumn structure (Casanova et al. 2002, 2003, 2006; Buxhoeveden et al. 2006). Minicolumns are functional arrangements of neurons that span most neocortical layers of the brain and serve to organize neurons in a defined space and have similar response properties. The minicolumn volumes of ASD patients were found to be reduced, but the cell number per minicolumn appeared normal (Casanova et al. 2002; Buxhoeveden et al. 2006). However, more recently, a study (Casanova et al. 2006) reported an excess of minicolumns packed closer together. This abnormal development could be explained by a precocious and fast minicolumn formation, leaving a shorter time window for experience-dependent inputs to influence the development of long-distance connections and local dendritic arbors (Courchesne and Pierce 2005; Blatt 2012). Furthermore, underdevelopment of inhibitory interneurons, important for isolating specific information processed by a single minicolumn, has been reported (Courchesne and Pierce 2005; Casanova et al. 2003; Polsek et al. 2011) which could lead to hyperactivation of neighboring minicolumns resulting in hyperstimulation by simple outside stimuli which would normally activate one or a small group of minicolumns (Levitt et al. 2004; Polsek et al. 2011). On the clinical level, this would result in weakened awareness of surrounding context and hyperexcitation by seemingly minor external influences, both often reported as a feature of ASD (Polsek et al. 2011). Furthermore, analyses of the basal ganglia have suggested increased volume of the caudate in ASD and changes in cortico-caudate connectivity circuits, which have been correlated with severity of repetitive behaviors (Sears et al. 1999; Hollander et al. 2005; Chen et al. 2015; Ismail et al. 2016). Linking the neuroanatomical findings to behavioral symptoms is vital to understanding the role of the structural changes in the etiology of ASD.

Researchers using functional MRI have designed tasks to directly assess each of the core symptoms of ASD, social interaction, language and communication, and executive function and repetitive symptoms. Unfortunately, fMRI studies have also shown wide variations in the findings leading to a lack of consensus in interpreting the results. Through the large number of studies, some degree of consistency has emerged allowing for a few conclusions to be drawn (Dichter 2012). Studies of social processes have generally found evidence of hypoactivation in nodes of the "social brain," including the medial prefrontal cortex, the inferior frontal gyrus and the anterior insula, the posterior superior temporal sulcus, the interparietal sulcus, the amygdala, and the fusiform gyrus. These brain areas are involved in facial recognition, emotion, evaluation, empathy, social cognition, and behavior (Kennedy and Adolphs 2012). Functional MRI research on language and communication impairments in ASDs has suggested differential patterns of language function lateralization, decreased synchrony of brain regions processing language, and recruitment of brain regions that do not typically process language including the right hemisphere. Research also suggests that individuals with ASD demonstrate a reliance on visualization for language processing. Studies investigating cognitive control, designed to address neural mechanisms underlying restricted and repetitive behaviors and interests, have converged on aberrant frontostriatal functioning in ASDs, specifically in inferior and middle frontal gyri, anterior cingulate cortex, and the basal ganglia. Reward processing studies have highlighted mesolimbic and mesocortical impairments when processing both social and nonsocial incentives in ASDs (Dichter 2012). In summary, there is a convergence of evidence for decreased cortical–cortical connectivity, with possibly increased connectivity between the subcortical regions and cortex and within primary sensory areas such as the visual cortex. These results, in combination with findings of decreased cortical specialization, and supported by structural imaging studies that indicate abnormal growth and organization of both gray and white matter, reinforce the model of atypical connectivity in ASD, possibly focusing on brain regions involved in social behavior, language, and motor stereotypies (Abrahams and Geschwind 2008; Ismail et al. 2016; Belmonte et al. 2004b).

Inconsistencies across studies are likely due to a number of variables including a lack of correlation with genetic information, variable methodologies, large age ranges, different populations, and small sample sizes. Oftentimes, imaging studies include patients with similar age groups, sex, and IQs but with diverse genetic and environmental factors that lead to the ASD diagnosis. Defined phenotypes in larger samples of children and well-characterized brain tissue will be necessary for clarification of the neuroanatomy of autism. However, obtaining such specific groups of participants for studies is very slow and difficult. Despite the evolving resolution of imaging studies, the easiest method is to analyze animal models of ASD. Mouse models display some of the brain anatomical and behavioral abnormalities detected in ASD patients but provide unprecedented access to manipulation of specific neurons or individual circuits providing insight into human neuropsychiatric disorders that will contribute to the screening of novel treatments.

2.3 Genetics

ASD is a complex end product of gene–environment interaction, mediated by changes in brain physiology, function, and morphology causing cognitive and behavioral dysfunction (Yoo 2015). Although the exact etiology of the condition is not known, family and twin studies strongly indicated genetic factors behind ASD. In fact, studies in mono- and dizygotic twins have shown that the estimated heritability of ASD is almost 90 %, which far exceeds the estimated heritability of other common polygenic diseases (e.g., cancer, heart disease, schizophrenia, and depression) (Levitt and Campbell 2009; Miles 2011; Tick et al. 2016).

Therefore, the greatest progress toward understanding the causes of ASD has come from identifying genetic mutations and other disorders that predispose a person to develop autism. Important technical advances in the late 1990s led to the first candidate gene association studies followed by whole-genome linkage studies to identify loci of potential interest and to assess copy number variation (CNV) (Abrahams and Geschwind 2008; Jacquemont et al. 2006; Sebat et al. 2007;

Szatmari et al. 2007). These studies identified a large number of potentially important novel candidate loci and showed that 20–25 % of ASD cases are accounted for by defined mutations, genetic syndromes, and de novo CNVs (Miles 2011). Single mutations account for no more than 1 % of cases, mainly due to phenotypic heterogeneity and variable penetrance. Several of these are described in Table 2.1. Though the prevalence is not strikingly high, syndromic autism helps to understand core deficits of ASD that specific genetic mutations carry and acts as a gateway to explore the genetic etiology of ASD (Yoo 2015). However, the field is beginning to focus more on defining unique phenotypic features of stratified populations of children, adolescents, and adults that may relate to specific genetic etiologies, such as increased risk due to common allelic variations, rare mutations, or copy number variation (Levitt and Campbell 2009).

It is important to note, however, that while there are genetic variants that are enriched in populations with particular dysfunctions, such as language, there are no single genes that directly regulate social behavior or language. Instead, genetic vulnerability resides in the disruption of cellular processes, due to the disruption of proteins encoded by genes, in specific brain circuits that may also be influenced by mechanisms of gene–environment interaction (Levitt and Campbell 2009; Miles 2011). Single-gene disorders, including fragile X (mutations in *FMR1*), tuberous sclerosis complex (mutations in *TSC1* and *TSC2*), duplication 15q syndrome, deletions in the *16p11.2* region, Rett syndrome (mutation in *MeCP2*), and neurofibromatosis (mutations in *NF1*), are well known as having an ASD phenotype as well as comorbid intellectual disabilities and epilepsy (Table 2.1). Behavioral manifestations of these disorders even within the autism spectrum vary greatly from one individual to another. Given the great heterogeneity, it is not clear whether the same etiological factors can explain such different phenotypes.

Recent studies are elucidating a few common neurobiological traits, including abnormal brain connectivity (Geschwind and Levitt 2007; Abrahams and Geschwind 2008), and defective synaptic function (Zoghbi 2003; Spooren et al. 2012; Zoghbi and Bear 2012; Bourgeron 2015), which have been hypothesized to link rare and common variants at the level of biological function (Abrahams and Geschwind 2008). In fact, recent genetic studies have identified a large number of candidate genes for ASD, many of which encode synaptic proteins (Won et al. 2013; Levitt and Campbell 2009). Of the genetic variations studied, the most consistently reported abnormalities are mutations in the synaptic genes, *neuroligin-3* (*NLGN3*) and *neuroligin-4 X-linked* (*NLGN4X*) (Jamain et al. 2003; Tabuchi et al. 2007; Abrahams and Geschwind 2008), *SHANK* (Wang et al. 2011; Uchino and Waga 2013; Zhou et al. 2016; Durand et al. 2007; Arons et al. 2012), and *contactin-associated protein-like 2* (*CNTNAP2*) (Rodenas-Cuadrado et al. 2014; Peñagarikano et al. 2011; Peñagarikano and Geschwind 2012). The identification of rare ASD-linked mutations, such as *NLGN3*, *NLGN4X*, and *Shank3* (Table 2.1), was an important advancement linking the ASDs to specific molecules that are involved in synaptic function (Jamain et al. 2003) providing a salient example of how the study of rare disease-linked variants can inform our understanding of disease mechanisms. This work also demonstrates the successful use of patients with structural chromosomal variation to guide gene choice in resequencing in large case–control cohorts (Abrahams and Geschwind 2008).

Overall, none of these molecules associated with ASDs have been shown to selectively cause autism. Instead, each seems to result in an array of abnormal neurobehavioral phenotypes, including autism, Asperger syndrome, non-syndromic mental retardation and other neurodevelopmental abnormalities (Abrahams and Geschwind 2008). For example, Laumonnier et al. reported a large French family in which ten males had nonspecific X-linked mental retardation, two had autism, and one had pervasive developmental disorder. All affected patients were found to have the same frameshift mutation in the *NLGN4* gene. One obligate female carrier had mild mental retardation (Laumonnier et al. 2004; Yan et al. 2005). Similarly, an extensive study of the 16p11 CNV in multiple clinical populations showed that it is at least as prevalent in a clinical population with global developmental delay or language delay as it is in autism (Weiss et al. 2008). Given this apparent lack of specificity for the ASDs, it will not be surprising if variation in some of these genes contributes to other neuropsychiatric disorders.

Linkage and association studies have not found "the autism gene" but have unequivocally demonstrated that more sophisticated solutions will be required to explain this group of disorders. The availability of new technology will permit the initiation of population-based strategies that are likely to provide more satisfying answers. An understanding of the contribution of common variation, the manner by which rare variants could modulate presentation, is an important future step (Abrahams and Geschwind 2008). ASDs are the product of the interplay between multiple common and rare genetic variants, and genetic diagnosis should involve a combination of multiple genetic markers as a form of targeted gene panels. Multiple parallel approaches will be necessary to advance our understanding of the genetic factors underlying ASDs, including whole-genome and pathway-based association studies, dense resequencing to identify mutations, and the continued collection of large well-characterized patient cohorts and their relatives for genotype–phenotype studies (Abrahams and Geschwind 2008). The ultimate goal of the evaluation of genetic etiology is the discovery of biomarkers for risk assessment, diagnosis, and prediction of therapeutic responses and prognoses and the development of therapeutic components (Yoo 2015), but despite many genes having been identified that lead to the predisposition of ASDs, the biological mechanisms remain unclear.

2.4 Animal Models and Validity

ASDs reflect an extremely complex and heterogeneous syndrome not only by their inherent variability but also by the core features (Veenstra-VanderWeele and Blakely 2012). From a clinical perspective, the fundamental symptoms of ASD are aberrant reciprocal social interactions (e.g., limited or absent response when calling the name or joint attention), stereotyped behaviors or unusual handling of objects (e.g., intensive observation of objects and stereotyped movements of hands and tapping, spinning, or flapping), and poor communications skills. Advances in the fields of genetics and molecular biology have led to the creation of mouse models with targeted genetic mutations of candidate genes found in human clinical disorders. In the case of ASDs, determining which genes to target has proven problematic, with research in humans showing several *loci* associated with ASD, suggesting a complex multigenetic cause (Levitt and Campbell 2009; Szatmari et al. 2007). However, animal models can be tremendously beneficial for determining disease etiology, effects on circuit and cellular function, and therapeutic efficacy of novel treatment strategies. Importantly, the ASD core symptoms can also be modeled, namely, repetitive behaviors and deficits in social interaction and communication (Table 2.2) (Silverman et al. 2010a; Williams 2011; Moy and Nadler 2008). Although it is difficult to reflect human pathophysiology in animal models, some aspects of molecular pathways, brain anatomy, and cognitive and behavioral phenotypes can be addressed, providing insight into human neuropsychiatric disorders that may contribute to the screening of novel drugs. Mouse models are advantageous in many respects, primarily because they are genetically developed and appropriate for invasive studies and offer invaluable opportunities to test the functional and behavioral repercussions of manipulating a particular aspect of the nervous system.

Mouse models of ASDs have been based on manipulations of loci that mediate single-gene human disorders characterized by ASD symptoms or that have been identified through association or linkage studies in human genetics. Other mouse models involve mutations in proteins along pathways thought to be altered in ASDs (Moy and Nadler 2008; Moy et al. 2006). The most common strategy for genetic modification is to generate a null allele, or targeted disruption, which deletes a portion of the locus and generally prevents the production of a functional protein, although a serious drawback of this approach is that the null allele may not be consistent with the allele in the ASD population (Moy et al. 2006); moreover, a complete removal of a protein in the brain can lead to several impairments or early death on several models. Additionally, in the case of ASD, most alleles already identified, are heterozygous mutations. A second common approach to creating relevant animal models is to engineer conditional knockouts using Cre–*loxP* recombination (van Duyne 2015) which allows for targeted and conditional deletion of the gene to specific cell types or after a certain time point. These are especially useful to circumvent issues of embryonic lethality or target the mutation to specific neurons or circuits for a better understanding of the molecular pathways and behavioral impact. Either way, it is important to understand which method is being used when evaluating the validity of the model and extrapolating the data to ASD phenotypes.

While translational research is needed to discover pharmacological targets and treatments of ASDs, animal models with phenotypic relevance to diagnostic criteria offer clear experimental strategies to test the efficacy and safety of novel treatments (Tania et al. 2014). In fact, a number of mouse models based on the genetic variants have been developed that are associated with ASD, and some of the most commonly used are highlighted in Table 2.3 and discussed below. While model systems are necessary to test hypotheses and better understand the underlying neurobiology, rodent models are inherently limited and cannot fully recapitulate the human disorder. Therefore, each system needs to be assessed on how well it mirrors the human

Table 2.2 ASD-relevant behavioral tasks for rodents

Behavioral test	Test description
Social defects	
Reciprocal social interaction	Fine-grained measures of interactions between pairs or groups of juvenile or adult mice placed together in standard cages or specialized arenas. Can measure nose-to-nose sniffing, nose-to-anogenital sniffing, following, pushing past each other with physical contact, crawling over and under each other with physical contact, chasing, mounting, wrestling, and grooming or licking each other. Behavioral profiles during social interaction can provide an index of social reciprocity
Three-chamber social approach test	A more standardized, higher-throughput assay to measure time spent (i.e., preference) with a novel mouse versus time spent with a nonsocial novel object. This task assesses social motivation as a measure of social novelty preference and social recognition
Social conditioned place preference	This choice task provides a measure of the reward value for a given context, without direct presentation of the motivating stimuli during the test. In the conditioning phase, mice learn to associate one set of unique environmental stimuli with social isolation and another set with a social context (group housing). Mice are then given a choice between the environmental stimuli paired with the social versus nonsocial contexts
Communication deficits	
Social transmission of food preference	Interaction with a cagemate who has eaten a novel-flavored food will confer familiarity with the flavor. Mice can learn to prefer a novel food that has previously been consumed by a "demonstrator" mouse through the social transfer of olfactory and other information, probably by sniffing food odors on the breath and mouth of the demonstrator
Olfactory habituation to social odors	Mice demonstrate high-level interest in urinary scents from other mice which deposit urinary steroidal pheromones as territorial markings. Quantification of this task includes doing a discrimination operant task or measuring bouts and duration of sniffing. Time to habituate to the same odor can also be measured
Ultrasonic vocalizations (USVs)	Mice emit complex ultrasonic vocalizations in social situations, especially pups separated from the dam and nest, juvenile interactions, resident females in a resident–intruder task, and males responding to female urinary pheromones
Repetitive behavior	
Stereotyped behaviors	Mice can exhibit abnormal preservative responses such as over grooming (sometimes to the point of self-injury), "jackhammer" jumping, cage-lid back flipping, wall climbing, locomotor circling, and increased digging in the bedding or in a marble burying assay
Restricted interests	Reduce interest can be measured by a lack of exploration in a novel environment, restricted pattern of poking in a nose poke task, and lack of preference for novel objects
Reversal learning	This task can be used to assess insistence on sameness or perseverative behaviors. Cognitive flexibility or rigidity can be assessed in the Morris water maze task. Mice learn to find the hidden platform in a fixed location in a circular pool. For reversal learning, the location of the platform is changed, and mice are then evaluated for their ability to adapt to the new learning condition. Reversal learning can also be tested in a Barnes maze or T-maze

Adapted from Buxbaum and Hof (2013), Silverman et al. (2010a)

Table 2.3 ASD mouse models and their ASD-relevant phenotypes

Mouse model	Social defects	Communication deficits	Repetitive behavior	Anatomy	Intervention
Fmr1	Inconsistent results from reduced to normal social behaviors	Increased USVs in pups	Increased stereotypies and perseveration	Abnormal spine morphology, altered synaptic plasticity, altered GABAergic transmission, and loss of GABAergic interneurons	Environmental enrichment, mGluR, GABAergic
Mecp2	Social avoidance, impaired social recognition	Increased USVs in pups (in Jae)	Limb stereotypies	Smaller brains with smaller cells that are more densely packed especially in cortex, hippocampus, cerebellum	Environmental enrichment, IGF-1, BDNF
TSC1 (+/-)	Decreased social interaction	n/a	n/a	Normal spine number and dendritic branching	n/a
TSC1 (cKO)	Reduced reciprocal social interactions, impaired nest-building behavior	Increased USVs in pups (cKO)	Increased grooming, increased inflexibility (cKO)	Abnormal spine density and morphology	Rapamycin
TSC2 (+/-)	Normal sociability	Increased USVs in pups	Normal inflexibility, normal perseveration	Dendritic spine pruning defect	Rapamycin, lovastatin
TSC2 (cKO)	Decreased sociability, decreased novelty	n/a	Increased perseveration, normal inflexibility	Neuronal disorganization and megalencephaly	Rapamycin
Dup15q11–q13	Low sociability	Ultrasonic vocalizations elevated in pups and reduced in adults	Increased inflexibility	Altered serotonergic signaling	n/a
Gabrb3 null	Low sociability, decreased preference for social novelty, impaired nest-building behavior, impaired social interaction	n/a	Repetitive stereotyped circling patterns	Hypoplasia of the cerebellar vermis	n/a

(continued)

Table 2.3 (continued)

Mouse model	Social defects	Communication deficits	Repetitive behavior	Anatomy	Intervention
Dup15q11–q13 (paternal allele)	Decreased social interaction	Increased USVs in pups but decreased in adult males	Behavioral inflexibility	Smaller brain regions including dentate gyrus, medial striatum	n/a
Del15q11–q13 (maternal deletion)	n/a	Increased USVs in pups	n/a	Increased perseverance	n/a
Ube3a-null	Normal social-seeking behavior	Increased USVs in pups	Increased stereotyped behaviors, increased perseveration	Reduced brain size in juveniles with maternal deletion, reduced spine density, and altered morphology	n/a
Del16p11.2	Normal sociability, normal social novelty	Reduced USVs in adult males	Increased circling, climbing, cognitive inflexibility	Reduced brain size but increased relative volume in midline structures, reduced neuron # in upper cortical layers, increased D2-expressing MSNs	mGluR5
Shank3 (23q13.3 del)	Decreased social interaction, decreased social novelty recognition	Decreased USVs in pups and adult males	Increased grooming, normal or impaired MWM reversal learning, increased perseveration	Hyperactivation of cortico-striatal-thalamic axis, enlarged brain regions including basal ganglia and thalamus while hippocampus, amygdala, and white matter tracts (not fornix) were reduced in volume, reduced spine density	IGF-1, mGluR5
Pten	Reduced reciprocal social interactions, low sociability, impaired social recognition	n/a	Increased grooming	Increased brain size, increased spine density	Rapamycin

Cntnap2	Decreased sociability, decreased juvenile play	Decreased USVs in pups	Increased grooming and digging, increased inflexibility	Abnormal neuronal migration, reduced numbers of interneurons, abnormal neuronal synchrony, increased size of frontal lobes but decreased cerebellum	Risperidone
Met	n/a	n/a	Reduced reversal ability	Altered forebrain GABAergic interneurons, enlarged frontal cortical areas, hippocampus, striatum, and thalamus	n/a
Nlgn4	Reduced reciprocal social interaction, reduced sociability, reduced juvenile play	Reduced to normal USVs in adult males	Increased stereotypies, increased perseveration, normal inflexibility	Reduced brain volume, especially in cerebellum and brainstem	n/a
Nlgn3 R451C	Slight deficit to normal social interaction and preference	Reduced ultrasonic vocalizations	Normal perseveration, normal inflexibility	Decreased total forebrain volume, smaller hippocampus, striatum, and thalamus	n/a
Neurexin 1α	Normal social interactions, impaired nest-building behavior	n/a	Increased repetitive grooming	n/a	n/a

Silverman et al. (2010a), Bey and Jiang (2014), Ellegood and Crawley (2015)

Fig. 2.1 Assessing the validity of an animal model

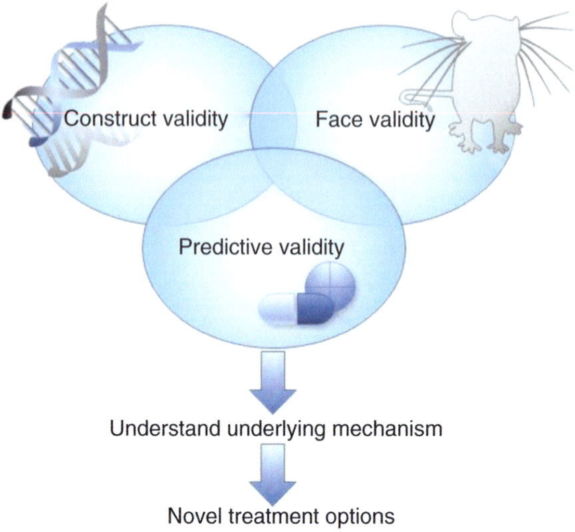

condition so we can better understand and contextualize the significance of any findings. Commonly, three criteria are used to assess the potential of a given system as a model of ASD: (1) construct validity, (2) face validity, and (3) predictive validity (Fig. 2.1) (Willner 1984; Chadman et al. 2009).

Construct validity is likely the most important criterion for assessing the validity of an animal model. Construct validity constitutes the similarity of the etiological factors underlying the disorder between the animal and the human disease that it models. In this case, construct validity is best understood in the context of genetic models, where a putative susceptibility gene is manipulated in mice to observe the behavioral and neurobiological consequences (Willner 1984; Chadman et al. 2009).

Face validity compares the symptoms of the human disease to the model system. The most common measure of face validity is usually based on the emergence of observable behaviors reminiscent of typical ASD-related behaviors such as repetitive behaviors, poor social interaction, and problems in communication (see Table 2.2). This task can be difficult due to breaking down complex behaviors into simpler aspects of rodent behavior. For example, one of the most commonly observed rodent behaviors that support face validity of ASD models is excessive grooming, which corresponds to an increase in a behavior that follows a stereotyped pattern (Moy et al. 2008; Silverman et al. 2010a; Peñagarikano et al. 2011; Peça et al. 2011; Ahmari et al. 2013). Face validity can also be established by analyzing the neuropathology, neurophysiological functioning, and neurochemical alterations in the rodent models (Chadman et al. 2009). Brain development can be measured by structural changes to forebrain neurons, alterations in GABAergic interneuron numbers, and changes in connectivity between brain areas.

Finally, predictive validity evaluates the treatment responses that are effective in humans. Drugs that ameliorate the human symptoms should also reverse the rodent symptoms and vice versa. Importantly, the rodent model can also be used to identify drugs beneficial to humans. For example, a rationale for developing metabotropic glutamate receptor 5 (mGluR5) antagonists as therapeutics has been provided by studies showing that a genetic reduction of mGluR5 reversed some of the symptoms in *Fmr1* mouse models of fragile X syndrome, in addition to studies showing that an mGluR5 antagonist treatment reversed *Fmr1* phenotypes and repetitive self-grooming in BTBR mice (Silverman et al. 2010a, b; Dolen et al. 2007; Dolen and Bear 2008; Michalon et al. 2012). Furthermore, a recent study tested various compounds and showed that the acute administration of the neuropeptide oxytocin improved social deficits in the *Cntnap2* mouse model of autism (Peñagarikano et al. 2015).

In the face of several genes clearly implicated in ASD and with corresponding mouse models that mimic the human risk variants, we are beginning to be able to analyze the phenotypes of those animals to understand the true range of ASD-like behavior in the rodent (Table 2.3). We are often restricted to behaviors that fit our expectations for how they may present in a mouse. But with standardization of behavioral tasks (Silverman et al. 2010a; Williams 2011) including assessment of cognitive function, a number of mouse models are moving toward an understanding of circuits and molecular pathways underlying neuropsychiatric disorders.

2.4.1 VPA

Environmental factors such as exposure to certain chemicals including thalidomide, misoprostol, and valproic acid (VPA) in early pregnancy are believed to contribute to autism (Tania et al. 2014). VPA is a medication primarily used to treat epilepsy and bipolar disorder and to prevent migraine headaches. In fact, one of the most robust models in rats for ASD is based on the fact that treatment of epilepsy or bipolar disorder in pregnant women during 20–24 days post conception with VPA is linked to an increased incidence of ASD in their children (Hyman et al. 2005; Gogolla et al. 2009).

Rodier et al. (1996) first reported that the brains of rats exposed to valproic acid in utero in early gestation had similar hypoplasia of brain stem nuclei to that found in a case of idiopathic autism (Rodier et al. 1996). The brains of animals exposed at the time of neural tube closure not only had decreased cellularity of the brain stem nuclei but had a subsequent decreased number of Purkinje cells in the cerebellum as a downstream event (Hyman et al. 2005; Ingram et al. 2000). A series of studies have reported that VPA-exposed rats display significantly fewer neurons and significant alterations in neuronal morphology including decreased dendritic branching and decreased spine density particularly in prefrontal cortical regions and cerebellum (Mychasiuk et al. 2012; Tania et al. 2014). Favre and colleagues (2013) reported that rat offspring exposed to VPA leads to hyper-connectivity between the neurons of the neocortex and amygdala. Various pathways in which VPA can induce impairments in neural development have been analyzed, and many led to increased glutamatergic neuronal density of the rat brain. This finding was evidenced by macrocephaly, increased neuronal number, and increased glutamatergic protein markers such as PSD95, α-CaMKII, NMDA, and AMPA receptors in postnatal VPA rat brains (Kim et al. 2013a; Mabunga et al. 2015). Furthermore, these rats showed downregulation of genes responsible for GABAergic inhibitory neuronal development and subsequent reduction in expression of GABAergic neuronal marker, GAD (Kim et al. 2013a; Tania et al. 2014; Fukuchi et al. 2009; Mabunga et al. 2015) The VPA animal model, aside from genetic models, is shedding light on the excitatory/inhibitory (E/I) imbalance observed in autism and offers good ground for therapeutic development. Importantly, VPA rat models have shown impairments in social behavior and abnormal nest seeking (Kim et al. 2013a; Favre et al. 2013). Therefore prenatal VPA exposure in rats appears to produce similar endophenotypes as reported in the autistic patients (Tania et al. 2014).

In rats, a single dose of VPA at an equivalent gestational time point recapitulates the human ASD phenotype (Gogolla et al. 2009; Tania et al. 2014; Mabunga et al. 2015). Prenatal exposure of VPA in rodents produces neuroanatomical and behavioral deficits and alters social behaviors. The VPA model of ASD is a direct example of construct validity as VPA induces ASD both in humans and animals. The etiological mechanism may involve changes in epigenetic marks, expression level of genetic determinants, as well as brain lesions (Mabunga et al. 2015). Similarly, in the VPA model, the disease endophenotypes are recapitulated and biologic markers were assessed for face validity, showing consistency with human ASD phenotypes (Mabunga et al. 2015). The VPA animal model also has strong construct validity as known drugs, and many drug candidates have been assessed for the applicability as potential therapeutics (Mabunga et al. 2015). Prenatal valproate exposure is not a major cause of autism, because few mothers of children with autism are treated with this agent for seizures, migraine prophylaxis, or mood disorders, but neurologists, internists, psychiatrists, obstetricians, and other practitioners treating adults must be aware of the teratogenicity of this agent when they prescribe it to women of child-bearing age (Hyman et al. 2005).

2.4.2 Fmr1

Fragile X syndrome (FXS), primarily affecting males, is one of the leading genetic causes for autism spectrum disorder. FXS is caused by extended CGG trinucleotide repeats, expanding the 5′ noncoding region of the fragile X mental retardation 1 (*FMR1*) gene on the X chromosome (Verkerk et al. 1991; Pieretti et al. 1991; Bassell and Warren 2008). This mutation leads to hypermethylation of the *FMR1* promoter, an epigenetic mechanism which transcriptionally silences *FMR1* and reduces levels of FMRP (fragile X mental retardation protein), an RNA-binding protein involved in suppressing activity-dependent translation of synaptic proteins, many of which have been independently implicated in ASDs (Ashley et al. 1993; Bassell and Warren 2008). However, mice with extended CGG repeats in *Fmr1* do not recapitulate the hypermethylation and transcriptional silencing of FMRP that is characteristic of human FXS (Brouwer et al. 2007; Hulbert and Jiang 2016). Instead, researchers have mimicked the molecular consequences of the human mutation by deleting exon 5 of *Fmr1* (Dutch-Belgian Fragile X Consortium 1994). The *Fmr1*-null mouse is one of the best characterized animal models associated with ASD. These mice mimic the genetic mutation underlying FXS patients who are characterized by intellectual disability, increased anxiety, hyperarousal to stimuli, physical abnormalities, and, in most cases, ASD (Hagerman et al. 1986, 2010; Moy et al. 2006).

FMRP is enriched postsynaptically in the brain, particularly at synapses that use the major excitatory neurotransmitter glutamate, so much attention has been focused on synaptic dysfunction in FXS. Many studies have reported differences in dendritic spines in *Fmr1* knockout mice with the main consistent finding indicating defects in activity-dependent spine plasticity and maturation (He and Portera-Cailliau 2013; Hulbert and Jiang 2016). Dendritic spines are the principal recipients of excitatory synaptic inputs and the basic units of neural computation in the mammalian brain. Alterations in the density, size, shape, and turnover of mature spines, or defects in how spines are generated and establish synapses during brain development, could all result in neuronal dysfunction and lead to cognitive and/or behavioral impairments. Both FXS patients and the *Fmr1* knockout mouse display abnormal spine development, but the exact nature of the defect is still controversial due to conflicting reports (He and Portera-Cailliau 2013). Using in vivo two-photon imaging, researchers recently found increased turnover in dendritic spines in the cortex of juvenile *Fmr1*-null mice (Cruz-Martin et al. 2010; Pan et al. 2010). Alterations in synaptic plasticity have also been well characterized (Chung et al. 2012; Sidorov et al. 2013), but the electrophysiological consequences of the *Fmr1* knockout vary across brain regions and development (He and Portera-Cailliau 2013; Hulbert and Jiang 2016). Nevertheless, these experiments have demonstrated an increase in mGluR-dependent synaptic plasticity (long-term depression (LTD)) (Huber et al. 2002). Normally, FMRP is dephosphorylated after activation of metabotropic glutamate receptors (mGluRs), leading to derepression of local translation (reviewed in Bassell and Warren 2008), a mechanism necessary for synaptic plasticity (Sutton and Schuman 2006). These data have paved the way for the mGluR theory for FXS pathogenesis: FXS symptoms are caused by overactivation of mGluR5 signaling leading to deregulated mRNA translation in the absence of FMRP (Bear et al. 2004). This theory has been supported by the effectiveness of genetic depletion of mGluR5 (Dolen et al. 2007) and mGluR5-negative allosteric modulators (e.g., CTEP; Michalon et al. (2012)) in alleviating behavioral and synaptic abnormalities in *Fmr1* knockout mice (Hulbert and Jiang 2016).

Total mGluR5 levels are normal in the forebrain of *Fmr1*-null mice; however, there is less mGluR5 in the postsynaptic density (PSD) fraction and an altered balance of mGluR5 association with short and long isoforms of the postsynaptic scaffolding protein, Homer (Giuffrida et al. 2005). Homer proteins bind to the intracellular C-terminal tail of group 1 mGluRs (mGluR5 and mGluR1a) and affect their trafficking, localization and function (Shiraishi-Yamaguchi and Furuichi 2007). Long, constitutively expressed forms of Homer (Homer1b, 1c, 2 and 3) multimerize through their C-terminal coiled-coil domain and localize mGluRs to the PSD through interactions with Shank (see Sect. 2.4.6), as well as scaffold mGluRs to signaling pathways. On the other hand, *Homer1a* (*H1a*), a short, activity-inducible form of Homer lacks the coiled-coil domain and cannot multimerize with other Homers, consequently, disrupting mGluR5–long Homer complexes, altering mGluR signaling and causing constitutive, agonist-independent activity of mGluR1/5 (Shiraishi-Yamaguchi and Furuichi 2007; Ango et al. 2001). In *Fmr1* KO mice mGluR5 is less associated with the long Homer isoforms and more associated with *H1a* (Giuffrida et al. 2005). Genetic deletion of *Homer1a* in *Fmr1*-null mice restored mGluR5–long Homer scaffolds and corrects multiple phenotypes in *Fmr1*-null mice including altered mGluR5 signaling, neocortical circuit dysfunction, and behavior (Ronesi et al. 2012). In contrast, *Homer1a* deletion does not rescue altered mGluR-dependent long-term synaptic depression or translational control of FMRP target mRNAs (Ronesi et al. 2012). Modulation and restoration of mGluR5–Homer interactions may represent a novel therapeutic strategy for fragile X and related cognitive and autistic disorders.

The *Fmr1* knockout mice also show decreased GABA subunit receptors, decreased synthesis of GABA, increased catabolism of GABA, and overall decreased GABAergic interneurons and inputs in many regions of the brain (D'Hulst et al. 2006; Hagerman et al. 2010; Selby et al. 2007; Curia et al. 2009; D'Hulst et al. 2009; Gogolla et al. 2009; Lozano et al. 2014). GABA is a major inhibitory neurotransmitter receptor in the brain, which is important in anxiety, depression, epilepsy, insomnia, and learning and memory (see Sect. 2.5). There are two main subtypes of GABA receptors: $GABA_A$ and $GABA_B$. The more abundant $GABA_A$ receptors are ligand-gated Cl^- channels that give fast inhibition, whereas the $GABA_B$ receptors are G-protein-coupled receptors which give slower and more prolonged inhibitory signals (Bormann 2000). The ionotropic $GABA_A$ receptors are usually localized postsynaptically, and their activation leads to opening of Cl^- channels and hyperpolarization of the membrane potential, thus making it difficult for excitatory neurotransmitters such as glutamate to generate an action potential. The metabotropic $GABA_B$ receptors, however, can be found either presynaptically and inhibit release of neurotransmitters through downregulation of high-voltage-activated Ca^{2+} channels or postsynaptically and decrease neuronal excitability through its influence on K^+ channels. FMRP can bind directly to the mRNA of the delta subunit of the $GABA_A$ receptor, suggesting that deficits in GABA-mediated inhibition may underlie many of the key symptoms in FXS, including the seizures, anxiety, and autistic-like behaviors (D'Hulst et al. 2006; Selby et al. 2007; Kooy 2003; Hagerman et al. 2010; Lozano et al. 2014). As $GABA_A$ receptors are the major inhibitory receptors in the brain, and are specifically involved in processes that are disturbed in FXS, including neuronal excitability (leading to enhanced seizure susceptibility), anxiety, sleep, and learning, enhancement of the function of $GABA_A$ receptors may have major therapeutic benefits for FXS. Heulens and colleagues (2012) have demonstrated that the use of the $GABA_A$ agonist ganaxolone (3α-hydroxy-3β-methyl-5α-pregnan-20-one) improved seizures in the KO mouse model of FXS (Heulens et al. 2012; Lozano et al. 2014). A randomized, phase II, double-blind, placebo-controlled crossover trial to investigate the efficacy of ganaxolone for the treatment of anxiety and attention deficits in children with FXS aged 6–17 years (http://www.

ClinicalTrials.gov; NCT01725152) is currently under way. Ganaxolone should increase and normalize $GABA_A$-mediated signaling—by boosting the signaling capacity of existing receptors—and improve behavior, particularly anxiety and attention (Lozano et al. 2014).

$GABA_B$ receptor agonists such as baclofen or arbaclofen, the more potent, right-sided isomer of baclofen, inhibit both presynaptic release of glutamate and postsynaptic transmission and/or intracellular signaling downstream from mGluR5. In *Fmr1* KO mice, arbaclofen corrected elevated protein synthesis in the hippocampus, reduced elevated AMPA (α-amino-3-hydroxy-5-methyl-4-isoxazolepropionic acid) receptor internalization to wild-type values, decreased mRNA translation in the cortex, and corrected the increased spine density prevalent in the mouse phenotype (Henderson et al. 2012; Hagerman et al. 2010; Lozano et al. 2014).

Curiously, minocycline, a widely used antibiotic for treating acne and skin infections, is another promising drug that may target core symptoms of FXS and autism. Minocycline inhibits matrix metalloproteinase (MMP)-9 which is elevated in FXS. This is an enzyme involved in synaptic plasticity, and is associated with immature dendritic spine morphology (Bilousova et al. 2009; Hagerman et al. 2010). Administration of minocycline to *Fmr1*-null mice leads to hippocampal neurons with mature dendritic spines and decreased levels of anxiety and improved exploration skills (Bilousova et al. 2009). Off-label use of minocycline to treat 50 individuals with FXS resulted in two-thirds of families noticing positive improvements in their child's language and attention and/or behavioral improvements while on the medication (Utari et al. 2010), and an open-label, double-blind trial for individuals with FXS aged 3.5–16 years showed similar mild improvements (Leigh et al. 2013).

The behavioral phenotype of the fragile X-model mice reflects symptoms associated with the human disorder. The *Fmr1*-null mice show cognitive deficits, including impaired reversal learning in the Morris water maze, and changes in social behavior (Moy et al. 2006; Santos et al. 2014). These differences may be attributed, in part, to the effect of the different genetic backgrounds of the mouse strains used for the *Fmr1*-null mice, suggesting that there are multiple genetic interactions, which can modulate complex behavioral phenotypes, even in a defined, single-locus disease (Moy et al. 2006). Research on FXS over the past few years has identified several hundred putative FMRP mRNA targets (for review, see Fernandez et al. (2013)). This large number of FMRP mRNA targets might explain the extensive and heterogeneous behavioral deficits in FXS, suggesting that FMRP loss influences different circuitries and causes alterations in various receptor pathways. Although, it is very well established that FMRP loss alters the glutamatergic signaling (mGluR theory), many other molecular pathways such as BDNF, mTOR, ERK1/2, cAMP, and PKC cascades are affected. In addition, different neuronal circuits, such as the GABAergic, cholinergic, dopaminergic, and serotonergic systems, are modified by FMRP loss (Fish et al. 2013; Santos et al. 2014). Finally, *Fmr1*-deficient mice demonstrate cytoarchitectonic and physiological aberrations, including altered dendritic spine morphology and macroorchidism, similar to changes in fragile X patients.

2.4.3 Mecp2

The X-linked methyl-CpG-binding protein 2 gene encodes for MeCP2 which binds to methylated CpG islands in genomic DNA, downregulating gene expression. A single gene mutation of the locus encoding for *MeCP2* causes Rett syndrome, on the autism spectrum, and is characterized by mental retardation, slowed growth rate, hypoactivity, motor abnormalities, seizures, and ASD-related behaviors including repetitive behaviors. Partial or complete genetic deletion of *MeCP2* in the mouse brain leads to the emergence of motor impairment, tremors, hypoactivity, repetitive behaviors, and deficits in social interaction (Chen et al. 2001; Moretti et al. 2005, 2006; Moretti and Zoghbi 2006; Fyffe et al. 2008). The global knockout of *Mecp2* in mice led to embryonic lethality (Tate et al. 1996). Since then, several lines have been generated including the best studied mice with an exon 3 deletion (Mecp2 tm1.1Jae; Chen et al. 2001), with deletions of exons 3 and 4 (Mecp2 tm1.1Bird; Jacky Guy et al. 2001), and mice with a 308X point mutation (Mecp2 tm1Hzo; Shahbazian et al. 2002), which introduces a premature stop codon that leads to truncation of the MeCP2 protein. The complete loss of both MeCP2 protein isoforms were revealed in hemizygous males (Mecp2 /y) of Mecp2tm1.1Jae and Mecp2tm1.1Bird mutants, whereas the female heterozygous mice (Mecp2 /+) are the model with best construct validity, as Rett syndrome primarily affects females and is lethal in males in most cases (Hulbert and Jiang 2016). However, most studies use hemizygous male mice because they develop more severe phenotypes, a phenomenon found in several other mouse models including those for Angelman syndrome (Sect. 2.4.4). An important question that remains is why humans are more sensitive than rodents to MeCP2 mutations.

To determine potential brain regions, cell types, and developmental time periods involved in Rett syndrome pathogenesis, several research groups moved to using Cre–*loxP* technology to generate conditional knockout mice with spatial and temporal manipulation of *MeCP2* (Jacky Guy et al. 2001; reviewed in Calfa et al. 2011). This allowed us to understand that postnatal expression of *MeCP2* in neurons is sufficient to recapitulate the Rett phenotype (Chen et al. 2001; Jacky Guy et al. 2012; Luikenhuis et al. 2004; Calfa et al. 2011). Interestingly, the deletion of *Mecp2* in either excitatory forebrain neurons or GABAergic inhibitory interneurons is sufficient to produce ASD-like features (Gemelli et al. 2006; Chao et al. 2010). However, it remains unclear if the mechanisms of Mecp2 function are the same in these circuits. Furthermore, it is likely that the Rett syndrome phenotypes can be induced in fully adult mice, underscoring the ongoing role of MeCP2 in adult neurological function. In fact, unlike the effects of other epigenetic instructions programmed during early life, the effects of early MeCP2 function are lost soon after its deletion (McGraw et al. 2011). These findings suggest that therapies for RTT must be maintained throughout life. Similarly, breakthrough studies have demonstrated that the major symptoms of Rett in mice caused by lack of *Mecp2* are also still reversible in adulthood upon activation of the endogenous gene (Moretti and Zoghbi 2006; Giacometti et al. 2007; Guy et al. 2007; Jugloff et al. 2008; Pitcher et al. 2015). Importantly, *Mecp2* rescue can be effective in a fully symptomatic adult stage. However, a gene therapy approach to restoring *Mecp2* copies presents significant difficulties in humans due to the dosage-sensitive nature of the gene involved in neuronal function (Collins et al. 2004; Calfa et al. 2011; Katz et al. 2016). These studies suggest that ASDs may not be purely developmental disorders but also arise from persistent abnormal neural functioning, rather than disrupted development. However, this hypothesis needs to be tested in other models of ASD, as the phenotypes reported in these studies are not necessarily generalizable (Hulbert and Jiang 2016).

While many of these studies have focused on the behavioral endophenotype, some anatomical and electrophysiological analyses have also been performed. Both *Mecp2 tm1.1Bird* and *Mecp2 tm1.1Jae* mice have cortical neurons with decreased spine density (Belichenko et al. 2009) and decreased dendritic complexity (Fukuda et al. 2005; Smrt et al. 2007), but this could vary across development (Chapleau et al. 2009; Hulbert and Jiang 2016). Moreover, adult *Mecp2tm1Hzo* mice have normal spine density and dendritic complexity in both the cortex and hippocampus (Moretti et al. 2006). Electrophysiologically, altered synaptic plasticity has been reported in hippocampal CA1 synapses in these three mouse lines (Asaka et al. 2006; Moretti et al. 2006). Recordings from sensory and motor cortex from Mecp2tm1Hzo mice also revealed reduced LTP (Moretti et al. 2006). Whole-cell patch-clamp recordings revealed reduced spontaneous activity due to a significant reduction in the amplitude of miniature excitatory postsynaptic currents (Dani et al. 2005), which are associated with decreased numbers of glutamatergic synapses on individual neurons (Chao et al. 2007). How the deficiency of Mecp2 results in abnormal functioning of neuronal synapses as well as ASD-like phenotypes is still not fully understood. One of the hundreds of genes deregulated in the brains of *Mecp2* mice is BDNF, a neurotrophic factor that is downregulated in Mecp2-deficient neurons. Not only do decreases in BDNF expression correlate with symptom severity (Chang et al. 2006), but treatments that increase BDNF also improve symptoms (Ogier et al. 2007; Kline et al. 2010).

Given the low penetrance of BDNF across the blood–brain barrier, other studies have focused on similar growth factors that might be more clinically tractable. Specifically, administration of the tripeptide insulin-like growth factor 1 (IGF1) to KO animals resulted in an extension of lifespan similar to that observed with BDNF overexpression and partially rescues locomotor activity, breathing variability, spine density, and synaptic amplitude (Tropea et al. 2009). Further, IGF1 treatment increased the number of glutamatergic synapses in neurons derived from induced pluripotent stem cells (iPSCs) from Rett syndrome patients (Marchetto et al. 2010). A phase I clinical trial (NCT identifier 01253317) is underway to administer IGF1 to Rett patients (Khwaja et al. 2014). The efficacy of this treatment will be clearer upon completion of the current phase II trials (NCT identifier 01777542) (Lombardi et al. 2015).

The great majority of ASD research has focused on brain-specific mechanisms and circuits, with little attention to potential contributions of the peripheral nervous system to ASD phenotypes. Recently, David Ginty's group was prompted to investigate the role of peripheral nervous system deficiencies caused by the disruption of

Mecp2 or other ASD-associated genes in cutaneous tactile sensitivity (Orefice et al. 2016). Interestingly, tactile hypersensitivity is common in patients with Rett syndrome (Badr et al. 1987; Amir et al. 1999). Similarly, abnormalities in tactile perception are observed in patients with fragile X syndrome (Rogers et al. 2003). Although abnormalities in touch perception are commonly reported in ASDs, the underlying neural mechanisms are unknown. The sensation of touch starts in the peripheral nervous system with receptors at the surface of the skin and travels along nerves in the spinal cord that connect into the brain. So Orefice and colleagues (2016) introduced mutations that silenced *MeCP2* specifically in the peripheral somatosensory neurons. The resulting *Mecp2* mutant mice were more sensitive to light touch: the mice startled more to a small puff of air on their backs than normal mice. Additionally, the mutants were unable to distinguish between rough and smooth textures. Just like normal mice—which love novelty—they played with new objects whenever given a choice between familiar and new ones that differed in shape and size. Interestingly, these mice also displayed autism-like behaviors beyond touch: the conditional knockout mice were also more anxious and less social, traits generally attributed to the central nervous system. For example, when mice are given the option to interact with another mouse or an object like an empty cup, the mutant mice spent just as much time with the object as with the other mouse, unlike normal mice, which prefer a living companion.

The researchers (Orefice et al. 2016) then silenced *Mecp2* in the peripheral nerves only during adulthood and found that while the mice were still hypersensitive to light touch, they did not display the behavioral abnormalities seen in the animals that had the gene silenced from birth. These data suggest that there is a developmental window of time when touch influences behavior. Early childhood tactile experiences are critical for the acquisition of normal social behavior and communication skills in humans and rodents (Hertenstein et al. 2006). Orefice suggests that if a light touch from another mouse is uncomfortable or the environment feels abrasive, a mouse might learn to avoid its peers and reduce exploration of the environment.

Mechanistically, Ginty's group went on to show that the deletion of *Mecp2* selectively in peripheral somatosensory neurons resulted in aberrant tactile sensitivity due to a loss of presynaptic inhibition of somatosensory neuron transmission in the spinal cord. They go on to suggest that this is due to loss of expression of GABRB3, the $GABA_A$ receptor subunit β3, in the spinal cord of *Mecp2* mutant mice (Orefice et al. 2016). Mutations to *Gabrb3* are associated with ASD in humans, and mice harboring a *Gabrb3* mutation exhibit social behavior deficits, hypersensitivity to both thermal and mechanical stimuli, and sensorimotor impairments (DeLorey et al. 1998, 2008, 2011). Moreover, *Gabrb3* conditional mutant mice (whereby *Gabrb3* was ablated from peripheral somatosensory neurons during development or adulthood) from each group exhibited enhanced tactile sensitivity (Orefice et al. 2016). However, only the mice with the conditional deletion of *Gabrb3* during development demonstrated impairments in social and cognitive behaviors. Thus, mice lacking *Gabrb3* in primary somatosensory neurons phenocopy mice lacking *Mecp2* in somatosensory neurons, implicating a functional link between these ASD-associated genes. These findings revealed an essential, cell-autonomous requirement for the ASD-associated genes *Mecp2* and *Gabrb3* for mechanosensory neuron synaptic transmission and tactile sensitivity, and they implicate developmental somatosensory dysfunction in the genesis of anxiety and aberrant social behaviors in patients with ASDs (Orefice et al. 2016). Low GABA levels in the brain have previously been linked to autism (see Sect. 2.4.5), but these findings further push for the need of treatments that restore GABA function in the periphery.

But a majority of people with autism spectrum disorders also have an altered tactile sense; they are often hypersensitive to light touch and can be overwhelmed by certain textures. It would be interesting to assess whether these findings apply to other genetic forms of autism spectrum disorders. MeCP2 has been shown to have unique effects on GABA in the brain; perhaps its peripheral effects are unique as well. Orefice and colleagues (2016) did begin to address this question by testing tactile sensitivity and texture discrimination in *Mecp2* (*Mecp2R306C*) mice, a common mutation found in human RTT patients (Lyst et al. 2013) and mice harboring mutations in *Shank3* (Peça et al. 2011) and *Fmr1* (Spencer et al. 2005), which in humans are associated with forms of ASDs and fragile X syndrome, respectively. Interestingly, these mice all exhibited enhanced tactile pre-pulse inhibition responses, compared to control littermates. However, mechanism was not further addressed, begging the question if pharmacological enhancement of GABA in the spinal cord could ameliorate these symptoms. Because of studies like these, there are several recent advances in preclinical and clinical trials (Katz et al. 2016). Interestingly, a recent study has demonstrated a link between deficient MECP2 expression in human brains and in mouse models and expression deficits in UBE3A and GABRB3, two genes linked to Angelman syndrome (Samaco et al. 2005).

2.4.4 15q11–13

Mutations on chromosome 15 are typically found along the 15q11.2–q13.1 region and can arise as deletions (Angelman syndrome or Prader–Willi syndrome) or as a duplication. Genes within the 15q11–13 region are typically expressed from a single parental chromosome (imprinted). Imprinted genes show expression from only one inherited copy of a gene; therefore, if there is a mutation or deletion of the gene copy that should be expressed, the second copy cannot compensate resulting in loss of function. When these genes are mutated, diverse phenotypes result depending on the parent of origin for the mutation. Prader–Willi syndrome occurs when part or the whole region of 15q11–q13 is deleted. These patients are characterized by polyphagia, mild to moderate developmental delay, hypogonadism resulting in delayed to no puberty, and hypotonia. Angelman syndrome (AS), on the other hand, results from a loss of gene activity in the maternal allele of the 15q11–q13 region and is characterized by severe mental retardation, ataxia, lack of speech, excessively happy demeanor, and display of autistic-like behaviors (Veltman et al. 2005). Genes found within the 15q11–13 locus include the maternally expressed *UBE3A* and several $GABA_A$ receptor (GABR) subunit genes including the *GABRB3*, *GABRA5*, and

GABRG3 genes, thought to be associated with ASD (DeLorey et al. 2008; Buxbaum et al. 2002). Angelman syndrome is thought to result from the loss of the maternal copy of Ube3A (ubiquitin protein ligase, E3A), a ubiquitin ligase (Clayton-Smith and Laan 2003). Interestingly, decreased Ube3A expression has also been observed in a small number of cases of ASD and Rett syndrome (Samaco et al. 2005).

One of the most widely used models for autism is the *Ube3A* maternal-deficient mouse that recapitulates most of the essential features of autism, including cognitive and motor abnormalities (Jana 2012). These mice have significantly low or no detectable Ube3a protein, further conferring high construct validity, and display motor dysfunction, enhanced seizure susceptibility, impaired synaptic plasticity, and a context-dependent learning deficit (Jiang et al. 1998; Miura et al. 2002). As with other ASD-related disorders, Ube3a also appears to be modulating experience-dependent synaptic development and plasticity (Weeber et al. 2003; Dindot et al. 2008; Yashiro et al. 2009; Greer et al. 2010).

Recent work returned a wild-type *Ube3a* allele to a mouse model of AS at different times in development using an inducible Cre model (Silva-Santos et al. 2015). This work demonstrated that the later Ube3a expression resulted in fewer rescued phenotypes. For instance, marble burying and rotarod deficits were returned to wild-type levels only when Ube3a was re-expressed at birth; Ube3a expression in adolescence or adulthood no longer rescued these phenotypes. Interestingly, despite the lack of behavioral rescue, LTP in the Schaffer collateral was reinstated in both juveniles and adults (Silva-Santos et al. 2015; Sell and Margolis 2015). Interestingly, these results are in contrast with those reported in Mecp2 mice models of Rett syndrome (2.4.3). This could be due to the different behaviors reported in each study, or it could indicate that some ASD susceptibility genes have tightly regulated functions during development whereas others are required during the entire lifespan (Hulbert and Jiang 2016).

Due to brain-specific genetic imprinting at this locus, the paternal *UBE3A* is silenced by a long antisense transcript, Ube3a-ATS. Inhibition of the antisense transcript could lead to "unsilencing" of paternal *UBE3A*, thus providing a therapeutic approach for AS and ASDs. Utilizing antisense oligonucleotides to disrupt the *Ube3a-ATS* and induce paternal expression of Ube3a protein, some phenotypes, such as fear conditioning and body weight, were ameliorated even upon treatment as juveniles; however, many phenotypes, including the robust and reproducible motor phenotypes and marble burying, were not rescued (Meng et al. 2014). Recently, Bailus and colleagues (2016) reported an engineered zinc finger-based artificial transcription factor (ATF) that, when injected intraperitoneal or subcutaneously, crossed the blood–brain barrier and increased *Ube3a* expression in the brain of an adult mouse model of AS (Bailus et al. 2016). The factor displayed widespread distribution throughout the brain, thus presenting an injectable engineered protein that can cause widespread activation of an endogenous gene in the brain. However, this study and others using pharmacological methods of expressing paternal UBE3A, while successful at initiating protein expression, have not been characterized to ameliorate Angelman syndrome phenotypes in vivo (Huang et al. 2011; King et al. 2013; Powell et al. 2013; Sell and Margolis 2015).

These studies, among others, have illustrated the importance of the timing of UBE3A expression in the intact animal. While re-expression of UBE3A later in development is capable of positively impacting synaptic plasticity, it less effectively rescues behavioral deficits. Such results question whether the clinically relevant phenotypes in AS mice are those related to cellular or behavioral changes. Given the complex nature by which UBE3A affects nervous system development, it is likely that studying UBE3A interactions and downstream effects relevant to AS pathogenesis can be best understood through in vivo studies. Systems such as neuronal culture are more apt to answer questions about general UBE3A function in the neuron, as developmental-dependent UBE3A effects are stripped of meaning in context of in vivo AS pathogenesis (Sell and Margolis 2015).

Gabrb3-null mice have high rates of neonatal mortality (Homanics et al. 1997), but those that do survive show enhanced seizure susceptibility, abnormal motor coordination, impaired learning and memory, impaired social interaction and nesting behaviors, hyperactivity, and repetitive, stereotyped circling in the contextual fear conditioning and passive avoidance test (Homanics et al. 1997; DeLorey et al. 1998, 2008).

Although patients with *UBE3A* mutations have a wide spectrum of neurological phenotypes, their features are usually milder than Angelman syndrome patients with deletions of 15q11–q13. Therefore, Jiang et al. (2010) generated mutant mice with a 1.6 Mb chromosomal deletion that included inactivation of both *Ube3a* and *Gabrb3* genes (Jiang et al. 2010). Homozygous deletion mutant mice died in the perinatal period due to a cleft palate resulting from the null mutation in *Gabrb3* gene. However, mice with a maternal deletion were viable and did not have any obvious developmental defects. Expression analysis of the maternal and paternal deletion mice confirmed that the *Ube3a* gene is maternally expressed in the brain and showed that the *Gabrb3* gene is bi-allelically expressed in all brain regions studied. Consistently, the maternal, but not paternal, deletion mice had increased spontaneous seizure activity and abnormal EEG, significant impairment in motor function, learning and memory tasks, and anxiety-related measures. Furthermore, the maternal deletion pups emitted significantly more ultrasonic vocalizations than wild-type littermates (Jiang et al. 2010). Thus, mutant mice with a maternal deletion from *Ube3a* to *Gabrb3* provide an Angelman syndrome mouse model that is molecularly more similar to the contiguous gene deletion form in humans than mice with the *Ube3a* mutation alone. These mice will be valuable for future comparative studies to mice with maternal deficiency of *Ube3a* alone.

Duplication of the 15q11–13 chromosomal region is present in up to 5 % of ASD cases and is most commonly maternally derived although evidence for paternally derived duplications is accumulating (Dykens et al. 2004; Bolton et al. 2004). On the basis of conserved human/mouse linkage, a transgenic mouse was generation carrying a 6.3 Mb duplication of mouse chromosome 7 mirroring the human chromosome 15q11–13 (Nakatani et al. 2009). Mice carrying a paternally derived 15q11–13 duplication resulted in reduced social interaction in the three-chamber social approach test, behavioral inflexibility in the Morris water maze and Barnes maze test, abnormal ultrasonic vocalizations in both neonatal pups and adult mice

(Nakatani et al. 2009), and cerebellar-dependent motor learning impairments (Piochon et al. 2014). However, mice carrying a maternally derived duplication did not display any behavioral abnormalities (Nakatani et al. 2009). Thus, while in humans the 15q11–13 duplication is usually maternally derived, these mice do mimic a chromosomal duplication found in human ASD patients, and several autistic-like behaviors are present in the paternally derived mice suggesting this could be a good model for studying mechanisms in ASD-like behavior (Robertson and Feng 2011). However, triplicating just the *Ube3a* maternal allele leads to a reconstitution of the three core autism traits in mice: defective social interaction, impaired communication, and increased repetitive stereotypic behavior (Smith et al. 2011). The penetrance of these autism traits depended on *Ube3a* gene copy number as mice with only a duplicate copy of *Ube3a* had an intermediate to normal phenotype. In animals with increased *Ube3a* gene dosage, glutamatergic, but not GABAergic, synaptic transmission was suppressed as a result of reduced presynaptic release probability, synaptic glutamate concentration, and postsynaptic action potential coupling. These results suggest that *Ube3a* gene dosage may contribute to the autism traits of individuals with maternal 15q11–13 duplication and support the idea that increased E3A ubiquitin ligase gene dosage results in reduced excitatory synaptic transmission (Smith et al. 2011).

To date, no conditional knockouts of any of these mouse models have been reported, so there is limited knowledge about regional and neuronal specificity correlated with the behavioral phenotypes. Numerous targets of Ube3a-dependent ubiquitination have been identified in attempts to dissect the molecular mechanisms underlying AS (Sell and Margolis 2015; Hulbert and Jiang 2016; Jana 2012). Specifically, one target is activity-regulated cytoskeleton protein (Arc), which promotes the internalization of AMPA receptors; in the *Ube3a*-null mice, the excitatory postsynaptic AMPARs are internalized, which impairs synaptic transmission (Greer et al. 2010). Interestingly, genetic reduction of ARC in mice with the maternal deletion of *Ube3a* is sufficient to decrease seizure-like activity in juvenile mice (Mandel-Brehm et al. 2015), possibly through restoring AMPARs and subsequently balancing E/I synaptic transmission. Recent findings also indicate that in *Drosophila*, Ube3a acts as a cofactor for some MeCP2 functions, and in fact, reduced Ube3a expression was able to rescue some cellular phenotypes induced by Mecp2 overexpression (Kim et al. 2013b). Additionally, *Ube3a* mice have presynaptic vesicle cycling defects specifically in inhibitory interneurons (Wallace et al. 2012). These observations clearly demand further investigation into some very basic questions (Hulbert and Jiang 2016). Importantly, it is critical to compare gene dosage effects of each of these genes and in combination in a more methodical and consistent manner to better understand the function of each gene and the full ASD-associated mutation.

2.4.5 Del16p11.2

A copy number variation on human chromosome 16p11.2 was found in 1 % of patients with autism and developmental delay (Weiss et al. 2008). Patients with a recurrent microdeletion display motor deficits, speech and language delay, cognitive impairments, hearing disorders, and seizures and are accompanied by ASD (Weiss et al. 2008; Hanson et al. 2015). A reciprocal microduplication has been associated with schizophrenia (McCarthy et al. 2009) and ASD (Weiss et al. 2008; Duyzend and Eichler 2015; Maillard et al. 2015). A set of anatomical, behavioral, and electrophysiological phenotypes were identified in the *16p11.2* deletion syndrome that provides insights into the developmental consequences of this mutation in agreement with ASD features. To date, three mouse models of 16p11.2 heterozygous deletions have been independently generated (Horev et al. 2011; Portmann et al. 2014; Arbogast et al. 2016). Mice with the heterozygous deletion (*Del16p11.2*) exhibited normal general health, neurological reflexes, responses to social and non-social odors, normal motor learning, social approach, and juvenile reciprocal social interaction (Portmann et al. 2014). However, *Del16p11.2* mice of all the lines exhibited low body weight, perinatal mortality, increased spontaneous locomotor activity in a novel home cage environment, a deficit in novel object recognition, sporadic motor stereotypies (Portmann et al. 2014; Horev et al. 2011; Arbogast et al. 2016), and learning deficits and cognitive inflexibility (Yang et al. 2015b), core symptoms of ASDs. Mice further revealed an elevated expression of DA receptors in the striatum (specifically D2-type receptors), suggesting abnormal basal ganglia circuitry functioning which correlated with the movement control problems and repetitive behaviors (Portmann et al. 2014). Furthermore, mice normally emit vocalizations in the ultrasonic range in response to olfactory and social cues; however, the *Del16p11.2* mice are deficient in their initial ultrasonic vocalization responses to novel social cues (Yang et al. 2015c). In contrast, the duplication of *16p11.2* in mice has a rather mild phenotype. Evaluation of the *16p11.2* deletion or duplication mouse allows for investigation of the impact of changes in the number of copies on the phenotypes. These *16p11.2* CNV models have dosage-dependent changes in gene expression, viability, brain architecture, and behavior (Horev et al. 2011; Arbogast et al. 2016).

These findings indicate that mutations to *16p11.2* cause brain and behavioral anomalies, providing insight into human autism spectrum disorders. However, the most common deletion in the 16p11.2 locus causes a loss of 550 kb of DNA that encodes for 26–29 different genes (Bey and Jiang 2014; Arbogast et al. 2016). Dissociating the role of each gene in ASD, or if it is a combinatorial effect, will be a significant undertaking. One of the genes in this region is the *MAPK3* gene which encodes the MAP kinase ERK1. ERK signaling has been genetically linked to ASD and other disorders of cognition (Kalkman 2012; Rauen 2013). ERK signaling pathways are critical in regulating the cell cycle in proliferating cortical progenitors. In fact, the *Del16p11.2* mice exhibit a smaller brain and alterations in cortical cytoarchitecture. Specifically, these mice have fewer pyramidal neurons in the upper layers and an increase in layer VI projection neurons due to a premature depletion of the progenitor pool due to a premature cell cycle exit (Pucilowska et al. 2015). Decreased ERK pathway activity could also explain a decrease in protein synthesis in hippocampal slices of *Del16p11.2* mice (Tian et al. 2015).

Interestingly, four genes that are deleted in this 16p11.2 locus are actually targets of FMRP, the protein absent in fragile X syndrome (Darnell et al. 2011). Consistent with this and several other ASD animal models, the *Del16p11.2* mice also exhibit deficits in metabotropic glutamate receptor 5 (mGluR5)- dependent synaptic plasticity and impaired hippocampal-dependent memory. The groups of Mark Bear and Alea Mills collaborated to further show that chronic treatment with a negative allosteric modulator of mGluR5 reversed the cognitive deficit in the *Del16p11.2* mice (Tian et al. 2015). These data suggest that some cognitive and neuropsychiatric symptoms of the *16p11.2* microdeletion disorder arise from altered synaptic signaling that is amenable to targeted drug therapy. This further strengthens the hypothesis that multiple causes of ASD converge on common pathophysiological processes, including synaptic function (Kelleher and Bear 2008; Zoghbi and Bear 2012).

Under traditional behavioral protocols, wild-type and mutant animals are raised together as part of the same litters. However, in the interest of paying careful attention to the role of social dominance in rodent behaviors, Yang and colleagues wondered whether behavioral outcomes of the mutation differ when mutants are housed in mixed genotype cages versus housing only mutants together in one group cage or only wild-type littermates after weaning (Yang et al. 2015a). *Del16p11.2* mice present a particularly good model organism to investigate this question, due to the smaller size of the heterozygotes relative to their wild-type littermates, and may therefore become subordinate to their larger cagemates. In contrast to the previous results, heterozygotes that lived in same-genotype cages emitted normal numbers of vocalizations during male–female interactions, and displayed normal novel object recognition, indicating that the deletion of *16p11.2* per se was not sufficient to cause cognitive or social deficits (Yang et al. 2015a). These findings suggest that elements of the home cage social environment could interact with genotype to impact aspects of disease phenotypes which could arise from social stress.

Given the prevalence of *16p11.2* CNVs and their frequent association with ASD in genetic studies, the *16p11.2* deletion and duplication mice clearly have strong molecular construct validity. However, these model mice are only now being validated across the ASD-relevant behavioral domains, and their utility as preclinical models hinges on whether and how robustly they recapitulate social, communicative, and repetitive behaviors. In addition, identification of the dose-sensitive genes within this locus and why both duplications and deletions can manifest in ASD diagnoses remain critical areas of future study (Bey and Jiang 2014).

2.4.6 Shank3

The *SHANK/ProSAP* genes (*SHANK1*, *SHANK2*, and *SHANK3*) have recently been identified to be mutated in ASDs, particularly *SHANK2* and *SHANK3* (Durand et al. 2007; Berkel et al. 2010; Sato et al. 2012; Nemirovsky et al. 2015). Additionally, loss of one copy of *SHANK3* in Phelan-McDermid syndrome is thought to contribute to the neurobehavioral features of the disorder, including ASDs (Table 2.1) (Bonaglia et al. 2001; Wilson et al. 2003). *SHANK* genes encode synaptic proteins that function as molecular scaffolds in the postsynaptic density of excitatory synapses and can form multimeric complexes with postsynaptic receptors, signaling molecules, and cytoskeletal proteins present in dendritic spines and postsynaptic regions. SHANKs can bind to the cell adhesion protein neuroligins, including *NLGN3* and *NLGN4*, and have been implicated in spinogenesis and synapse development (Leblond et al. 2014; Berkel et al. 2010; Durand et al. 2007; Hulbert and Jiang 2016). Mouse models for each of the three Shank proteins have been created to better understand the role of these proteins in vivo and their contributions to ASDs (Hulbert and Jiang 2016). While there are currently no studies using conditional knockouts of the Shank genes in different cells types or brain regions, the Shanks are differentially expressed: Shank1 and Shank2 are predominantly expressed in the cerebral cortex, hippocampus, and cerebellum, whereas Shank3 is predominantly found in the striatum (Peça et al. 2011), giving some specialization to the function of each of these proteins. A considerable amount of work has characterized the neurobiological and behavioral phenotypes that result from the loss of these proteins.

Mice with a null mutation in *Shank1* displayed smaller, thinner postsynaptic densities, an altered composition of postsynaptic density proteins, and reduced size of dendritic spines in the hippocampus (Hung et al. 2008). Behaviorally, adult *Shank1*-null mice have impaired motor functions but do not show ASD-relevant social interaction problems nor repetitive grooming directly (Silverman et al. 2011). Conversely, mice carrying a mutation identical to the ASD-associated microdeletion in the human *SHANK2* gene (Berkel et al. 2010) exhibit ASD-like behaviors including reduced social interaction, reduced social communication by ultrasonic vocalizations, and repetitive jumping (Won et al. 2012). These mice have normal synapse numbers and morphology but show a marked decrease in the NMDA (N-methyl-D-aspartate) glutamate receptor (NMDAR) function. Interestingly, direct stimulation of NMDARs with D-cycloserine, a partial agonist of NMDARs, normalized NMDAR function and improved social interaction in *Shank2*-null mice. Furthermore, treatment of in *Shank2*-null mice with a positive allosteric modulator of metabotropic glutamate receptor5 (mGluR5), which enhances NMDAR function via mGluR5 activation, also normalized NMDAR function and markedly enhanced social interaction (Won et al. 2012). Taken together, these results suggest a causal link between mutations in *SHANK2*, reduced NMDAR function and impaired social behavior. Reduced NMDAR function may contribute to the development of ASD-like phenotypes in *Shank2*-null mice, and mGluR modulation of NMDARs offers a potential strategy to treat ASD (Won et al. 2012).

SHANK3 is the most widely studied of the *SHANK* genes. In fact, 11 different lines of *Shank3* mutant mice have been reported, but due to the transcriptional complexity of *Shank3* (Wang et al. 2014; Hulbert and Jiang 2016), only one of the published lines disrupts all isoforms, but all result in ASD-like behaviors to various degrees (reviewed in Bey and Jiang 2014; Hulbert and Jiang 2016; Wang et al. 2016). *SHANK3* is located on chromosome 22q13.3 and identified in families with ASD in many studies (Durand et al. 2007). The transmission pattern of *SHANK3* mutations is variable, but inheritance from healthy parents or existence of affected siblings has been reported. However, it was recently reported a case of germ line mosaicism for a heterozygous cytosine deletion in exon 21 of *SHANK3* by whole-genome sequencing, exhibiting phenotypes of severe intellectual disability, the absence of language, and autism spectrum symptoms. Whereas humans with SHANK3-related ASDs are either haploinsufficient due to a large chromosomal deletion or have point mutations in one copy of their SHANK genes, many of the studies utilizing mouse models only report behavioral abnormalities in homozygous mutants. This, along with the fact that until this year no model existed in which all Shank3 isoforms are disrupted, limits the construct validity of these models (Hulbert and Jiang 2016). Furthermore, as with other potential candidates, the associated phenotypes of *SHANK3* mutations are not specific for ASD, but *SHANK3* is regarded as one of the potential causative genes and therapeutic targets of ASD, based on animal and cellular model studies (Yoo 2015; Durand et al. 2007).

In mice, the *Shank3* mutation leads to synaptic disruptions that can produce ASD-like symptoms, including abnormal social behaviors, excessive grooming, and self-injurious repetitive behaviors (Peça et al. 2011; Duffney et al. 2015; Jaramillo et al. 2016). The mechanism through which deletion of Shank proteins leads to synaptic dysfunction is likely due to impaired interactions between glutamate receptors and postsynaptic density proteins leading to impaired signaling in dendritic spines. For instance, *Shank3b*-null mice also exhibit defects at the cortical–striatal circuits and changes in medium spiny neuron morphology with reduced spine density within the striatum. This mutation resulted in reduced expression of a number of proteins from the striatal postsynaptic machinery, including SAPAP3 (see Sect. 2.6), Homer, PSD-93, and glutamatergic receptor subunits in striatal synaptosomal fractions (Peça et al. 2011; Wang et al. 2016; Jaramillo et al. 2016), and significantly diminished NMDA receptor synaptic function and synaptic distribution in the prefrontal cortex (Duffney et al. 2015). Like in the *Shank2* model, pharmacological enhancement of mGluR5 rescued behavioral deficits in the *Shank3*-null mouse (Vicidomini et al. 2016). Concomitantly, *Shank3*-deficient mice have a marked loss of cortical actin filaments, which is associated with increased activity of cofilin, the major actin depolymerizing factor. Interestingly, altering actin polymerization with peripheral administration of an actin stabilizer rescued prefrontal cortical synaptic deficits and rescued social deficits and reduced repetitive grooming (Duffney et al. 2015). These results indicate that the aberrant regulation of synaptic actin filaments and loss of synaptic NMDARs contribute to the manifestation of autism-like phenotypes. Thus, targeting actin regulators provides a strategy for autism treatment.

In a follow-up study to Peça et al. (2011), Guoping Feng's group have now shown that they can reverse some of the behavioral symptoms by turning the gene back on later in life, allowing the brain to properly rewire itself. In the new study, Mei and colleagues genetically engineered mice using a tamoxifen-induced Cre-dependent conditional knock-in strategy (Mei et al. 2016). In these mice, the *Shank3* gene was turned off during embryonic development but was turned back on later in life when tamoxifen was added to the mice's diet. When *Shank3* was turned on in adult mice, the mice's repetitive behavior and their tendency to avoid social interaction was reduced. At the cellular level, the density of dendritic spines dramatically increased in the striatum of treated mice, demonstrating the structural plasticity in the adult brain. However, the mice's anxiety and some motor coordination symptoms that only disappeared in Shank3 were turned on earlier in life: by 20 days after birth (Mei et al. 2016). These findings suggest that the adult brain can display plasticity to some degree allowing for the behavioral defects to be reversible, giving hope that we can develop treatment for autistic patients in the future. Clearly there are different critical periods for the formation of the different circuits, and work to define these will prove extremely useful to not only understand which circuits control which behaviors but also to help determine the best time to intervene therapeutically. For the small population of people with *SHANK3* mutations, these findings suggest that genome-editing techniques could, one day, in theory be used to repair the defective *Shank3* gene and improve individuals' symptoms, even later in life (Mei et al. 2016).

Although it is difficult to directly correlate mouse behaviors with patient symptoms and diagnosis, recent studies provide neurobiological evidence that *SHANK3* mutations associated with ASD cause common and differential defects at molecular, synaptic, and behavioral levels. More broadly, different mutations of the same gene may elicit neurobiological changes at different developmental stages, brain regions, and cell types through a variety of potential brain mechanisms including differential mRNA stability, differential regulation of compensatory gene expression, and different degrees of signaling complex disruption (Zhou et al. 2016). Wang and colleagues recently described the first *Shank3* complete knockout mice with the deletion of the protein-coding exons 4–22 (Wang et al. 2016). These mice demonstrate a similar phenotype to the other Shank3 mouse models but in a more complete analysis of the neurobiology and better construct validity. In these mice, both mGluR5-Homer scaffolds and mGluR5-mediated signaling were selectively altered in striatal neurons. These changes were associated with perturbed function at striatal synapses, abnormal brain morphology, aberrant structural connectivity, and ASD-like behavior. In vivo recording revealed that the corticostriatal–thalamic circuit is tonically hyperactive in mutants but becomes hypoactive during social behavior. Furthermore, this study was also able to show that manipulation of mGluR5 activity attenuates excessive grooming and rescues impaired striatal synaptic plasticity in *Shank3Δe4–22*-null mice (Wang et al. 2016). These findings show that deficiency of Shank3 can impair mGluR5–Homer scaffolding, resulting in corticostriatal circuit abnormalities that underlie deficits in learning and ASD-like behaviors. These data suggest causal links between genetic, molecular, and circuit mechanisms underlying the pathophysiology of ASDs. These studies further highlight the role of glutamatergic signaling and synaptic function as common factors in ASDs and solidify the role for the corticostriatal circuit in mediating ASD behaviors.

Recently, the idea of faulty channels, rather than synaptic problems, was thrown into the mix. Using human neurons with conditional *SHANK3* mutations, Yi et al. (2016) found that *SHANK3* mutations severely and specifically impaired hyperpolarization-activated cation (I_h) channels, thereby increasing neuronal input resistance and enhancing neuronal excitability (Yi et al. 2016) as seen in various *Shank3* mouse models. This impairment in intrinsic electrical properties accounted, at least in part, for the decreased dendritic arborization and synaptic transmission of *SHANK3*-mutant neurons since chronic pharmacological blockage of I_h channels reproduced these phenotypes (Yi et al. 2016). The reduced I_h current phenotype manifests early in neuronal development and is similarly observed in immature *Shank3*-mutant mouse neurons. SHANK3 protein interacted with hyperpolarization-activated cyclic nucleotide-gated channel proteins (HCN proteins) that form I_h channels; therefore, SHANK3 may perform a general role during neurodevelopment by scaffolding HCN channels that mediate I_h currents in neurons. Here, instead of affecting synapses, *SHANK3* mutations primarily caused a channelopathy that may be amenable to pharmacological intervention.

Finally, targeted deletion of Shank3 in the ventral tegmental area (VTA) during the first postnatal week impaired the maturation of excitatory synapses onto both VTA dopaminergic and GABAergic neurons (Bariselli et al. 2016). These synaptic changes were concomitant with reduced in vivo burst activity of dopaminergic neurons, increased activity of GABA neurons, and behavioral deficits including impaired social preference that persisted into adulthood. In order to provide a causal link between altered dopaminergic neuronal activity and social behavior, Bariselli et al. found that systemic treatment with a positive allosteric modulator of mGluR1 during the postnatal period of synapse maturation normalized social preference defects into adulthood, owing to a specific partial rescue of dopamine neuron excitatory transmission and activity. Moreover, optogenetic activation of VTA dopamine neurons increased social preference in *Shank3*-deficient mice, confirming sufficiency of dopamine neuron activity to support social interactions (Bariselli et al. 2016). Collectively, these data reveal the contribution of impaired ventral tegmental area function to social behaviors and highlighting, once again, glutamatergic (via mGluR1) modulation during postnatal development as a potential treatment strategy. Importantly, this is the first demonstration of how *Shank3* insufficiency affects specific neural circuits and how it relates to specific symptoms.

2.4.7 Cntnap2

CNTNAP2 is another candidate gene associated with ASD by human and animal model studies (Peñagarikano and Geschwind 2012). The molecular function of *cntnap2* is relatively unclear, but it is known to encode a neuronal transmembrane protein member of the neurexin superfamily that is involved in neural–glia interactions and clustering of potassium channels in myelinated axons (Poliak et al. 1999, 2001, 2003) that increases risk for abnormal functional brain connectivity (Peñagarikano and Geschwind 2012; Peñagarikano et al. 2011; Scott-Van et al. 2010; Rodenas-Cuadrado et al. 2014). The model mouse lacks a functional gene for contactin-associated protein-like 2 (*Cntnp2*). In humans, mutation of this gene causes cortical dysplasia and focal epilepsy (CDFE) syndrome, epilepsy, and intellectual disability, and almost 70 % of CDFE patients also display symptoms characteristic of ASDs. Importantly, the characteristics of the mice—including their deficiencies in social behavior—are highly similar to those of humans with the *CNTNAP2* mutation (Table 2.2). Interestingly, the *Cntnap2* knockout mice also show behavioral inflexibility as measured by the Morris water maze and increased grooming, a hallmark for excessive repetitive behaviors. A nonsedating dose of risperidone, an atypical antipsychotic medication frequently used in ASD, significantly reduced hyperactivity and grooming behavior (Peñagarikano et al. 2011). Furthermore, these mice have altered striatal structure and function, reduced GABAergic interneuron numbers in the striatum and cortex and abnormal cortical neuron migration (Peñagarikano et al. 2011), and reduced spine stability in the cortex (Amos Gdalyahu et al. 2015).

Cntnap2 knockout mice are strongly associated with ASD and neurodevelopment disorders. Mice show deficits in the three core ASD behavioral domains (Tables 2.2 and 2.3), as well as hyperactivity and epileptic seizures, as have been reported in humans with *CNTNAP2* mutations (Peñagarikano et al. 2011). Neuropathological and physiological analyses of these mice reveal neuronal migration and network abnormalities, demonstrating a functional role for *CNTNAP2* in brain development.

More recently, Geschwind's research team tested different drugs in the *Cntnp2* mutant mice in an effort to find a compound that could ameliorate the social behavior impairment. Only two drugs increased the number of social interactions of the *Cntnap2*-null mice: oxytocin and, its structural relative, vasopressin (Peñagarikano et al. 2015). Oxytocin is a neuropeptide produced in the hypothalamus that plays a crucial role in childbirth, stimulating milk production for breastfeeding, and more recently associated with social bonding (Insel and Shapiro 1992). The team went on to show that vasopressin most likely exerts its effect by cross-reacting with the oxytocin receptor: blocking the oxytocin receptor prevented the behavioral improvements seen with either compound, while blocking the vasopressin receptor did not. Furthermore, the brains of *Cntnp2*-mutant mice had fewer oxytocin-expressing neurons than those of wild-type animals and, as a result, lower levels of the hormone. Administering a single dose of oxytocin to the *Cntnap2*-null mice increased sociability for just a few hours. However, daily doses of oxytocin for 2 weeks in young pups increased the number of neurons expressing oxytocin, and the social behavior improvement lasted at least 9 days after treatments were stopped.

This suggests that there might be a window of treatment opportunity soon after birth for obtaining such long-lasting effects. Given the heterogeneity of ASD, a more beneficial course of treatment might also be seen if clinical trials for oxytocin were targeted to the patients most likely to benefit, for example, those shown to have oxytocin deficits. Research already exists that suggests that oxytocin could help humans with autism spectrum disorders (Yatawara et al. 2015), but Peñagarikano and colleagues directly demonstrated the role of oxytocin in social behavior: they were also able to improve social behavior in the mice by pharmacologically increasing the release of the animals' own oxytocin. This result is critical to target treatments that are directly based on a clear mechanism (Peñagarikano et al. 2015).

Finally, FOXP2 binds to and dramatically downregulates CNTNAP2 (Vernes et al. 2008). *FOXP2* encodes a transcription factor belonging to the Forkhead-box superfamily and was the first identified gene implicated in a speech and language disorder characterized by difficulties in the production of coordinated orofacial movements, developmental verbal dyspraxia, and impaired linguistic processing

(French and Fisher 2014; Rodenas-Cuadrado et al. 2014). Analysis of *CNTNAP2* polymorphisms in children with typical specific language impairment detected significant quantitative associations with nonsense-word repetition, a heritable behavioral marker of this disorder. Intriguingly, this region coincides with one associated with language delays in children with autism (Vernes et al. 2008). The *FOXP2–CNTNAP2* pathway provides a mechanistic link between clinically distinct syndromes involving disrupted language and a possible common pathway for ASDs.

2.4.8 HGF/SF-Met

Met is a tyrosine kinase receptor which binds with high affinity to the ligand, HGF/SF (hepatocyte growth factor/scatter factor) (Naldini et al. 1991). Genetic studies have shown that *Met* is encoded on human chromosome 7q31, a susceptibility region for autism and Tourette syndrome (Gutknecht 2001; Kroisel et al. 2001; Díaz-Anzaldúa et al. 2004; Campbell et al. 2006; Sousa et al. 2009; Thanseem et al. 2010; Levitt and Campbell 2009). In fact, autistic patients have significantly decreased levels of Met protein in the cerebral cortex (Campbell et al. 2006).

In the nervous system, HGF/SF and Met participate in axonal guidance, dendritic outgrowth, and cellular proliferation, differentiation, migration, and survival (Birchmeier and Gherardi 1998; Maina et al. 1997; Powell et al. 2001, 2003b). Interestingly, impaired Met signaling specifically in the cerebral cortex and hippocampus during development leads to enlarged forebrain structures in adult mice, specifically the frontal cortical areas, hippocampus, striatum, and thalamus (Smith et al. 2012). These mice further display an imbalance in excitation/inhibition in the thalamocortical transmission in somatosensory cortex due to decreased expression of the $GABA_A$ receptor (Lo et al. 2016). Furthermore, HGF/SF signaling has been shown to modulate the development of forebrain GABAergic interneurons (Powell et al. 2001, 2003a; Martins et al. 2007, 2011; Bissonette et al. 2010), suggesting a mechanism for the involvement of HGF/SF-Met function and GABAergic interneuron development underlying ASD. Behavioral characterization of some of these mice demonstrated delayed procedural learning and reversal learning, with otherwise normal activity and emotionality (Martins et al. 2011). These deficits are common endophenotypes reported in patients with ASDs including Tourette syndrome; however, these mutations are all conditional mutations due to the embryonic lethality of *Met*- and HGF/SF-null mutants (Bladt et al. 1995; Schmidt et al. 1995; Uehara et al. 1995). While in a way, this limits the construct validity of these models, the temporal and spatial specificity of Met deletion allows for more targeted analysis of the importance of Met signaling in development.

Consistently, decreased HGF/SF signaling in the *Plaur* (*uPAR*; urokinase plasminogen activator receptor)-null mouse leads to reduced numbers of cerebral cortical and striatal GABAergic interneurons leading to seizures and impaired cognition (Bissonette et al. 2010; Bae et al. 2010; Powell et al. 2003a). However, it remains unclear what mechanism underlies this deficit since *uPAR* can mediate several molecular interactions, including the activation of HGF/SF, and HGF/SF itself can also modulate several aspects of cellular development. A complementary study demonstrated that reversal learning (Table 2.2) is in part dependent upon proper numbers of GABAergic interneurons. Using a genetic approach to supplement HGF/SF postnatally in the *Plaur*-null mice, both the interneuron population in the forebrain and the reversal learning impairments were restored (Bissonette et al. 2010). These results showed that GABAergic local circuitry in the orbitofrontal cortex and striatum are critical for modulating behavioral flexibility and that birth defects can be corrected by replenishing crucial growth factors. In the absence of *Plaur*, reduced levels of HGF/SF and Met in the forebrain appear to limit embryonic cell migration and survival (Powell et al. 2001; Bae et al. 2010). Thus, postnatal supplementation of HGF/SF may prevent the GABAergic interneuron loss and rescue the functional deficits, suggesting a possible mechanism to correct deficits in neuropsychiatric disorders (Bissonette et al. 2010).

2.5 GABAergic Imbalance

As discussed throughout the animal models, one of the common themes in ASDs is an imbalance between excitatory and inhibitory (E/I) neurotransmission. This imbalance can occur through two contrasting mechanisms: altered glutamatergic signaling or altered GABAergic signaling. While this is a simplistic view, each brain region can independently vary in the E/I balance, and there can be alterations in both systems leading to a normal E/I ratio. Regardless, GABA has a common role arising in many cases of ASD. The amino acid, GABA (γ-aminobutyric acid), is the main inhibitory neurotransmitter in the central nervous system of mammals. The primary inhibitory function of GABA is to control, dampen, and coordinate the excitability of principal excitatory neurons, which provide the main pathways of neuronal communication within and between neuronal networks of the brain (Purpura et al. 1957; Kuffler 1960; Ben-Ari 2001; McBain and Fisahn 2001; Ben-Ari et al. 2004; Markram et al. 2004). Although GABAergic interneurons represent only about 20 % of neurons in various forebrain regions, inhibitory neurons are highly divergent, strategically positioned, and physiologically tuned to exert functional control over excitatory communication (R. Miles et al. 1996; Kawaguchi and Kubota 1997; McBain and Fisahn 2001).

Long-term deficits in the GABAergic system in rodent and primate forebrains can lead to behavioral and cognitive symptoms commonly associated with mental retardation, mood disorders, schizophrenia, Tourette syndrome (TS), and other autism spectrum disorders (Keverne 1999; Benes and Berretta 2001; Andres 2002; Noebels 2003; Gross and Hen 2004; Levitt et al. 2004; Polleux and Lauder 2004; Kalanithi et al. 2005; Steriade 2005; DiCicco-Bloom et al. 2006; Leckman et al. 2006; Cristo 2007). Hussman (2001) initially hypothesized that individuals with ASD have a suppression of GABA in the brain, and therefore there is a favoring of the excitatory pathways (Hussman 2001). In fact, autistic patients show deficits in the GABAergic system, with decreased levels of GABA receptors in the hippocampus and the GABA-synthesizing enzymes in both the cerebral cortex and cerebellum (Blatt et al. 2001; Gutknecht 2001; Hussman 2001; Fatemi et al. 2002; Casanova et al. 2003; Polleux and Lauder 2004). Similarly, TS patients demonstrate altered expression patterns of interneurons in the basal ganglia (Kalanithi et al. 2005; Kataoka et al. 2010; Leckman et al. 2006). Furthermore, the genes encoding for GABA receptors are located on chromosome 15, an autism susceptibility locus (Andres 2002; Dykens et al. 2004; see Table 2.1).

Disruption of GABAergic interneuron development can alter the balance of excitatory to inhibitory neurotransmission, leading to behavioral deficits. However, alterations in numbers of GABAergic interneurons and the associated cognitive consequences are only beginning to be elucidated. In fact, the loss of GABAergic interneurons in the forebrain such as those seen in *Dlx1*-null mice shows generalized electrographic seizures and histological evidence of seizure-induced reorganization, linking the *Dlx1* mutation to delayed-onset epilepsy associated with interneuron loss (Cobos et al. 2005). Similarly, mice with altered GABAergic tone, such as those lacking the GABA synthetic enzyme, Gad65, or *GABAA* receptor-null mice (including the α1, β3 and δ subunit "knockouts"), are more susceptible to seizures (Asada et al. 1996; Kash et al. 1997; DeLorey et al. 1998, 2008; Wong and Carter 2001; Kralic et al. 2002; Möhler 2007). Deficits in GABAergic circuitry may lead to learning and memory disabilities (Keverne 1999) and may underlie cases of temporal lobe epilepsy (Noebels 2003). Decreases in GABAergic interneurons in the mouse forebrain have also been associated with increased anxiety levels (Powell et al. 2003a), as have alterations in GABAergic transmission (Depino et al. 2008) or changes in expression of the GABA receptors or transporter (Chiu et al. 2005; Möhler 2007; Partyka et al. 2007).

Approximately one-third of autistic individuals develop clinically apparent seizures, and, of those, more than 50 % develop "sharpspike" activity during sleep when recorded by EEG or magnetoencephalography (Lewine et al. 1999; Ballaban-Gil and Tuchman 2000; Polleux and Lauder 2004). These observations led several researchers to hypothesize that the cortex of autistic individuals is characterized by an imbalance between excitation and inhibition, leading to hyperexcitability and an unstable activity of cortical networks following normal sensory stimulation (Hussman 2001; Rubenstein and Merzenich 2003; Belmonte et al. 2004b). Most interestingly, functional imaging studies in humans and nonhuman primates have revealed that rhythmic synchronization of neural discharges in the gamma frequency band (20–60 Hz) may provide the necessary spatial and temporal links that bind together the processing in different brain areas to construct an object representation, or perception (Tallon-Baudry and Bertrand 1999; Polleux and Lauder 2004), suggesting that gamma oscillation resulting from synchronized neuronal activity at the cortical and subcortical levels not play an essential role in sensory perception and attention-based cognitive tasks. Neuronal synchrony in hippocampal, cortical, and thalamic networks has been shown to be critically dependent on the integrity of the discharge of interneurons in relation to the activity of the pyramidal neuron. Therefore, a slight disruption of the balance between excitation and inhibition in the cortex could have dramatic consequences on the function of the neuronal networks underlying perception and attention (Polleux and Lauder 2004).

A number of established mouse models of ASD do in fact show a reduction in GABAergic interneurons throughout the brain. In a meta-analysis study, Gogolla and colleagues (2009) found that VPA model and even the genetic models including *FMRP*, *NL-3*, *Cntnap2, Met*, *uPAR* (*Plaur*) and *MeCP2* have a loss of interneurons predominantly in the cortex. Specifically, the conditional deletion of *MeCP2* in forebrain GABAergic interneurons leads to a significant reduction in GAD and GABA immunoreactivity. Subsequently, these mice display features of ASD including repetitive behaviors (Chao et al. 2010). Furthermore, *Mecp2* deficiency leads to decreased expression of *Gabrb3* in brains of both humans and mice (Samaco et al. 2005) with various cognitive and behavioral consequences (see Sect. 2.4.3). The *Gabrb3* gene encodes for the $GABA_A$ receptor subunit beta-3, whose activation leads to opening of Cl^- channels and hyperpolarization of the membrane potential, reducing the probability of an action potential.

2.6 Corticostriatal Circuits

One of the core symptom domains of ASD is restricted interests and repetitive behaviors (American Psychiatric Association 2013). Previous studies have examined heterogeneity in repetitive behaviors and found support for two different factors: repetitive sensorimotor behaviors (e.g., hand/finger mannerisms, unusual sensory interests, repetitive use of objects, and complex mannerisms) and insistence on sameness (e.g., difficulties with change in routine, compulsions/rituals, and unusual attachment to objects) (Bishop et al. 2006). Some of these behaviors overlap with symptoms of other disorders, including obsessive–compulsive disorder (Leyfer et al. 2006). ASD patients have difficulties maintaining an appropriate problem-solving set for attainment of a future goal (executive function) and have little common sense about set shifting or behavior inhibition and holding mental representations (Griffith et al. 1999; Van Eylen et al. 2011; Landry and Al-Taie 2016). Patients with ASD often display circumscribed interests, which included behaviors such as intense, focused hobbies, strong preoccupations with particular topics, and unusually strong attachment to certain objects. However, research has been limited in this area, and the results from different studies have varied by sample and analytical methods; thus, replication is needed.

Neuroimaging studies have correlated abnormal activity in corticostriatal circuits with repetitive behaviors that underlie symptoms of ASD and obsessive–compulsive disorders (OCDs) (Lehmkuhl et al. 2008; Dichter et al. 2012; Kates et al. 2005; Reiss et al. 1995), but a causal link or the precise neural circuitry involved has yet to be established. The corticostriatal circuit has been closely associated with the development of habitual behaviors which are important for us to efficiently and rapidly respond to our environment. However, taken to the extreme, a habit can become so repetitive that it impacts daily function. We learn to perform certain actions to obtain specific outcomes in our lives, e.g., to press a button of an elevator to get to a particular floor. These actions are goal-directed, and their performance is highly sensitive to changes in both the incentive value of the outcome and to changes in the contingency between the action and the outcome. However, with practice and over time, these actions can become automated and habitual (Balleine et al. 2007; Dickinson 1985; Yin and Knowlton 2006). Habits are assembled routines that link sensory cues with motor actions but are less sensitive to outcome devaluation and changes in contingency (and can lead us to press the same button in a new elevator).

Understanding the neural substrates of habit formation and procedural learning may lead to a better understanding of ASD (Solomon et al. 2011; Sears et al. 2009; Sasson et al. 2008; Mostofsky et al. 2000; Marsh et al. 2004; Esch et al. 2009). Individuals with autism exhibit impairments in executive functioning, including deficits in planning, organization, flexibility of mental functioning, and self-regulation which can prompt self-injurious behaviors, and psychomotor coordination problems (Dawson et al. 2004; Walker 2008). These behavior challenges prevent acquisition of appropriate behavior throughout development. They can potentially cause the learners to harm themselves and others, to restrict motivation, to constrain ability to attend to stimuli and instruction, or to make conditional discriminations across sensory modalities. These human studies have thus begun to demonstrate the importance of proper striatal function in mediating repetitive and habitual behaviors (Knowlton et al. 1996; Tricomi et al. 2009).

Interestingly, studies in both rats and mice have shown that extensive training on an instrumental task where animals lever press for particular food reinforcements can lead to a shift from goal-directed to habitual responding (Adams and Dickinson 1981; Adams 1982). The neuroanatomical circuits that support the learning and the performance of goal-directed actions are different from those supporting the formation of habits (Yin and Knowlton 2006; Balleine and Dickinson 1998). The acquisition of goal-directed actions appears to rely on the associative corticobasal ganglia circuit involving the dorsomedial or associative striatum (Yin et al. 2005a, b), the pre-limbic cortex (Balleine and Dickinson 1998), the premotor cortex (akin to pre-supplementary motor area in primates) (Gremel and Costa 2013b), the orbitofrontal cortex (Gremel and Costa 2013a), and the mediodorsal thalamus (Corbit et al. 2003). On the other hand, the formation of habits depends upon the dorsolateral or sensorimotor striatum (Yin et al. 2004) and the infralimbic cortex (Killcross and Coutureau 2003). Repetitive, stereotyped behaviors are also believed to rely on the same neural circuits as habit formation (Graybiel 2008; Gillan et al. 2016), suggesting that such behaviors may be habits gone awry. Several of the mouse models discussed here including the *CNTNAP2* and *Shank3* mutant mice normally have altered striatal function if for no other reason than that protein is strongly expressed in the striatum likely leading to altered striatal–cortical activity (Peñagarikano et al. 2011; Peça et al. 2011). Mice with deletions in each of these genes demonstrate stereotypic movements such as self-injurious repetitive grooming behavior. But unfortunately, these mice have not been carefully studied at the level of correlating corticostriatal function with repetitive behaviors.

Mice with the maternal deletion of *Ube3a* have been assessed in instrumental conditioning, a striatum-dependent task (Hayrapetyan et al. 2014). *Ube3a* mice were severely impaired in initial acquisition of lever pressing, and whereas the lever pressing of wild-type controls was reduced by outcome devaluation and instrumental contingency reversal, the performance of *Ube3a* mice were more habitual, impervious to changes in outcome value and action–outcome contingency (Hayrapetyan et al. 2014). This effect is similar to what has been observed with manipulations to dorsomedial striatum (DMS) (Yin et al. 2005a, b; Lee et al. 2014). Ube3a mice in a 7.0 Tesla MRI showed a slightly smaller medial region of the striatum relative to wild-type littermates (Ellegood et al. 2015). Hayrapetyan and colleagues (2014) performed whole-cell patch-clamp recordings to measure glutamatergic transmission in the DMS and dorsolateral striatum (DLS). Interestingly, only the DMS, not the DLS, of *Ube3a* mice showed reduced amplitude and frequency of miniature excitatory postsynaptic currents, implying impaired glutamatergic synaptic transmission in DMS (Hayrapetyan et al. 2014). These results show for the first time a selective deficit in instrumental conditioning in the *Ube3a*-deficient mouse model and suggest a specific impairment in glutamatergic transmission in the associative corticostriatal circuit in AS.

A few studies have begun to dissect the influence of these circuits on repetitive behaviors directly by using optogenetic manipulation, whereby the neurons of interest are engineered to express the light-activated ion channel channelrhodopsin 2 (ChR2), such that when the cells are exposed to light—by means of a fiber optic cable pointing a laser at the relevant brain region—the channels open, ions flood in, and nerve impulses fire (Boyden et al. 2005; Lenz and Lobo 2013). In a seminal study, ChR2 was expressed in orbitofrontal cortical glutamatergic neurons and then photostimulated the axon terminals in the VMS that came from the OFC (Ahmari et al. 2013). The goal of Ahmari and colleagues was to hyperactivate the corticostriatal inputs to induce repetitive behaviors. However, it took regular photostimulation of once a day for 5 days to mimic this hyperactivity. The repeated stimulation resulted in a progressive increase in grooming (a behavior that commonly assessed in rodents and likened to human repetitive behaviors; see Table 2.2) that lasted for up to 2 weeks after the final episode of photostimulation. Importantly, Ahmari (2013) showed that the increase in grooming corresponded to electrophysiological changes in VMS neurons: their rate of firing in response to light stimulation increased after the hyperstimulation protocol. Furthermore, treatment with fluoxetine both reversed the changes in grooming behavior and normalized the light-evoked activity in VMS neurons (Ahmari et al. 2013).

Interestingly, a second study took an opposite approach using a transgenic mouse that exhibited repetitive behaviors and used optogenetics to stop it (Burguière et al. 2013). Burguière used a model of ASD and more commonly used to study OCD, the *Sapap3* (SAP90/PSD95-associated protein 3)-mutant mice. This study trained *Sapap3* which exhibits several OCD-related behaviors, including repetitive grooming to associate an audible tone with the delivery of a water drop to the forehead. Both controls and mutant mice developed a conditioned response (facial grooming) to the tone. As training continued, the control mice eventually stopped responding to the tone and delayed grooming until after delivery of the water drop. *Sapap3* mutant mice, however, continued to respond to the tone and displayed increased firing of striatal medium spiny neurons (MSNs) likely due to a loss of GABAergic interneurons. The authors then expressed ChR2 in cortical pyramidal neurons and photostimulated the axon terminals of lateral OFC neurons in the striatum to drive feedforward inhibition of MSNs. This both normalized the activity of MSN neurons and reversed the deficits in inhibition of the conditioned response (Burguière et al. 2013).

Basal ganglia circuits contain several cell types and subcircuits. More specifically, they encompass two major pathways linking input (striatum) to output: a monosynaptic GABAergic projection from dopamine D1 receptors-expressing striatal medium spiny projection neurons (striatonigral MSNs) to the output nuclei like the substantia nigra pars reticulata (SNr), called "direct pathway" (Gerfen et al. 1990), and a polysynaptic projection from dopamine D2 receptors-expressing striatal medium spiny projection neurons (striatopallidal MSNs) to output nuclei through the external globus pallidus and subthalamic nucleus, named "indirect pathway" (Gerfen et al. 1990). Classical models of basal ganglia circuit function suggest that the direct and indirect pathway are differentially modulated by dopamine and work in an antagonistic manner to facilitate or inhibit movement, respectively (Albin et al. 1989; DeLong 1990; DeLong and Wichmann 2009; Kravitz et al. 2012). However, other models propose that the coordinated activity of both direct and indirect pathways is critical for actions (Hikosaka et al. 2000; Mink 2003; Tecuapetla et al. 2016). Still, although these models make some predictions about how direct and indirect pathways could behave during an action, they are much less clear about the role of these basal ganglia subcircuits in the execution of repetitive and habitual behaviors. Furthermore, most of the existing models ignore the possibility that different subsets of basal ganglia output neurons could be modulating different regions/targets.

In humans, neuroligin-3 mutations are associated with autism, whereas in mice, the corresponding mutations produce robust synaptic and behavioral changes. However, different neuroligin-3 mutations cause largely distinct phenotypes in mice, and no causal relationship links a specific synaptic dysfunction to a behavioral change. Using rotarod motor learning as a proxy for acquired repetitive behaviors in mice, Rothwell et al. (2014) found that different *neuroligin-3* (*Nlgn3*) mutations uniformly enhanced formation of repetitive motor routines. Specifically, depletion of Nlgn3 in the D1-MSNs of the nucleus accumbens (using a localized injection of AAV-Cre) was sufficient to drive repetitive motor routines on the rotarod test, whereas depletion of Nlgn3 in D2-MSNs or in the dorsal striatum was not (Rothwell et al. 2014). Interestingly, depletion of Nlgn3 in Purkinje cells of the cerebellum or GABAergic interneurons did not affect motor performance but increased and decreased activity in the open field, respectively (Rothwell et al. 2014). These data thus suggest that different autism-associated neuroligin-3 mutations cause a common increase in acquired repetitive behaviors by impairing a specific striatal synapse and thereby provide a plausible circuit substrate for autism pathophysiology.

In a more recent study, the subcircuits of the dorsal striatum were more clearly dissected for their role in repetitive behaviors (Tecuapetla et al. 2016). This study optogenetically manipulated the activity of the direct or indirect pathway neurons of the dorsolateral striatum during a learned repetitive behavior. Mice were trained on a fixed ratio task (FR8; whereby only the eighth lever press is rewarded) until they were performing sequences of more than one press, and then direct striatonigral or indirect striatopallidal pathway neurons were activated after sequence initiation. Tecuapetla's findings demonstrate that subtle activation of dorsolateral striatonigral neurons after sequence initiation was sufficient to support the performance of well-learned actions and that this effect was not due to reinforcement but likely due to the stimulation of the specific ongoing motor pattern because it was not observed in animals with low levels of training and was impaired (but not aborted) by more frequency of activation of these neurons or by the activation of more neurons (Tecuapetla et al. 2016). Conversely, stimulation of striatopallidal pathway neurons after sequences was initiated and many sequences were aborted, with animals abandoning the usual zone of performance. There was a decrease in the total number of sequences during the stimulation block and an increase in the number of trials where mice performed single lever presses. These data complement the striatopallidal inhibition findings and indicate that proper activity of striatopallidal neurons during sequence performance permits ongoing actions to continue, while too little or too much activity of the striatopallidal pathway leads to sequence abortion and to animals switching to different behaviors (Tecuapetla et al. 2016).

Together, these studies confirm the involvement of corticostriatal circuitry in repetitive behaviors and suggest a model in which sustained hyperactivity in striatal neurons, possibly resulting from altered inhibitory input or an imbalance between direct and indirect pathways, induces changes in neuroplasticity that have behavioral consequences. These studies really delineate a pathway for repetitive behaviors in a more refined manner than anything possible in humans, pointing us in the direction of the pathophysiology of the disorder and new targets for potential intervention. Further development of new techniques will be key to dissecting and understanding the alterations in the circuits underlying ASD symptoms.

2.7 Concluding Remarks

Autism spectrum disorders affect millions of individuals worldwide. Despite increased autism diagnoses over the past 30 years, therapeutic intervention is still limited. Monogenetic disorders (e.g., fragile X syndrome, Rett syndrome, and neurofibromatosis) that have phenotypic overlap with autism provide insights into ASD pathology through the identification novel drug targets, such as glutamatergic or GABAergic receptors. Other novel targets include oxytocin, BDNF, and IGF and open up the ideal of gene therapy. However, widespread delivery of gene regulators to the brain remains challenging. Bone marrow transplantation may be a possible approach: Derecki et al. (2012) transplanted wild-type bone marrow into irradiation-conditioned Mecp2-null murine model and reported that wild-type Mecp2-expressing microglia within the context of a Mecp2-null mouse arrested disease development and improved locomotor activity (Derecki et al. 2012). And as previously discussed, Bailus and colleagues (2016) reported an engineered zinc finger-based artificial transcription factor (ATF) that, when injected intraperitoneal or subcutaneously, crossed the blood–brain barrier and increased *Ube3a* expression in the brain of an adult mouse model of AS (Bailus et al. 2016). While this study and many others using pharmacological methods are often successful at initiating protein expression, very few are checking to see if there is an improvement in the behavioral phenotypes. Regardless, these observations have important implications for the study and treatment of neurological disorders. Encouragingly, some of these novel drug targets provide symptomatic improvement, even in patients who have lived with ASDs for protracted periods of time (Spooren et al. 2012).

While rodent models cannot perfectly replicate a human disease, fundamental symptoms can be approximated for the purpose of testing theories about the biochemical, circuit, and genetic causes of the human condition. Hypotheses about genes underlying neuropsychiatric disorders are addressed by applying these targeted gene mutations and comparing the behavioral and anatomical endophenotypes. The development of rodent models and corresponding behavioral tasks has constituted a unique challenge to neuroscientists. However, through genetic linkage studies that attribute specific genes to the prevalence of ASD, candidate genes can then be similarly mutated or deleted in a mouse. Rodent models subsequently allow for hypothesis testing and probe the underlying neurobiology through careful behavioral and anatomical analysis, with detailed probing of molecular and circuitry changes that may underlie the pathophysiology of ASD. Furthermore, rodent models allow for immediate access to the brain and allow for the manipulation of specific neuronal circuits through pharmacogenetic approaches or direct optogenetic stimulation or inhibition of cells. As described in Sect. 2.6, optogenetic manipulations of rodent circuits are beginning to elucidate the functional importance of the corticostriatal circuit in repetitive behaviors. Other studies are also beginning to look at the circuits involved in social interaction. For example, Gunaydin et al. showed that the activity of the ventral tegmental area to the nucleus accumbens D1-expressing projections could encode and predict key features of social interaction (Gunaydin et al. 2014). Similarly, inhibition of projections from the basolateral complex of the amygdala to the ventral hippocampus significantly increased social interaction whereas activation of these same projections significantly reduced social behaviors (Felix-Ortiz and Tye 2014). Only now are studies beginning to investigate the circuit-level mechanisms underlying autism-like behaviors in genetically modified autism models with strong construct validity. With the advent of CRISPR/Cas9 genome editing (Sander and Joung 2014), it should be much faster and easier to generate more ASD mouse models. The combination of optogenetics and CRISPR/Cas9 genome editing tools in ASD models should produce significant insight into whether there are common circuits disrupted in ASD models with different genetic defects. New imaging technologies should also help unravel circuit functions. One- and two-photon imaging techniques are pushing the imaging field allowing for in vivo imaging of various neurons in a fully awake and behaving mouse (Ziv et al. 2013; Grutzendler et al. 2002). These imaging techniques in rodents have the added advantage of being able to target the imaging to specific neuronal populations due to Cre–*loxP* technology. Furthermore, CRISPR/Cas9 should allow for generating mice with mutations along the various signaling pathways to begin to dissect the molecular pathways. These emerging techniques to analyze specific circuits offer the possibility of working back and forth between genetic and pharmacological models that perturb specific circuits and optogenetic models that can evaluate whether an observed change in circuit function is necessary and specific to generate the observed behavior. We can also expect that optogenetic and imaging findings will direct the attention of human neuroimaging studies to specific circuits or nodes that may otherwise have been ignored. Importantly, we should continue to pursue models with clear construct validity to focus on factors that impact ASD humans. In summary, basic science and the clinic need to be brought closer together, to incentivize better human studies and optimize rodent studies to parallel the human pathology and thus better address the underlying neurobiological dysfunctions.

There are some glaring missing links in our understanding of the pathophysiology of ASDs. Specifically, it remains unclear how the mutation of an individual gene, a disrupted molecular pathway, and dysfunctional synapses affect the circuitry and produce ASD-like behavioral manifestations. Understanding the circuitry underlying autism, both anatomically and functionally, is critical to the development of effective clinical intervention. Several competing hypotheses regarding the circuit-level mechanisms have been proposed in the human literature; however, methodological and conceptual controversy, likely due to the substantial molecular and genetic heterogeneity of human patients for whom the etiologies are mostly unknown, demonstrate a need for animal research because of homogenous genetic defects (Hulbert and Jiang 2016). As imaging technology rapidly evolves, studies that take genetics and age into account are critical for the advancement of imaging results. Imaging studies are slowly beginning to show consistency in altered connectivity between brain structures and even structural abnormalities within brain regions. Therefore, it will be critical to always compare the rodent and human data. Evidence that the same neural circuitry and neuropharmacology underlies the mouse and the human behavioral domains will increase confidence that a pharmacological intervention, which reverses deficits in the animal model, will similarly reverse deficits in the human condition. To this end, several labs are implementing MRI and DTI studies to the mouse models to compare structural changes with those found in humans, further adding not only to our knowledge of the model but increasing its validity. The use of multiple methods for investigating the differences and phenotypes in these ASD mouse models, determining the behavioral, neuroanatomical, and histological phenotypes, allows one to localize the difference, establish the cellular mechanism, and directly relate these differences to the behavior, all of which will be required for an accurate assessment of both the model and possible rescues by interventions (Ellegood and Crawley 2015).

Given the highly variable genetics and phenotypes observed in ASD patients, it would appear unlikely the existence of any convergence in biology, yet recent studies using different methods have identified some common themes underlying ASD etiologies. A growing body of evidence from human genetics, neuropathology, animal models, and systems biology has identified a large degree of convergence at various biological levels. Studies from these disciplines generally corroborate a "many genes, common pathways" hypothesis (Geschwind 2008; Chen et al. 2015). In fact, many genetic studies of ASD have identified several risk genes that are key regulators of synaptic plasticity. Indeed, many of the risk genes that have been linked to these disorders encode synaptic scaffolding proteins, receptors, cell adhesion molecules or proteins that are involved in chromatin remodeling, transcription, protein synthesis or degradation, or actin cytoskeleton dynamics. Specifically, in ASD cases, rare mutations and CNVs have been identified in genes encoding neuroligins, neurexins, contactin-associated protein-like 2 (CNTNAP2), and SH3 and multiple ankyrin repeat domains (SHANKs) and even in syndromic ASD genes such as *FMR1*. Changes in any of these proteins can increase or decrease synaptic strength or number and, ultimately, neuronal connectivity in the brain. In addition, when deleterious mutations occur, inefficient genetic buffering and impaired synaptic homeostasis may increase an individual's risk for ASD (Bourgeron 2015). Therapies targeted toward these specific points of convergence have already been attempted; for example, the mGluR5 modulators, which are thought to normalize aberrant synaptic protein synthesis, have already blocked ASD-like phenotypes in the *Fmr1* and *TSC2* mouse models as well as in the valproic acid (Mehta et al. 2011) mouse model, which are not based on monogenic human disorders, speaking to the potential generalizability of mechanism in the face of diverse genetic and environmental etiologies. The possibility of other pharmaceutical agents targeted toward common pathways of convergence, such as synaptic gene regulation, excitation–inhibition balance, and other pathways identified in an unbiased manner using genetic screens, is likely to soon arise (Chen et al. 2015). However, it is necessary to state that mutations in synaptic genes are not specific to ASD and are also found in other neuropsychiatric disorders, such as schizophrenia, Alzheimer's disease, and epilepsy. However, as these neuropsychiatric conditions share common features with ASD, such as cognitive dysfunction, limited emotional expression, and lack of social reciprocity, synaptic dysfunction is still considered a common pathway of these major, chronic neuropsychiatric illnesses.

During normal brain development, a burst of synapse formation occurs in infancy, particularly in the cortex, a region involved in autistic behaviors; pruning eliminates about half of these cortical synapses by late adolescence. Synapses are known to be affected by many genes linked to autism, and some researchers have hypothesized that people with autism may have more synapses. Spine density is an important aspect of network function. As the number of spines increases, so do the number of neuronal connections and the computational power of the brain (Yuste 1995; He and Portera-Cailliau 2013). It follows, then, that alterations in the numbers of spines would result in significant network dysfunction. Analysis of tissue in the temporal lobe of children and adolescents with autism showed a surplus of synapses in the brain (Tang et al. 2014); however, due to methodological parameters, this data is controversial (He and Portera-Cailliau 2013; Nimchinsky et al. 2001). Regardless, Tang et al. show that the surplus synapses are likely due to a slowdown in a normal brain "pruning" process during development that was correlated with hyperactivated mTOR and impaired autophagy (Tang et al. 2014). Interestingly, rapamycin, an mTOR inhibitor, corrected ASD-like behaviors and similar spine pruning defects in the ASD mouse model, *Tsc2* (Tang et al. 2014), and various other models (Table 2.3). The brains of children with ASD tend to be larger than those of age-matched controls, but by adulthood, they tend to be smaller than controls. Brain enlargement seems to be postnatal as newborns show few or no differences with controls. Many mechanisms have been hypothesized to explain these observations, such as increase in neurogenesis, decrease in neuronal apoptosis, increase in glial cell production, diminished synaptic pruning, or myelin abnormalities, but all of these remain to be confirmed (Bernardet and Crusio 2006).

A final note of caution on animal models comes with the issue of reproducibility—this is not an issue unique to the human studies. Animal behavior is inherently variable, and the literature is filled with conflicting behavioral measures likely due to differences in genetic background or lack of standardization of behavioral tasks to assess the core ASD symptoms. A fundamental question for preclinical discovery of treatment targets for ASD is the predictive value of phenotypes detected in the animal models. High replicability of a strong phenotype is essential to evaluate therapeutic efficacy of an intervention. However, it could also be interesting to assess this inherent variability as it could explain some of the human variability in twin studies. Mouse littermates with varying degrees of the same behavior could display epigenetic changes in utero, critical to our understanding of genetic control in ASDs. Finally, it will be critical to always compare the rodent and human data. Evidence that the same neural circuitry and neuropharmacology underlies the mouse and the human behavioral domains will increase confidence that a pharmacological intervention, which reverses deficits in the animal model will similarly reverse deficits in the human condition. To this end, several labs are implementing MRI and DTI imaging studies to the mouse models to compare with the available human data and the use of multiple methods for investigating the differences and phenotypes in these ASD mouse models. Determining the behavioral, neuroanatomical, and histological phenotypes allows one to localize the difference, establish the cellular mechanism, and directly relate these differences to the behavior, all of which will be required for an accurate assessment of both the model and possible rescues by interventions (Ellegood and Crawley 2015).

The brain mechanisms responsible for autism are only beginning to be understood properly, and animal models paralleling related emotional and cognitive impairments are proving helpful in unraveling them. Better animal models may play a critical role in understanding the etiology of autism and develop more effective therapies. Through careful behavioral analyses, most of the core characteristics of autism, that is, impairments in social interaction, difficulty with language, and repetitive and stereotyped motor behaviors can be modeled in mice (Silverman et al. 2010a). Integrating clinical studies on humans with genetic manipulations in mice that allow for in-depth, careful neurobiological analysis will offer the most promising approach for understanding the biology of autism and allowing the development and testing of therapeutic agents.

References

Abrahams BS, Geschwind DH (2008) Advances in autism genetics : on the threshold of a new neurobiology. Nat Rev Genet 9:341–356. doi:10.1038/nrg2346

Adams CD (1982) Variations in the sensitivity of instrumental responding to reinforcer devaluation. Q J Exp Psychol Comp Physiol Psychol 34B:77–98

Adams CD, Dickinson A (1981) Instrumental responding following reinforcer devaluation. The Q J Exp Psychol Sect B: Comp Physiol Psychol 33(2):109–121. doi:10.1080/14640748108400816

Ahmari SE, Spellman T, Douglass NL, Kheirbek MA, Simpson HB, Karl D, Gordon JA, Hen R (2013) Repeated cortico-striatal stimulation generates persistent OCD-like behavior. Science 340(6137):1234–1239
Albin RL, Young AB, Penney JB (1989) The functional anatomy of basal ganglia disorders. Trends Neurosci 12(10):366–375
Amaral DG, Schumann CM, Nordahl CW (2008) Neuroanatomy of Autism. Trends Neurosci 31:137–145
American Psychiatric Association (2013) Diagnostic and statistical manual of mental disorders: DSM-5, 5th edn. APA, Washington, D.C
Amir RE, Van den Veyver IB, Wan M, Tran CQ, Francke U, Zoghbi HY (1999) Rett syndrome is caused by mutations in X-linked MECP2, encoding methyl-CpG-binding protein 2. Nat Genet 23:185–188
Andres C (2002) Molecular genetics and animal models in autistic disorder. Brain Res Bull 57(1):109–119. http://www.sciencedirect.com/science/article/B6SYT-451DHNS-G/2/c94b64aad77b24b2df04f2a8205d2445
Ango F, Prezeau L, Muller T, Tu JC, Xiao B, Worley PF, Pin JP, Bockaert J, Fagni L (2001) Agonist-independent activation of metabotropic glutamate receptors by the intracellular protein homer. Nature 411(6840):962–965
Arbogast T, Ouagazzal A-M, Chevalier C, Kopanitsa M, Afinowi N, Migliavacca E, Cowling BS et al (2016) Reciprocal effects on neurocognitive and metabolic phenotypes in mouse models of 16p11.2 deletion and duplication syndromes. PLoS Genet 12(2):e1005709
Arons MH, Thynne CJ, Grabrucker AM, Li D, Schoen M, Cheyne JE, Boeckers TM, Montgomery JM, Garner CC (2012) Autism-associated mutations in ProSAP2 / Shank3 impair synaptic transmission and neurexin-neuroligin-mediated transsynaptic signaling. J Neurosci 32(43):14966–14978. doi:10.1523/JNEUROSCI.2215-12.2012
Asada H, Kawamura Y, Maruyama K, Kume H, Ding R-g, Ji FY, Kanbara N et al (1996) Mice lacking the 65 kDa isoform of glutamic acid decarboxylase (GAD65) maintain normal levels of GAD67 and GABA in their brains but are susceptible to seizures. Biochem Biophys Res Commun 229(3):891. http://www.sciencedirect.com/science/article/B6WBK-45MH34T-17/2/5d796a838c6bae89c6f2602238ea6dd1
Asaka Y, Jugloff DG, Zhang L, Eubanks JH, Fitzsimonds RM (2006) Hippocampal synaptic plasticity is impaired in the Mecp2-null mouse model of Rett syndrome. Neurobiol Dis 21(1):217–227
Ashley CT Jr, Wilkinson KD, Reines D, Warren ST (1993) FMR1 protein: conserved RNP family domains and selective RNA binding. Science 262(5133):563–566
Badr GG, Witt-Engerstrom I, Hagberg B (1987) Brain stem and spinal cord impairment in Rett syndrome: somatosensory and auditory evoked responses investigations. Brain Dev 9:517–522
Bae M, Bissonette GB, Mars WM, Michalopoulos GK, Achim CL, Depireux DA, Powell EM (2010) Hepatocyte growth factor (HGF) modulates GABAergic inhibition and seizure susceptibility. Exp Neurol 221:129–135
Bailus BJ, Pyles B, McAlister MM, O'Geen H, Lockwood SH, Adams AN, Nguyen JTT, Yu A, Berman RF, Segal DJ (2016) Protein delivery of an artificial transcription factor restores widespread Ube3a expression in an Angelman syndrome mouse brain. Mol Ther 24(3):548–555
Ballaban-Gil K, Tuchman R (2000) Epilepsy and epileptiform EEG: association with autism and language disorders. Ment Retard Dev Disabil Res Rev 6:300–308
Balleine BW, Dickinson A (1998) Goal-directed instrumental action: contingency and incentive learning and their cortical substrates. Neuropharmacology 37(4–5):407–419. doi:10.1016/S0028-3908(98)00033-1
Balleine BW, Delgado MR, Hikosaka O (2007) The role of the dorsal striatum in reward and decision-making. J Neurosci Off J Soc Neurosci 27(31):8161–8165. doi:10.1523/JNEUROSCI.1554-07.2007
Bariselli S, Tzanoulinou S, Glangetas C, Prévost-Solié C, Pucci L, Viguié J, Bezzi P et al (2016) SHANK3 controls maturation of social reward circuits in the VTA. Nat Neurosci. doi:10.1038/nn.4319

Bassell GJ, Warren ST (2008) Fragile X syndrome: loss of local mRNA regulation alters synaptic development and function. Neuron 60(2):201–214

Bear MF, Huber KM, Warren ST (2004) The mGluR theory of fragile X mental retardation. Trends Neurosci 27:370–377

Belichenko PV, Wright EE, Belichencko NP, Masliah E, Li HH, Mobley WC, Francke U (2009) Widespread changes in dendritic and axonal morphology in Mecp2-mutant mouse models of Rett syndrome: evidence for disruption of neuronal networks. J Comp Neurol 514(3): 240–258

Belmonte MK, Cook EH Jr, Anderson GM, Rubenstein JLR, Greenough WT, Beckel-Mitchener A, Courchesne E et al (2004a) Autism as a disorder of neural information processing: directions for research and targets for therapy[ast]. Mol Psychiatry 9(7):646–663. http://dx.doi.org/10.1038/sj.mp.4001499

Belmonte M, Allen G, Beckel-Mitchener L, Boulanger A, Carper R, Webb S (2004b) Autism and abnormal development of brain connectivity. J Neurosci 24:9228–9231

Ben-Ari Y (2001) Developing networks play a similar melody. Trends Neurosci 24(6):353. http://www.sciencedirect.com/science/article/B6T0V-4313P77-Y/2/5ed98404eb14804e9c1fdb4164eb2193

Ben-Ari Y, Khalilov I, Represa A, Gozlan H (2004) Interneurons set the tune of developing networks. Trends Neurosci 27(7):422. http://www.sciencedirect.com/science/article/B6T0V-4CDS2CG-1/2/9dc4d10ba1a1e4467a92a5a567da2097

Benes FM, Berretta S (2001) GABAergic interneurons: implications for understanding schizophrenia and bipolar disorder. Neuropsychopharmacology 25(1):1–27

Berkel S, Marshall CR, Weiss B, Howe J, Roeth R, Moog U, Endris V et al (2010) Mutations in the SHANK2 synaptic scaffolding gene in autism spectrum disorder and mental retardation. Nat Genet 42:489–491

Bernardet M, Crusio WE (2006) Fmr1 KO mice as a possible model of autistic features. ScientificWorldJournal 6:1164–1176

Bey AL, Jiang Y-h (2014) Overview of mouse models of autism spectrum disorders. Curr Protoc Pharmacol 66(5):1–26

Bilousova TV, Dansie L, Ngo M, Aye J, Charles JR, Ethell DW, Ethell IM (2009) Minocycline promotes dendritic spine maturation and improves behavioural performance in the fragile X mouse model. J Med Genet 46:94–102

Birchmeier C, Gherardi E (1998) Developmental roles of HGF/SF and its receptor, the c-Met tyrosine kinase. Trends Cell Biol 8(10):404. http://www.sciencedirect.com/science/article/B6TCX-3TXT178-B/2/d1eb156d610390256cb10c761b69648a

Bishop S, Richler J, Lord C (2006) Association between restricted and repetitive behaviors and nonverbal IQ in children with autism spectrum disorders. Child Neuropsychol 12:247–267

Bissonette GB, Bae M, Suresh T, Jaffe DE, Powell EM (2010) Astrocyte-mediated HGF/SF supplementation restores GABAergic interneurons and corrects reversal learning deficits in mice. J Neurosci 30(8):2918–2923

Bladt F, Riethmacher D, Isenmann S, Aguzzi A, Birchmeier C (1995) Essential role for the c-Met receptor in the migration of myogenic precursor cells into the limb bud. Nature 376(6543):768–771. http://dx.doi.org/10.1038/376768a0

Blatt GJ (2012) The neuropathology of autism. Scientifica 2012:16

Blatt GJ, Fitzgerald CM, Guptill JT, Booker AB, Kemper TL, Bauman ML (2001) Density and distribution of hippocampal neurotransmitter receptors in autism: an autoradiographic study. J Autism Dev Disorders 31(6):537–543. http://www.springerlink.com/openurl.asp?genre=article&id=doi:10.1023/A:1013238809666

Bolton PF, Veltman MW, Weisblatt E, Holmes JR, Thomas NS, Youings SA, Thompson RJ et al (2004) Chromosome 15q11-13 abnormalities and other medical conditions in individuals with autism spectrum disorders. Psychiatr Genet 14(3):131–137

Bonaglia MC, Giorda R, Borgatti R, Felisari G, Gagliardi C, Selicorni A, Zuffardi O (2001) Disruption of the ProSAP2 gene in a t(12;22)(q24.1;q13.3) is associated with the 22q13.3 deletion syndrome. Am J Hum Genet 69(2):261–268

Bormann J (2000) The 'ABC' of GABA receptors. Trends Pharmacol Sci 21(1):16–19

Bourgeron T (2015) From the genetic architecture to synaptic plasticity in autism spectrum disorder. Nat Rev Neurosci 16:551–563

Boyden ES, Zhang F, Bamberg E, Nagel G, Deisseroth K (2005) Millisecond-timescale, genetically targeted optical control of neural activity. Nat Neurosci 8(9):1263–1268

Brouwer JR, Mientjes EJ, Bakker CE, Nieuwenhuizen IM, Severijnen LA, Van der Linde HC, Nelson DL, Oostra BA, Willemsen R (2007) Elevated Fmr1 mRNA levels and reduced protein expression in a mouse model with an unmethylated Fragile X full mutation. Exp Cell Res 313(2):244–253

Burguière E, Monteiro P, Feng G, Graybielb AM (2013) Optogenetic stimulation of lateral orbitofrontostriatal pathway suppresses compulsive behaviors. Science 340(6137):1243–1246. http://science.sciencemag.org/content/340/6137/1243?iss=6137

Buxbaum JD, Hof PR (2013) The neuroscience of autism spectrum disorders, 1st edn. Elsevier Inc., Amsterdam

Buxbaum JD, Silverman JM, Smith CJ, Greenberg DA, Kilifarski M, Reichert J, Jr Cook EH, Fang Y, Song CY, Vitale R (2002) Association between a GABRB3 polymorphism and autism. Mol Psychiatry 7(3):311–316

Buxhoeveden DP, Semendeferi K, Buckwalter J, Schenker N, Switzer R, Courchesne E (2006) Reduced minicolumns in the frontal cortex of patients with autism. Neuropathol Appl Neurobiol 32:483–491

Calfa G, Percy AK, Pozzo-Miller L (2011) Experimental models of Rett syndrome based on Mecp2 dysfunction. Exp Biol Med 236:3–19. doi:10.1258/ebm.2010.010261

Campbell DB, Sutcliffe JS, Ebert PJ, Militerni R, Bravaccio C, Trillo S, Elia M et al (2006) A genetic variant that disrupts MET transcription is associated with autism. Proc Natl Acad Sci U S A 103(45):16834–16839. doi:10.1073/pnas.0605296103

Casanova MF, Buxhoeveden DP, Switala AE, Roy E (2002) Minicolumnar pathology in autism. Neurology 58(3):428–432

Casanova MF, Buxhoeveden D, Gomez J (2003) Disruption in the inhibitory architecture of the cell minicolumn: implications for autisim. Neuroscientist 9(6):496–507. doi:10.1177/1073858403253552

Casanova MF, van Kooten IA, Switala AE, Van Engeland H, Heisen H, Steinbusch HW, Hof PR, Trippe J, Stone J, Schmitz C (2006) Minicolumnar abnormalities in autism. Acta Neuropathol 112(3):287–303

Chadman KK, Yang M, Crawley JN (2009) Criteria for validating mouse models of psychiatric diseases. Am J Med Genet B Neuropsychiatr Genet 150B(1):1–11

Chang Q, Khare G, Dani VS, Nelson S, Jaenisch R (2006) The disease progression of Mecp2 mutant mice is affected by the level of BDNF expression. Neuron 49(3):341–348

Chao H-t, Zoghbi HY, Rosenmund C (2007) Report MeCP2 controls excitatory synaptic strength by regulating glutamatergic synapse number. Neuron 56:58–65. doi:10.1016/j.neuron.2007.08.018

Chao H-t, Chen H, Samaco RC, Xue M, Chahrour M, Yoo J, Neul JL et al (2010) Dysfunction in GABA signalling mediates autism-like stereotypies and Rett syndrome phenotypes. Nature 468(7321):263–269. doi:10.1038/nature09582

Chapleau CA, Calfa GD, Lane MC, Albertson AJ, Larimore JL, Kudo S, Armstrong DL, Percy AK, Pozzo-Miller L (2009) Dendritic spine pathologies in hippocampal pyramidal neurons from Rett syndrome brain and after expression of Rett-associated MECP2 mutations. Neurobiol Dis 35(2):219–233

Chen RZ, Akbarian S, Tudor M, Jaenisch R (2001) Deficiency of methyl-CpG binding protein-2 in CNS neurons results in a Rett-like phenotype in mice. Nat Genet 27(3):327–331

Chen R, Jiao Y, Herskovitz EH (2011) Structural MRI in autism spectrum disorder. Pediatr Res 69(5 Pt 2):63R–68R

Chen JA, Olga P, Grant Belgard T, Swarup V, Geschwind DH (2015) The emerging picture of autism spectrum disorder: genetics and pathology. Annu Rev Pathol Mech Dis 10:111–144

Chiu C-S, Brickley S, Jensen K, Southwell A, McKinney S, Cull-Candy S, Mody I, Lester HA (2005) GABA transporter deficiency causes tremor, ataxia, nervousness, and increased GABA-

induced tonic conductance in cerebellum. J Neurosci 25(12):3234–3245. doi:10.1523/jneurosci.3364-04.2005
Chugani DC (2004) Serotonin in autism and pediatric epilepsies. Ment Retard Dev Disabil Res Rev 10(2):112–116
Chung L, Bey AL, Jiang YH (2012) Synaptic plasticity in mouse models of autism spectrum disorders. Korean J Physiol Pharmacol 16:369–378
Clayton-Smith J, Laan L (2003) Angelman syndrome: a review of the clinical and genetic aspects. J Med Genet 40(2):87–95
Cobos I, Calcagnotto ME, Vilaythong AJ, Thwin MT, Noebels JL, Baraban SC, Rubenstein JLR (2005) Mice lacking Dlx1 show subtype-specific loss of interneurons, reduced inhibition and epilepsy. Nat Neurosci 8(8):1059. http://dx.doi.org/10.1038/nn1499
Collins AL, Levenson JM, Vilaythong AP, Richman R, Armstrong DL, Noebels JL, Sweatt JD, Zoghbi HY (2004) Mild overexpression of MeCP2 causes a progressive neurological disorder in mice. Hum Mol Genet 13(21):2679–2689. doi:10.1093/hmg/ddh282
Corbit LH, Muir JL, Balleine BW (2003) Lesions of mediodorsal thalamus and anterior thalamic nuclei produce dissociable effects on instrumental conditioning in rats. Eur J Neurosci 18(5):1286–1294
Courchesne E, Pierce K (2005) Brain overgrowth in autism during a critical time in development: implications for frontal pyramidal neuron and interneuron development and connectivity. Int J Dev Neurosci 23(2–3):153–170
Courchesne E, Campbell K, Solso S (2011) Brain growth across the life span in autism: age-specific changes in anatomical pathology. Brain Res 1380:138–145
Cristo G (2007) Development of cortical GABAergic circuits and its implications for neurodevelopmental disorders. Clin Genet 72(1):1–8. http://dx.doi.org/10.1111/j.1399-0004.2007.00822.x
Cruz-Martin A, Crespo M, Portera-Cailliau C (2010) Delayed stabilization of dendritic spines in Fragile X mice. J Neurosci 30:7793–7803
Curia G, Papouin T, Seguela P, Avoli M (2009) Downregulation of tonic GABAergic inhibition in a mouse model of Fragile X syndrome. Cereb Cortex 19:1515–1520
D'Hulst C, DeGreest N, Reeve SP, Van Dam D, De Deyen PP, Hassan BA, Kooy RF (2006) Decreased expression of the GABAA receptor in Fragile X syndrome. Brain Res 1121(1):238–245
D'Hulst C, Heulens I, Brouwer JR, Willemsen R, DeGreest N, Reeve SP, De Deyen PP, Hassan BA, Kooy RF (2009) Expression of the GABAergic system in animal models for Fragile X syndrome and Fragile X associated tremor/ataxia syndrome (FXTAS). Brain Res 1253:176–183
Dani VS, Chang Q, Maffei A, Turrigiano GG, Jaenisch R, Nelson SB (2005) Reduced cortical activity due to a shift in the balance between excitation and inhibition in a mouse model of Rett syndrome. Proc Natl Acad Sci U S A 102(35):12560–12565
Darnell JC, Van Driesche SJ, Zhang C, Hung KY, Mele A, Fraser CE, Stone EF et al (2011) FMRP stalls ribosomal translocation on mRNAs linked to synaptic function and autism. Cell 146(2):247–261
Dawson G, Toth K, Abbott R, Osterling J, Munson J, Estes A, Liaw J (2004) Early social attention impairments in autism: social orienting, joint attention, and attention to distress. Dev Psychol 40(2):271–283
DeLong MR (1990) Primate models of movement disorders of basal ganglia origin. Trends Neurosci 13(7):281–285
DeLong MR, Wichmann T (2009) Update on models of basal ganglia function and dysfunction. Parkinsonism Relat Disord 15(Supp 3):S237–S240
DeLorey TM, Handforth A, Anagnostaras SG, Homanics GE, Minassian BA, Asatourian A, Fanselow MS, Delgado-Escueta A, Ellison GD, Olsen RW (1998) Mice lacking the beta 3 subunit of the GABAA receptor have the epilepsy phenotype and many of the behavioral characteristics of angelman syndrome. J Neurosci 18(20):8505–8514. http://www.jneurosci.org/cgi/content/abstract/18/20/8505

DeLorey TM, Sahbaie P, Hashemi E, Homanics GE, Clark JD (2008) Gabrb3 gene deficient mice exhibit impaired social and exploratory behaviors, deficits in non-selective attention and hypoplasia of cerebellar vermal lobules: a potential model of autism spectrum disorder. Behav Brain Res 187:207–220

DeLorey TM, Sahbaie P, Hashemi E, Li WW, Salehi A, Clark DJ (2011) Somatosensory and sensorimotor consequences associated with the heterozygous disruption of the autism candidate gene, Gabrb3. Behav Brain Res 216:36–45

Depino AM, Tsetsenis T, Gross C (2008) GABA homeostasis contributes to the developmental programming of anxiety-related behavior. Brain Res 1210:189–199

Derecki NC, Cronk JC, Lu Z, Xu E, Abbot SBG, Guyenet PG, Kipnis J (2012) Wild-type microglia arrest pathology in a mouse model of Rett syndrome. Nature 484:105–109

Díaz-Anzaldúa A, Joober R, Rivière J-B, Dion Y, Lespérance P, Chouinard S, Richer F, Rouleau GA (2004) Association between 7q31 markers and Tourette syndrome. Am J Med Genet A 127A(1):17–20. http://dx.doi.org/10.1002/ajmg.a.20631

Dichter GS (2012) Functional magnetic resonance imaging of autism spectrum disorders. Dialogues Clin Neurosci 14(3):319–351

Dichter GS, Damiano CA, Allen JA (2012) Reward circuitry dysfunction in psychiatric and neurodevelopmental disorders and genetic syndromes: animal models and clinical findings. J Neurodev Disord 4(19):1–43

DiCicco-Bloom E, Lord C, Zwaigenbaum L, Courchesne E, Dager SR, Schmitz C, Schultz RT, Crawley J, Young LJ (2006) The developmental neurobiology of autism spectrum disorder. J Neurosci 26(26):6897–6906. doi:10.1523/jneurosci.1712-06.2006

Dickinson A (1985) Actions and habits: the development of behavioral autonomy. Philos Trans R Soc B Biol Sci 308(1135):67–78

Dindot SV, Antalffy BA, Bhattacharjee MB, Beaudet AL (2008) The Angelman syndrome ubiquitin ligase localizes to the synapse and nucleus, and maternal deficiency results in abnormal dendritic spine morphology. Hum Mol Genet 17(1):111–118

Dolen G, Bear MF (2008) Role for metabotropic glutamate receptor 5 (mGluR5) in the pathogenesis of Fragile X syndrome. J Physiol 586(6):1503–1508

Dolen G, Emily O, Shankaranarayana Rao BS, Smith GB, Auerbach BD, Chattarji S, Bear MF (2007) Correction of Fragile X syndrome in mice. Neuron 56(6):955–962

Duffney LJ, Zong P, Wei J, Matas E, Cheng J, Qin L, Ma K et al (2015) Autism-like deficits in Shank3-deficient mice are rescued by targeting actin regulators. Cell 11(9):1400–1413

Durand CM, Betancur C, Boeckers TM, Bockmann J, Chaste P, Fauchereau F, Nygren G et al (2007) Mutations in the gene encoding the synaptic scaffolding protein SHANK3 are associated with autism spectrum disorders. Nat Genet 39(1):25–27

Dutch-Belgian Fragile X Consortium, The (1994) Fmr1 knockout mice: a model to study Fragile X mental retardation. Cell 78(1):23–33

Duyzend MH, Eichler EE (2015) Genotype-first analysis of the 16p11.2 deletion defines a new type of 'autism'. Biol Psychiatry 77(9):769–771

Dykens EM, Sutcliffe JS, Levitt P (2004) Autism and 15q11-q13 disorders: behavioral, genetic, and pathophysiological issues. Mental Retard Dev Disabil Res Rev 10(4):284–291. http://dx.doi.org/10.1002/mrdd.20042

Ellegood J, Crawley JN (2015) Behavioral and neuroanatomical phenotypes in mouse models of autism. Neurotherapeutics 12(3):521–533

Ellegood J, Nakai N, Nakatani J, Henkelman M, Takumi T, Lerch J (2015) Neuroanatomical phenotypes are consistent with autism-like behavioral phenotypes in the 15q11-13 duplication mouse model. Autism Res 8(5):545–555

Esch BE, Carr JE, Grow LL (2009) Evaluation of an enhanced stimulus-stimulus pairing procedure to increase early vocalizations of children with autism. J Appl Behav Anal 42(2):225–241. doi:10.1901/jaba.2009.42-225

Fatemi SH, Halt AR, Stary JM, Kanodia R, Schulz SC, Realmuto GR (2002) Glutamic acid decarboxylase 65 and 67 kDa proteins are reduced in autistic parietal and cerebellar cortices. Biol

Psychiatry 52(8):805–810. http://www.sciencedirect.com/science/article/B6T4S-46WV67F-P/2/5fbfed89b3bf4942d1c788d0f12a7e61

Favre MR, Barkat TR, Lamendola D, Khazen G, Markram H, Markram K (2013) General developmental health in the VPA-rat model of autism. Front Behav Neurosci 7:88

Felix-Ortiz AC, Tye KM (2014) Amygdala inputs to the ventral hippocampus bidirectionally modulate social behavior. J Neurosci 34(2):586–595

Fernandez E, Rajan N, Bagni C (2013) The FMRP regulon: from targets to disease convergence. Front Neurosci 7:191

Fish EW, Krouse MC, Stringfield SJ, DiBerto JF, Elliott Robinson J, Malanga CJ (2013) Changes in sensitivity of reward and motor behavior to dopaminergic, glutamatergic, and cholinergic drugs in a mouse model of Fragile X syndrome. PLoS One 8(10):e77896

French CA, Fisher SE (2014) What can mice tell us about Foxp2 function? Curr Opin Neurobiol 28:72–79

Fukuchi M, Nii T, Ishimaru N, Minamino A, Hara D, Takasaki I, Tabuchi A, Tsuda M (2009) Valproic acid induces up- or down-regulation of gene expression responsible for the neuronal excitation and inhibition in rat cortical neurons through its epigenetic actions. Neurosci Res 65(1):35–43

Fukuda T, Yamashita Y, Nagamitsu S, Miyamoto K, Jin JJ, Ohmori I, Ohtsuka Y et al (2005) Methyl-CpG binding protein 2 gene (MECP2) variations in Japanese patients with Rett syndrome: pathological mutations and polymorphisms. Brain Dev 27(3):211–217

Fyffe SL, Neul JL, Samaco RC, Chao HT, Ben-Shachar S, Moretti P, McGill BE et al (2008) Deletion of Mecp2 in Sim1-expressing neurons reveals a critical role for MeCP2 in feeding behavior, aggression, and the response to stress. Neuron 59(6):947–958

Gdalyahu A, Lazaro M, Penagarikano PGO, Trachtenberg JT, Geschwind DH (2015) The autism related protein contactin-associated protein-like 2 (CNTNAP2) stabilizes new spines: an in vivo mouse study. PLoS One 10(5):e0125633

Gemelli T, Berton O, Nelson ED, Perrotti LI, Jaenisch R, Monteggia LM (2006) Postnatal loss of methyl-CpG binding protein 2 in the forebrain is sufficient to mediate behavioral aspects of Rett syndrome in mice. Biol Psychiatry 59(5):468–476

Gerfen CR, Engber TM, Mahan LC, Chase TN, Jr Monsma FJ, Sibley DR (1990) D1 and D2 dopamine receptor-regulated gene expression of striatonigral and striatopallidal neurons. Science 250(4986):1429–1432

Geschwind DH (2008) Autism: many genes, common pathways? Cell 135(3):391–395

Geschwind DH, Levitt P (2007) Autism spectrum disorders: developmental disconnection syndromes. Curr Opin Neurobiol 17:103–111

Giacometti E, Luikenhuis S, Beard C, Jaenisch R (2007) Partial rescue of MeCP2 deficiency by postnatal activation of MeCP2. Proc Natl Acad Sci U S A 104(6):1931–1936

Gillan CM, Robbins TW, Sahakian BJ, van den Heuvel OA, van Wingen G (2016) The role of habit in compulsivity. Eur Neuropsychopharmacol 26(5):828–840

Giuffrida R, Musumeci S, D'Antoni S, Bonaccorso CM, Giuffrida-Stella AM, Oostra BA, Catania MV (2005) A reduced number of metabotropic glutamate subtype 5 receptors are associated with constitutive homer proteins in a mouse model of Fragile X syndrome. J Neurosci 25(39):8908–8916

Gogolla N, Leblanc JJ, Quast KB, Südhof TC, Fagiolini M, Hensch TK (2009) Common circuit defect of excitatory-inhibitory balance in mouse models of autism. J Neurodev Disord 1:172–181. doi:10.1007/s11689-009-9023-x

Graybiel AM (2008) Habits, rituals, and the evaluative brain. Annu Rev Neurosci 31:359–387. doi:10.1146/annurev.neuro.29.051605.112851

Greer PL, Hanayama R, Bloodgood BL, Mardinly AR, Lipton DM, Flavell SW, Kim TK et al (2010) The Angelman syndrome protein Ube3A regulates synapse development by ubiquitinating arc. Cell 140(5):704–716

Gremel CM, Costa RM (2013a) Orbitofrontal and striatal circuits dynamically encode the shift between goal-directed and habitual actions. Nat Commun 4:2264

Gremel CM, Costa RM (2013b) Premotor cortex is critical for goal-directed actions. Front Comput Neurosci 7(110). doi:10.3389/fncom.2013.00110. eCollection 2013.
Griffith E, Penningon B, Wehner E, Rogers S (1999) Executive functions in young children with autism. Child Dev 70:817–832
Gross C, Hen R (2004) The developmental origins of anxiety. Nat Rev Neurosci 5(7):545–552. http://dx.doi.org/10.1038/nrn1429
Grutzendler J, Kasthuri N, Gan WB (2002) Long-term dendritic spine stability in the adult cortex. Nature 420(6917):812–816
Gunaydin LA, Grosenick L, Finkelstein JC, Kauvar IV, Fenno LE, Adhikari A, Lammel S et al (2014) Natural neural projection dynamics underlying social behavior. Cell 157(7):1535–1551
Gutknecht L (2001) Full-genome scans with autistic disorder: a review. Behav Genet 31(1):113–123. http://www.springerlink.com/openurl.asp?genre=article&id=doi:10.1023/A:1010218227600
Guy J, Hendrich B, Holmes M, Martin JE, Bird A (2001) A mouse Mecp2-null mutation causes neurological symptoms that mimic Rett syndrome. Nat Genet 27(3):322–326
Guy J, Gan J, Selfridge J, Cobb SR, Bird A (2007) Reversal of neurological defects in a mouse model of Rett syndrome. Science 315(5815):1143–1147
Guy J, Merusi C, De Sousa D, Selfridge J, Bird A (2012) Postnatal inactivation reveals enhanced requirement for MeCP2 at distinct age windows. Hum Mol Genet 21(17):3806–3814. doi:10.1093/hmg/dds208
Hagerman RJ, 3rd Jackson AW, Levitas A, Rimland B, Branden M (1986) An analysis of autism in fifty males with the Fragile X syndrome. Am J Med Genet 23(1–2):359–374
Hagerman R, Hoem G, Hagerman P (2010) Fragile X and autism: intertwined at the molecular level leading to targeted treatments. Mol Autism 1(1):12
Hanson E, Bernier R, Porche K, Jackson FI, Goin-kochel RP, Snyder LG, Snow AV et al (2015) Archival report the cognitive and behavioral phenotype of the 16p11 . 2 deletion in a clinically ascertained population. Biol Psychiatry 77(9):785–793. doi:10.1016/j.biopsych.2014.04.021. Elsevier
Hardan AY, Libove RA, Keshavan MS, Melhem NM, Minshew NJ (2010) Cortical thickness in autism. Biol Psychiatry 66(4):320–326. doi:10.1016/j.biopsych.2009.04.024.A
Hayrapetyan V, Stephen C, Sukharnikova T, Yu C, Cao X, Jiang Y-H, Yin HH (2014) Region-specific impairments in striatal synaptic transmission and impaired instrumental learning in a mouse model of Angelman syndrome. Eur J Neurosci 39:1018–1025
He CX, Portera-Cailliau C (2013) The trouble with spines in Fragile X syndrome: density, maturity and plasticity. Neuroscience 251:120–128
Henderson C, Wijetunge L, Kinoshita MN, Shumway M, Hammond RS, Postma FR, Brynczka C et al (2012) Reversal of disease-related pathologies in the Fragile X mouse model by selective activation of GABAB receptors with arbaclofen. Sci Transl Med 4(152):152ra128
Hertenstein MJ, Verkamp JM, Kerestes AM, Holmes RM (2006) The communicative functions of touch in humans, nonhuman primates, and rats: a review and synthesis of the empirical research. Genet Soc Gen Psychol Monogr 132:5–94
Heulens I, D'Hulst C, Van Dam D, De Deyen PP, Kooy RF (2012) Pharmacological treatment of Fragile X syndrome with GABAergic drugs in a knockout mouse model. Behav Brain Res 229(1):244–249
Hikosaka O, Takikawa Y, Kawagoe R (2000) Role of the basal ganglia in the control of purposive saccadic eye movements. Physiol Rev 80(3):953–978
Hollander E, Anagnostou E, Chaplin W, Esposito K, Haznedar MM, Licalzi E, Wasserman S, Soorya L, Buchsbaum M (2005) Striatal volume on magnetic resonance imaging and repetitive behaviors in autism. Biol Psychiatry 58(3):226–232. http://www.sciencedirect.com/science/article/B6T4S-4G9Y520-3/2/13635c9f4c58be5b630409c7e7ac1e6a
Homanics GE, DeLorey TM, Firestone LL, Quinlan JJ, Handforth A, Harrison NL, Krasowski MD et al (1997) Mice devoid of gamma-aminobutyrate type A receptor beta3 subunit have epilepsy, cleft palate, and hypersensitive behavior. Proc Natl Acad Sci U S A 94(8):4143–4148

Horev G, Ellegood J, Lerch JP, Son Y-e E, Muthuswamy L, Vogel H, Krieger A et al (2011) Dosage-dependent phenotypes in models of 16p11.2 lesions found in autism. Proc Natl Acad Sci U S A 108(41):17076–17081. doi:10.1073/pnas.1114042108/-/DCSupplemental. www.pnas.org/cgi/doi/10.1073/pnas.1114042108

Huang HS, Allen JA, Mabb AM, King IF, Miriyala J, Taylor-Blake B, Sciaky N et al (2011) Topoisomerase inhibitors unsilence the dormant allele of Ube3a in neurons. Nature 481(7380):185–189

Huber KM, Gallagher SM, Warren ST, Bear MF (2002) Altered synaptic plasticity in a mouse model of Fragile X mental retardation. Proc Natl Acad Sci U S A 99:7746–7750

Hulbert SW, Jiang YH (2016) Monogenic mouse models of autism spectrum disorders: common mechanisms and missing links. Neuroscience 321:3–23

Hung AY, Futai K, Sala C, Valtschanoff JG, Ryu J, Woodworth MA, Kidd FL et al (2008) Smaller dendritic spines, weaker synaptic transmission, but enhanced spatial learning in mice lacking Shank1. J Neurosci 28(7):1697–1708

Hussman J (2001) Letters to the editor: suppressed GABAergic inhibition as a common factor in suspected etiologies of autism. J Autism Dev Disorders 31(2):247. http://www.springerlink.com/openurl.asp?genre=article&id=doi:10.1023/A:1010715619091

Hyman SL, Arndt TL, Rodier PM (2005) Environmental agents and autism: once and future associations. Int Rev Res Ment Retard 30:171–194. doi:10.1016/S0074-7750(05)30005-X

Ingram JL, Peckham SM, Tisdale B, Rodier PM (2000) Prenatal exposure of rats to valproic acid reproduces the cerebellar anomalies associated with autism. Neurotoxicol Teratol 22(3):319–324

Insel TR, Shapiro LE (1992) Oxytocin receptor distribution reflects social organization in monogamous and polygamous voles. Proc Natl Acad Sci U S A 89(13):5981–5985

Ismail MM, Keynton RS, Mostapha MMMO, ElTanboly AH, Casanova MF, Gimel'farb GL, El-Baz A (2016) Studying autism spectrum disorder with structural and diffusion magnetic resonance imaging: a survey. Front Hum Neurosci 10:211

Jacquemont ML, Sanlaville D, Redon R, Raoul O, Cormier-Daire V, Lyonnet S, Amiel J et al (2006) Array-based comparative genomic hybridisation identifies high frequency of cryptic chromosomal rearrangements in patients with syndromic autism spectrum disorders. J Med Genet 43(11):843–849

Jamain S, Quach H, Betancur C, Råstam M, Colineaux C, Gillberg IC, Soderstrom H et al (2003) Mutations of the X-linked genes encoding neuroligins NLGN3 and NLGN4 are associated with autism. Nat Genet 34(1):27–29

Jana NR (2012) Understanding the pathogenesis of angelman syndrome through animal models. Neural Plast 2012:710943

Jaramillo TC, Speed HE, Xuan Z, Reimers JM, Liu S, Powell CM (2016) Altered striatal synaptic function and abnormal behaviour in Shank3 Exon4-9 deletion mouse model of autism. Autism Res 9(3):350–375

Jiang YH, Armstrong D, Albrecht U, Atkins JL, Noebels JL, Eichele G, Sweatt JD, Beaudet AL (1998) Mutation of the Angelman ubiquitin ligase in mice causes increased cytoplasmic p53 and deficits of contextual learning and long-term potentiation. Neuron 21(4):799–811

Jiang YH, Pan Y, Zhu L, Landa L, Yoo J, Spencer C, Lorenzo I, Brilliant M, Noebels JL, Beaudet AL (2010) Altered ultrasonic vocalization and impaired learning and memory in Angelman syndrome mouse model with a large maternal deletion from Ube3a to Gabrb3. PLoS One 5(8):e12278

Jugloff DG, Vandamme K, Logan R, Visanji NP, Brotchie JM, Eubanks JH (2008) Targeted delivery of an Mecp2 transgene to forebrain neurons improves the behavior of female Mecp2-deficient mice. Hum Mol Genet 17(10):1386–1396

Kalanithi PSA, Zheng W, Kataoka Y, DiFiglia M, Grantz H, Saper CB, Schwartz ML, Leckman JF, Vaccarino FM (2005) Altered parvalbumin-positive neuron distribution in basal ganglia of individuals with Tourette syndrome. Proc Natl Acad Sci U S A 102(37):13307–13312. doi:10.1073/pnas.0502624102

Kalkman HO (2012) Potential opposite roles of the extracellular signal-regulated kinase (ERK) pathway in autism spectrum and bipolar disorders. Neurosci Biobehav Rev 36(10): 2206–2213

Kana RK, Uddin LQ, Kenet T, Chugani D, Muller R-A (2014) Brain connectivity in autism. Front Hum Neurosci 8:349

Kash SF, Johnson RS, Tecott LH, Noebels JL, Mayfield RD, Hanahan D, Baekkeskov S (1997) Epilepsy in mice deficient in the 65-kDa isoform of glutamic acid decarboxylase. Proc Natl Acad Sci U S A 94(25):14060–14065. http://www.pnas.org/cgi/content/abstract/94/25/14060

Kataoka Y, Kalanithi PSA, Grantz H, Schwartz ML, Saper C, Leckman JF, Vaccarino FM (2010) Decreased number of parvalbumin and cholinergic interneurons in the striatum of individuals with Tourette syndrome. J Comp Neurol 518(3):277–291. doi:10.1002/cne.22206

Kates WR, Lanham DC, Singer HS (2005) Frontal white matter reductions in healthy males with complex stereotypies. Pediatr Neurol 32(2):109–112

Katz DM, Adrian B, Coenraads M, Gray SJ, Menon DU, Philpot BD, Tarquinio DC (2016) Rett syndrome: crossing the threshold to clinical translation. Trends Neurosci 39(2):100–113

Kawaguchi Y, Kubota Y (1997) GABAergic cell subtypes and their synaptic connections in rat frontal cortex. Cereb Cortex 7(6):476–486. doi:10.1093/cercor/7.6.476

Kelleher RJ, Bear MF (2008) The autistic neuron: troubled translation? Cell 135(3):401–406

Kennedy D, Adolphs R (2012) Perception of emotions from facial expressions in high-functioning adults with autism. Neuropsychologia 50(14):3313–3319

Keverne EB (1999) GABA-ergic neurons and the neurobiology of schizophrenia and other psychoses. Brain Res Bull 48(5):467. http://www.sciencedirect.com/science/article/B6SYT-3WH6444-2/2/32bb497a58c3412613d294fb46cd095d

Khwaja OS, Ho E, Barnes KV, O'Leary HM, Pereira LM, Finkelstein Y, Nelson CA III et al (2014) Safety, pharmacokinetics, and preliminary assessment of efficacy of mecasermin (recombinant human IGF-1) for the treatment of Rett syndrome. Proc Natl Acad Sci U S A 111(12): 4596–4601

Killcross S, Coutureau E (2003) Coordination of actions and habits in the medial prefrontal cortex of rats. Cereb Cortex 13(4):400–408

Kim K, Kim P, Go HS, Choi CS, Park JH, Kim HJ, Jeon SJ et al (2013a) Male-specific alteration in excitatory post-synaptic development and social interaction in pre-natal valproic acid exposure model of autism spectrum disorder. J Neurochem 124(6):832–843

Kim S, Chahrour M, Ben-Shachar S, Lim J (2013b) Ube3a/E6AP is involved in a subset of MeCP2 functions. Biochem Biophys Res Commun 437(1):67–73

King IF, Yandava CN, Mabb AM, Hsiao JS, Huang HS, Pearson BL, Calabrese JM et al (2013) Topoisomerases facilitate transcription of long genes linked to autism. Nature 501(7465): 58–62

Kline DD, Ogier M, Kunze DL, Katz DM (2010) Exogenous brain-derived neurotrophic factor rescues synaptic dysfunction in Mecp2-null mice. J Neurosci 30(15):5303–5310

Knowlton BJ, Mangels JA, Squire LR (1996) A neostriatal habit learning system in humans. Science (New York, N.Y.) 273(5280):1399–1402. doi:10.1126/science.273.5280.1399

Kooy RF (2003) Of mice and the Fragile X syndrome. Trends Genet 19:148–154

Kralic JE, Korpi ER, O'Buckley TK, Homanics GE, Morrow AL (2002) Molecular and pharmacological characterization of GABAA receptor alpha 1 subunit knockout mice. J Pharmacol Exp Ther 302(3):1037–1045. http://jpet.aspetjournals.org/cgi/content/abstract/302/3/1037

Kravitz A, Tye L, Kreitzer AC (2012) Distinct roles for direct and indirect pathway striatal neurons in reinforcement. Nat Neurosci 15:816–818

Kroisel PM, Petek E, Emberger W, Windpassinger C, Wladika W, Wagner K (2001) Brief clinical report candidate region for gilles de La Tourette syndrome at 7q31. Am J Med Genet 101(3):259–261. http://dx.doi.org/10.1002/1096-8628(20010701)101:3<259::AID-AJMG1374>3.0.CO;2-#

Kuffler SW (1960) Excitation and inhibition in single nerve cells. Harvey Lect 54:176–218

Landry O, Al-Taie S (2016) A meta-analysis of the wisconsin card sort task in autism. J Autism Dev Disord 46(4):1220–1235

Laumonnier F, Bonnet-Brilhault F, Gomot M, Blanc R, David A, Moizard MP, Raynaud M et al (2004) X-linked mental retardation and autism are associated with a mutation in the NLGN4 gene, a member of the neuroligin family. Am J Hum Genet 74(3):552–557

Leblond CS, Nava C, Polge A, Gauthier J, Huguet G, Lumbroso S, Giuliano F et al (2014) Meta-analysis of SHANK mutations in autism spectrum disorders: a gradient of severity in cognitive impairments. PLoS Genet 10(9):e1004580

Leckman JF, Vaccarino FM, Kalanithi PSA, Rothenberger A (2006) Annotation: Tourette syndrome: a relentless drumbeat – driven by misguided brain oscillations. J Child Psychol Psychiatry 47(6):537–550. http://dx.doi.org/10.1111/j.1469-7610.2006.01620.x

Lee AS, Andre JM, Pittenger C (2014) Lesions of the dorsomedial striatum delay spatial learning and render cue-based navigation inflexible in a water maze task in mice. Front Behav Neurosci 8:42

Lehmkuhl HD, Storch EA, Bodfish JW, Geffken GR (2008) Exposure and response prevention for obsessive compulsive disorder in a 12-year-old with autism. J Autism Dev Disord 38:977–981. doi:10.1007/s10803-007-0457-2

Leigh MJ, Nguyen DV, Winarni TI, Schneider A, Chechi T, Polussa J, Doucet P et al (2013) A randomized double-blind, placebo-controlled trial of minocycline in children and adolescents with Fragile X syndrome. J Dev Behav Pediatr 34(3):147–155

Lenz JD, Lobo MK (2013) Optogenetic insights into striatal function and behavior. Behav Brain Res 255:44–54. doi:10.1016/j.bbr.2013.04.018. Elsevier B.V

Levitt P, Campbell DB (2009) The genetic and neurobiologic compass points toward common signaling dysfunctions in autism spectrum disorders. J Clin Invest 119(4):747–754. doi:10.1172/JCI37934.the

Levitt P, Eagleson KL, Powell EM (2004) Regulation of neocortical interneuron development and the implications for neurodevelopmental disorders. Trends Neurosci 27(7):400. http://www.sciencedirect.com/science/article/B6T0V-4CJ472R-3/2/725b7cfcf8586bde21f02a7035256c1f file:///C:/Documents and Settings/Gabi/My Documents/DATA/Cre Project/GABAergic development in Hippocampus.doc

Lewine JD, Andrews R, Chez M, Patil AA, Devinsky O, Smith M, Kanner A et al (1999) Magnetoencephalographic patterns of epileptiform activity in children with regressive autism spectrum disorders. Pediatrics 104(3 Pt1):405–418

Leyfer OT, Folstein SE, Bacalman S, Davis NO, Dinh E, Morgan J, Tager-Flushberg H, Lainhart JE (2006) Comorbid psychiatric disorders in children with autism: interview development and rates of disorders. J Autism Dev Disord 36(7):849–861

Lo FS, Erzurumlu RS, Powell EM (2016) Insulin-independent GABAA receptor-mediated response in the barrel cortex of mice with impaired met activity. J Neurosci 36(13):3691–3697

Lombardi LM, Baker SA, Zoghbi HY (2015) MECP2 disorders: from the clinic to mice and back. J Clin Invest 125(8):2914–2923

Lozano R, Hare EB, Hagerman RJ (2014) Modulation of the GABAergic pathway for the treatment of Fragile X syndrome. Neuropsychiatr Dis Treat 10:1769–1779

Luikenhuis S, Giacometti E, Beard CF, Jaenisch R (2004) Expression of MeCP2 in postmitotic neurons rescues Rett syndrome in mice. Proc Natl Acad Sci U S A 101(16):6033–6038

Lyst MJ, Ekiert R, Ebert DH, Merusi C, Nowak J, Selfridge J, Guy J et al (2013) Rett syndrome mutations abolish the interaction of MeCP2 with the NCoR/SMRT co-repressor. Nat Neurosci 16(7):898–902

Mabunga DFN, Gonzales ELT, Kim J-W, Kim KC, Shin CY (2015) Exploring the validity of valproic acid animal model of autism. Exp Neurobiol 24(4):285–300

Maillard AM, Ruef A, Pizzagalli F, Migliavacca E, Hippolyte L, Adaszewski S, Dukart J et al (2015) The 16p11.2 locus modulates brain structures common to autism, schizophrenia and obesity. Mol Psychiatry 20(1):140–147

Maina F, Hilton MC, Ponzetto C, Davies AM, Klein R (1997) Met receptor signaling is required for sensory nerve development and HGF promotes axonal growth and survival of sensory neurons. Genes Dev 11(24):3341–3350. doi:10.1101/gad.11.24.3341
Mandel-Brehm C, Salogiannis J, Dhamne SC, Rotenberg A, Greenberg ME (2015) Seizure-like activity in a juvenile Angelman syndrome mouse model is attenuated by reducing arc expression. Proc Natl Acad Sci U S A 112(16):5129–5134
Marchetto MC, Carromeu C, Acab A, Yu D, Yeo GW, Mu Y, Chen G, Gage FH, Muotri AR (2010) A model for neural development and treatment of Rett syndrome using human induced pluripotent stem cells. Cell 143(4):527–539
Markram H, Toledo-Rodriguez M, Wang Y, Gupta A, Silberberg G, Caizhi W (2004) Interneurons of the neocortical inhibitory system. Nat Rev Neurosci 5(10):793–807. http://dx.doi.org/10.1038/nrn1519
Marsh R, Alexander GM, Packard MG, Zhu H, Wingard JC, Quackenbush G, Peterson BS (2004) Habit learning in Tourette syndrome: a translational neuroscience approach to a developmental psychopathology. Arch Gen Psychiatry 61(12):1259–1268. doi:10.1001/archpsyc.61.12.1259
Martins GJ, Plachez CC, Powell EM (2007) Loss of embryonic met signaling alters profiles of hippocampal interneurons. Dev Neurosci 29(1–2):143–158. doi:10.1159/000096219
Martins GJ, Shahrokh M, Powell EM (2011) Genetic disruption of met signaling impairs GABAergic striatal development and cognition. Neuroscience 10(176):199–209
McBain CJ, Fisahn A (2001) Interneurons unbound. Nat Rev Neurosci 2(1):11–23
McCarthy S, Makarov V, Kirov G, Addington A, McClellan J, Yoon S, Perkins D et al (2009) Microduplications of 16p11.2 are associated with schizophrenia. Nat Genet 41(11):1223–1227
McGraw CM, Samaco RC, Zoghbi HY (2011) Adult neural function requires MeCP2. Science 333(6039):186
Mehta MV, Gandal MJ, Siegel SJ (2011) mGluR5-antagonist mediated reversal of elevated stereotyped, repetitive behaviors in the VPA model of autism. PLoS One 6:e26077
Mei Y, Monteiro P, Yang Z, Kim J-A, Gao X, Zhanyan F, Feng G (2016) Adult restoration of Shank3 expression rescues selective autistic-like phenotypes. Nature 530:481–484
Meng L, Ward AJ, Chun S, Bennett CF, Beaudet AL, Rigo F (2014) Towards a therapy for Angelman syndrome by targeting a long non-coding RNA. Nature 518:409–412
Michalon A, Sidorov M, Ballard RM, Ozmen L, Spooren W, Wettstein JG, Jaeschke G, Bear MF, Lindemann L (2012) Chronic pharmacological mGlu5 inhibition corrects Fragile X in adult mice. Neuron 74(1):49–56
Miles JH (2011) Autism spectrum disorders—a genetics review. Genet Med 13:278–294
Miles R, Tóth K, Gulyás AI, Hájos N, Freund TF (1996) Differences between somatic and dendritic inhibition in the hippocampus. Neuron 16(4):815–823. http://linkinghub.elsevier.com/retrieve/pii/S0896627300801014
Mink JW (2003) The basal ganglia and involuntary movements: impaired inhibition of competing motor patterns. Arch Neurol 60(10):1365–1368
Minshew NJ, Keller TA (2010) The nature of brain dysfunction in autism: functional brain imaging studies. Curr Opin Neurol 23(2):124–130
Miura K, Kishino T, Li E, Webber H, Dikkes P, Holmes GL, Wagstaff J (2002) Neurobehavioral and electroencephalographic abnormalities in Ube3a maternal-deficient mice. Neurobiol Dis 9(2):149–159
Möhler H (2007) Molecular regulation of cognitive functions and developmental plasticity: impact of GABAAreceptors.JNeurochem102(1):1–12.http://dx.doi.org/10.1111/j.1471-4159.2007.04454.x
Moretti P, Zoghbi HY (2006) MeCP2 dysfunction in Rett syndrome and related disorders. Curr Opin Genet Dev 16(3):276–281
Moretti P, Adriaan Bouwknecht J, Teague R, Paylor R, Zoghbi HY (2005) Abnormalities of social interactions and home-cage behavior in a mouse model of Rett syndrome. Hum Mol Genet 14(2):205–220
Moretti P, Levenson JM, Battaglia F, Atkinson R, Teague R, Antalffy B, Armstrong D, Arancio O, Sweatt JD, Zoghbi HY (2006) Learning and memory and synaptic plasticity are impaired in a mouse model of Rett syndrome. J Neurosci 26(1):319–327

Mostofsky SH, Goldberg MC, Landa RJ, Denckla MB (2000) Evidence for a deficit in procedural learning in children and adolescents with autism: implications for cerebellar contribution. J Int Neuropsychol Soc 6(7):752–759

Moy SS, Nadler JJ (2008) Advances in behavioral genetics : mouse models of autism. Mol Psychiatry 13:4–26. doi:10.1038/sj.mp.4002082

Moy SS, Nadler JJ, Magnuson TR, Crawley JN (2006) Mouse models of autism spectrum disorders: the challenge for behavioral genetics. Am J Med Genet C Semin Med Genet 142C:40–51

Moy SS, Nadler JJ, Poe MD, Nonneman RJ, Young NB, Koller BH, Crawley JN, Duncan GE, Bodfish JW (2008) Development of a mouse test for repetitive , restricted behaviors : relevance to autism. Behav Brain Res 188:178–194. doi:10.1016/j.bbr.2007.10.029

Mychasiuk R, Richards S, Nakahashi A, Kolb B, Gibb R (2012) Effects of rat prenatal exposure to valproic acid on behaviour and neuro-anatomy. Dev Neurosci 34(2–3):268–276

Nakatani J, Tamada K, Hatanaka F, Ise S, Ohta H, Inoue K, Tomonaga S et al (2009) Abnormal behavior in a chromosome-engineered mouse model for human 15q11-13 duplication seen in autism. Cell 137(7):1235–1246

Naldini L, Vigna E, Narsimhan RP, Gaudino G, Zarnegar R, Michalopoulos GK, Comoglio PM (1991) Hepatocyte growth factor (HGF) stimulates the tyrosine kinase activity of the receptor encoded by the proto-oncogene c-MET. Oncogene 6(4):54–501

Nemirovsky SI, Córdoba M, Zaiat JJ, Completa SP, Vega PA, González-Morón D, Medina NM et al (2015) Whole genome sequencing reveals a de novo SHANK3 mutation in familial autism spectrum disorder. PLoS One 10(2):e0116358

Nimchinsky EA, Oberlander AM, Svoboda K (2001) Abnormal development of dendritic spines in FMR1 knock-out mice. J Neurosci 21(14):5139–5146

Noebels JL (2003) The biology of epilepsy genes. Annu Rev Neurosci 26(1):599–625. http://arjournals.annualreviews.org/doi/abs/10.1146/annurev.neuro.26.010302.081210

Ogier M, Wang H, Hong E, Wang Q, Greenberg ME, Katz DM (2007) Brain-derived neurotrophic factor expression and respiratory function improve after ampakine treatment in a mouse model of Rett syndrome. J Neurosci 27(40):10912–10917

Orefice LL, Zimmerman AL, Chirila AM, Sleboda SJ, Head JP, Ginty DD (2016) Peripheral mechanosensory neuron dysfunction underlies tactile and behavioral deficits in mouse models of ASDs. Cell 166(2):299–313. http://dx.doi.org/10.1016/j.cell.2016.05.033

Palmen S, Engeland H, Hof P, Schmitz C (2004) Neuropathological findings in autism. Brain 127:2572–2583

Pan F, Aldridge GM, Greenough WT, Gan WB (2010) Dendritic spine instability and insensitivity to modulation by sensory experience in a mouse model of Fragile X syndrome. Proc Natl Acad Sci U S A 107:17768–17773

Partyka A, Kłodzińska A, Szewczyk B, Wierońska JM, Chojnacka-Wójcik E, Librowski T, Filipek B, Nowak G, Pilc A (2007) Effects of GABAB receptor ligands in rodent tests of anxiety-like behavior. Pharmacol Rep 59(6):757–762

Peça J, Feliciano C, Ting JT, Wang W, Wells MF, Venkatraman TN, Lascola CD, Fu Z, Feng G (2011) Shank3 mutant mice display autistic-like behaviours and striatal dysfunction. Nature 472(7344):437–442

Peñagarikano O, Geschwind DH (2012) What does CNTNAP2 reveal about autism spectrum disorder ? Trends Mol Med 18(3):156–163. doi:10.1016/j.molmed.2012.01.003

Peñagarikano O, Abrahams BS, Herman EI, Winden KD, Gdalyahu A, Dong H, Sonnenblick LI et al (2011) Absence of CNTNAP2 leads to epilepsy , neuronal migration abnormalities , and core autism-related deficits. Cell 147:235–246. doi:10.1016/j.cell.2011.08.040

Peñagarikano O, Lázaro MT, Lu X-h, Gordon A, Dong H, Lam HA, Peles E et al (2015) Exogenous and evoked oxytocin restores social behavior in the Cntnap2 mouse model of autism. Sci Transl Med 7(271):271ra8

Pieretti M, Zhang FP, Fu YH, Warren ST, Oostra BA, Caskey CT, Nelson DL (1991) Absence of expression of the FMR-1 gene in Fragile X syndrome. Cell 66(44):817–822

Piochon C, Kloth AD, Grasselli G, Titley HK, Nakayama H, Hashimoto K, Wan V et al (2014) Cerebellar plasticity and motor learning deficits in a copy number variation mouse model of autism. Nat Commun 5:5586

Pitcher MR, Herrera JA, Buffington SA, Kochukov MY, Merritt JK, Fisher AR, Schanen NC, Costa-Mattioli M, Neul JL (2015) Rett syndrome like phenotypes in the R255X Mecp2 mutant mouse are rescued by MECP2 transgene. Hum Mol Genet 24(9):2662–2672

Poliak S, Gollan L, Martinez R, Custer A, Einheber S, Salzer JL, Trimmer JS, Shrager P, Peles E (1999) Caspr2, a new member of the neurexin superfamily, is localized at the juxtaparanodes of myelinated axons and associates with K+ channels. Neuron 24(4):1037–1047

Poliak S, Gollan L, Salomon D, Berglund EO, Ohara R, Ranscht B (2001) Localization of Caspr2 in myelinated nerves depends on axon – glia interactions and the generation of barriers along the axon. J Neurosci 21(19):7568–7575

Poliak S, Salomon D, Elhanany H, Sabanay H, Kiernan B, Pevny L, Stewart CL et al (2003) Juxtaparanodal clustering of shaker-like K+ channels in myelinated axons depends on Caspr2 and TAG-1. J Cell Biol 162(6):1149–1160. doi:10.1083/jcb.200305018

Polleux F, Lauder JM (2004) Toward a developmental neurobiology of autism. Ment Retard Dev Disabil Res Rev 10(4):303–317. http://dx.doi.org/10.1002/mrdd.20044

Polsek D, Tomislav J, Cepanec M, Hof PR, Simic G (2011) Recent developmnets in neuropathology of autism spectrum disorders. Transl Neurosci 2(3):256–264

Portmann T, Yang M, Mao R, Panagiotakos G, Ellegood J, Dolen G, Bader PL et al (2014) Behavioral abnormalities and circuit defects in the basal ganglia of a mouse model of 16p11.2 deletion syndrome. Cell 7(4):1077–1092. doi:10.1016/j.celrep.2014.03.036. The Authors

Powell EM, Mars WM, Levitt P (2001) Hepatocyte growth factor/scatter factor is a motogen for interneurons migrating from the ventral to dorsal telencephalon. Neuron 30(1):79–89

Powell EM, Campbell DB, Stanwood GD, Davis C, Noebels JL, Levitt P (2003a) Genetic disruption of cortical interneuron development causes region- and GABA cell type-specific deficits, epilepsy, and behavioral dysfunction. J Neurosci 23(2):622–631. http://www.jneurosci.org/cgi/content/abstract/23/2/622

Powell EM, Mühlfriedel S, Bolz J, Levitt P (2003b) Differential regulation of thalamic and cortical axonal growth by hepatocyte growth factor/scatter factor. Dev Neurosci 25(2–4):197. http://www.karger.com/DOI/10.1159/000072268

Powell WT, Coulson RL, Gonzales ML, Crary FK, Wong SS, Adams S, Ach RA et al (2013) R-loop formation at Snord116 mediates topotecan inhibition of Ube3a-antisense and allele-specific chromatin decondensation. Proc Natl Acad Sci U S A 110(34):13938–13943

Pucilowska XJ, Vithayathil J, Tavares EJ, Kelly C, Karlo JC, Landreth GE (2015) The 16p11 . 2 deletion mouse model of autism exhibits altered cortical progenitor proliferation and brain cytoarchitecture linked to the ERK MAPK pathway. J Neurosci 35(7):3190–3200. doi:10.1523/JNEUROSCI.4864-13.2015

Purpura DP, Girado M, Grunsdfest H (1957) Selective blockade of excitatory synapses in the cat brain by gamma-aminobutyric acid. Science 125(3259):1200–1202

Rauen KA (2013) The RASopathies. Annu Rev Genomics Hum Genet 14:355–369

Redcay E, Courchesne E (2005) When is the brain enlarged in autism? A meta-analysis of all brain size reports. Biol Psychol 58(1):1–9

Reiss AL, Abrams MT, Greenlaw R, Freund L, Denckla MB (1995) Neurodevelopmental effects of the FMR-1 full mutation in humans. Nat Med 1(2):159–167

Robertson HR, Feng G (2011) Transgenic mouse models of childhood onset psychiatric disorders. J Child Psychol Psychiatry 52(4):442–475

Rodenas-Cuadrado P, Ho J, Vernes SC (2014) Shining a light on CNTNAP2: complex functions to complex disorders. Eur J Hum Genet 22:171–178. doi:10.1038/ejhg.2013.100. Nature Publishing Group

Rodier PM, Ingram JL, Tisdale B, Nelson S, Romano J (1996) Embryological origin for autism: developmental anomalies of the cranial nerve motor nuclei. J Comp Neurol 370:247–261

Rogers SJ, Hepburn S, Wehner E (2003) Parent reports of sensory symptoms in toddlers with autism and those with other developmental disorders. J Autism Dev Disord 33:631–642

Ronesi JA, Collins KA, Hays SA, Tsai N-P, Guo W, Birnbaum SG, Hu J-H, Worley PF, Gibson JR, Huber KM (2012) Disrupted mGluR5-Homer scaffolds mediate abnormal mGluR5 signaling, circuit function and behavior in a mouse model of Fragile X syndrome. Nat Neurosci 15(3):431–4S1

Rose'Meyer R (2013) A review of the serotonin transporter and prenatal cortisol in the development of autism spectrum disorders. Mol Autism 4:37

Rothwell PE, Fuccillo MV, Maxeiner S, Hayton SJ, Gokce O, Lim BK, Fowler SC, Malenka RC, Su TC (2014) Autism-associated neuroligin-3 mutations commonly impair striatal circuits to boost repetitive behaviors. Cell 158(1):198–212. doi:10.1016/j.cell.2014.04.045

Rubenstein JLR, Merzenich MM (2003) Model of autism: increased ratio of excitation/inhibition in key neural systems. Genes Brain Behav 2(5):255–267. http://dx.doi.org/10.1034/j.1601-183X.2003.00037.x

Samaco RC, Hogart A, LaSalle JM (2005) Epigenetic overlap in autism-spectrum neurodevelopmental disorders: MECP2 deficiency causes reduced expression of UBE3A and GABRB3. Hum Mol Genet 14:483–492

Sander JD, Joung JK (2014) CRISPR-Cas systems for editing, regulating and targeting genomes. Nat Biotechnol 32:347–355

Santos AR, Kanellopoulos AK, Bagni C (2014) Learning and behavioral deficits associated with the absence of the Fragile X mental retardation protein: what a fly and mouse model can teach us. Learn Mem 21:543–555

Sasson NJ, Turner-brown LM, Holtzclaw TN, Lam KSL, Bodfish JW (2008) Children with autism demonstrate circumscribed attention during passive viewing of complex social and nonsocial picture arrays. Autism Res 1(1):31–42. doi:10.1002/aur.4

Sato D, Lionel AC, Leblond CS, Prasad A, Pinto D, Walker S, O'Connor I et al (2012) SHANK1 deletions in males with autism spectrum disorder. Am J Hum Genet 90:879–887

Schmidt C, Bladt F, Goedecke S, Brinkmann V, Zschiesche W, Sharpe M, Gherardi E, Birchmeler C (1995) Scatter factor/hepatocyte growth factor is essential for liver development. Nature 373(6516):699–702. http://dx.doi.org/10.1038/373699a0

Scott-Van A, Abrahams B, Alvarez-Retuerto A, Sonnenblick L, Rudie J, Ghahremani D, Mumford JA, Poldrack RA, Dapretto M, Geschwind DH (2010) Altered functional connectivity in frontal lobe circuits is associated with variation in the autism risk gene CNTNAP2. Sci Transl Med 2(56):56ra80. http://stm.sciencemag.org/content/2/56/56ra80

Sears L, Vest C, Mohamed S, Bailey J, Ranson BJ, Piven J (1999) An MRI study of the basal ganglia in autism. Prog Neuropsychopharmacol Biol Psychiatry 23(4):613–624

Sears L, Mathai ÆG, Casanova MF (2009) Event-related potential study of novelty processing abnormalities in autism. Appl Psychophysiol Biofeedback 34(1):37–51. doi:10.1007/s10484-009-9074-5

Sebat J, Lakshmi B, Malhotra D, Troge J, Lese-Martin C, Walsh T, Yamrom B et al (2007) Strong association of de novo copy number mutations with autism. Science 316(5823):445–449

Selby L, Zhang C, Sun QQ (2007) Major defects in neocortical GABAergic inhibitory circuits in mice lacking the Fragile X mental retardation protein. Neurosci Lett 412:227–232

Sell GL, Margolis SS (2015) From UBE3A to Angelman syndrome: a substrate perspective. Front Neurosci 9:322

Shahbazian M, Young J, Yuva-Paylor L, Spencer C, Antalffy B, Noebels JL, Armstrong D, Paylor R, Zoghbi HY (2002) Mice with truncated MeCP2 recapitulate many Rett syndrome features and display hyperacetylation of histone H3. Neuron 35(2):243–254

Shiraishi-Yamaguchi Y, Furuichi T (2007) The homer family proteins. Genome Biol 8(2):206

Sidorov MS, Auerbach BD, Bear MF (2013) Fragile X mental retardation protein and synaptic plasticity. Mol Brain 8(6):15

Silva-Santos S, van Woerden GM, Bruinsma CF, Mientjes E, Jolfaei MA, Distel B, Kushner SA, Elgersma Y (2015) Ube3a reinstatement identifies distinct developmental windows in a murine Angelman syndrome model. J Clin Invest 125(5):2069–2076

Silverman JL, Yang M, Lord C, Crawley JN (2010a) Behavioural phenotyping assays for mouse models of autism. Nat Rev Neurosci 11(7):490–502. doi:10.1038/nrn2851. Nature Publishing Group

Silverman JL, Tolu SS, Barkan CL, Crawley JN (2010b) Repetitive self-grooming behavior in the BTBR mouse model of autism is blocked by the mGluR5 antagonist MPEP. Neuropsychopharmacology 35(4):976–989

Silverman JL, Turner SM, Barkan CL, Tolu SS, Saxena R, Hung AY, Sheng M, Crawley JN (2011) Sociability and motor functions in Shank1 mutant mice. Brain Res 1380:120–137. doi:10.1016/j.brainres.2010.09.026. Elsevier B.V

Smith SEP, Zhou Y-D, Zhang G, Jin Z, Stoppel DC, Anderson MP (2011) Increased gene dosage of Ube3a results in autism traits and decreased glutamate synaptic transmission in mice. Sci Transl Med 3(103):103ra97

Smith JM, Xu J, Powell EM (2012) Age dependent forebrain structural changes in mice deficient in the autism associated gene met tyrosine kinase. Neuroimage Clin 1(1):66–74

Smrt RD, Eaves-Egenes J, Barkho BZ, Santistevan NJ, Zhao C, Aimone JB, Gage FH, Zhao X (2007) Mecp2 deficiency leads to delayed maturation and altered gene expression in hippocampal neurons. Neurobiol Dis 27(1):77–89

Solomon M, Smith AC, Frank MJ, Ly S, Carter CS (2011) Probabilistic reinforcement learning in adults with autism spectrum disorders. Autism Res 4(2):109–20. doi:10.1002/aur.177.

Sousa I, Clark TG, Toma C, Kobayashi K, Choma M, Holt R, Sykes NH et al (2009) MET and autism susceptibility: family and case-control studies. Eur J Hum Genet 17:749–758

Spencer CM, Alekseyenko O, Serysheva E, Yuva-Paylor LA, Paylor R (2005) Altered anxiety-related and social behaviors in the Fmr1 knockout mouse model of fragile X syndrome. Genes Brain Behav 4:420–430

Spooren W, Lindemann L, Ghosh A, Santarelli L (2012) Synapse dysfunction in autism: a molecular medicine approach to drug discovery in neurodevelopmental disorders. Trends Pharmacol Sci 33(12):669–684

Steriade M (2005) Sleep, epilepsy and thalamic reticular inhibitory neurons. Trends Neurosci 28(6):317. http://www.sciencedirect.com/science/article/B6T0V-4FT6HKH-1/2/45157cfc8be5733821116e78249ac1e6

Stigler KA, McDonald BC, Anand A, Saykin AJ, McDougle CJ (2011) Structural and functional magnetic resonance imaging of autism spectrum disorders. Brain Res 1380:146–161. doi:10.1016/j.brainres.2010.11.076. Elsevier B.V

Sutton MA, Schuman EM (2006) Dendritic protein synthesis, synaptic plasticity, and memory. Cell 127:49–58

Szatmari P, Paterson AD, Zwaigenbaum L, Roberts W, Brian J, Liu X-Q, Vincent JB et al (2007) Mapping autism risk loci using genetic linkage and chromosomal rearrangements. Nat Genet 39:319–328

Tabuchi K, Blundell J, Etherton MR, Hammer RE, Liu X, Powell CM, Südhof TC (2007) A neuroligin-3 mutation implicated in autism increases inhibitory synaptic transmission in mice. Science 318(5847):71–76

Tallon-Baudry C, Bertrand O (1999) Oscillatory gamma activity in humans and its role in object representation. Trends Cogn Sci 3(4):151–162

Tang G, Gudsnuk K, Kuo S-H, Cotrina ML, Rosoklija G, Sonders MS, Sosunov A, Kanter E et al (2014) Loss of mTOR-dependent macroautophagy causes autistic-like synaptic pruning deficits. Neuron 83(5):1131–1143

Tania M, Ma K, Recent XK, Khan A (2014) Recent Advances in Animal Model Experimentation in Autism Research. Acta Neuropsychiatr 26(5):264–271. doi:10.1017/neu.2013.58

Tate P, Skarnes W, Bird A (1996) The methyl-CpG binding protein MeCP2 is essential for embryonic development in the mouse. Nature 12(2):205–208

Tecuapetla F, Jin X, Lima S, Costa RM (2016) Complementary but distinct contribution of striatal projection pathways to the initiation and execution of action sequences. Cell (in press)

Thanseem I, Nakamura K, Miyachi T, Toyota T, Yamada S, Tsujii M, Tsuchiya KJ et al (2010) Further evidence for the role of MET in autism susceptibility. Neurosci Res 68:137–141

Tian D, Stoppel LJ, Heynen AJ, Lindemann L, Jaeschke G, Mills AA, Bear MF (2015) Contribution of mGluR5 to pathophysiology in a mouse model of human chromosome 16p11.2 microdeletion. Nat Neurosci 18(2):16–19. doi:10.1038/nn.3911

Tick B, Bolton P, Happe F, Rutter M, Rijsdijk F (2016) Heritability of autism spectrum disorders: a meta-analysis of twin studies. J Child Psychol Psychiatry 57(5):585–595
Tricomi E, Balleine BW, O'Doherty JP (2009) A specific role for posterior dorsolateral striatum in human habit learning. Eur J Neurosci 29(11):2225–2232. doi:10.1111/j.1460-9568.2009.06796.x
Tropea D, Giacometti E, Wilson NR, Beard C, McCurry C, Fu DD, Flannery R, Jaenisch R, Sur M (2009) Partial reversal of Rett syndrome-like symptoms in MeCP2 mutant mice. Proc Natl Acad Sci U S A 106(6):2029–2034
Uchino S, Waga C (2013) SHANK3 as an autism spectrum disorder-associated gene. Brain Dev 35(2):106–110. doi:10.1016/j.braindev.2012.05.013. The Japanese Society of Child Neurology
Uddin LQ, Superkar K, Menon V (2013) Reconceptualizing functional brain connectivity in autism from a developmental perspective. Front Hum Neurosci 7:458
Uehara Y, Minowa O, Mori C, Shiota K, Kuno J, Noda T, Kitamura N (1995) Placental defect and embryonic lethality in mice lacking hepatocyte growth factor/scatter factor. Nature 373(6516):702–705. http://dx.doi.org/10.1038/373702a0
Utari A, Chonchaiya W, Rivera SM, Schneider A, Hagerman RJ, Faradz SMH, Ethell IM, Nguyen DV (2010) Side effects of minocycline treatment in patients with fragile X syndrome and exploration of outcome measures. Am J Intellect Dev Disabil 115(5):433–443
van Duyne GD (2015) Cre recombinase. Microbiol Spectr 3(1):MDNA3–0014 – 2014
Van Eylen, Lien BB, Steyaert J, Evers K, Wagemans J, Noens I (2011) Cognitive flexibility in autism spectrum disorder:explaining the inconsistencies? Res Autism Spectr Disord 5:1390–1401
Veenstra-VanderWeele J, Blakely RD (2012) Networking in autism : leveraging genetic , biomarker and model system findings in the search for new treatments. Neuropsychopharmacology 37(1):196–212. doi:10.1038/npp.2011.185. Nature Publishing Group
Veltman MW, Craig EE, Bolton PF (2005) Autism spectrum disorders in Prader-Willi and Angelman syndromes: a systematic review. Psychiatr Genet 15(4):243–254
Verkerk AJ, Pieretti M, Sutcliffe JS, Fu YH, Kuhl DP, Pizzuti A, Reiner O, Richards S, Victoria MF, Zhang FP (1991) Identification of a gene (FMR-1) containing a CGG repeat coincident with a breakpoint cluster region exhibiting length variation in fragile X syndrome. Cell 65(5):905–914
Vernes SC, Newbury DF, Abrahams BS, Winchester L, Nicod J, Groszer M, Alarcón M et al (2008) A functional genetic link between distinct developmental language disorders. N Engl J Med 359:2337–2345. http://www.nejm.org/doi/full/10.1056/NEJMoa0802828#t=abstr
Vicidomini C, Ponzoni L, Lim D, Schmeisser MJ, Reim D, Morello N, Orellana D et al (2016) Pharmacological enhancement of mGlu5 receptors rescues behavioral deficits in SHANK3 knock-out mice. Mol Psychiatry. doi:10.1038/mp.2016.30
Vissers ME, Cohen MX, Geurts HM (2012) Brain connectivity and high functioning autism: a promising path of research that needs refined models, methodological convergence, and stronger behavioral links. Neurosci Biobehav Rev 36(1):604–625
Walker G (2008) Constant and progressive time delay procedures for teaching children with autism: a literature review. J Autism Dev Disorders 38(2):261–275. doi:10.1007/s10803-007-0390-4
Wallace ML, Burette AC, Weinberg RJ, Philpot BD (2012) Maternal Loss of Ube3a Produces an Excitatory/inhibitory Imbalance through Neuron Type-Specific Synaptic Defects. Neuron 74(5):793–800
Wang X, Mccoy PA, Rodriguiz RM, Pan Y, Je HS, Roberts AC, Kim CJ et al (2011) Synaptic dysfunction and abnormal behaviors in mice lacking major isoforms of Shank3. Hum Mol Genet 20(15):3093–3108. doi:10.1093/hmg/ddr212
Wang X, Xu Q, Bey AL, Lee Y, Jiang Y-h (2014) Transcriptional and functional complexity of Shank3 provides a molecular framework to understand the phenotypic heterogeneity of SHANK3 causing autism and Shank3 mutant mice. Mol Autism 5:30
Wang X, Bey AL, Katz BM, Badea A, Kim N, David LK, Duffney LJ et al (2016) Altered mGluR5-Homer scaffolds and corticostriatal connectivity in a Shank3 complete knockout model of autism. Nat Commun 10(7):11459

Weeber EJ, Jiang YH, Elgersman Y, Varga AW, Carrasquillo Y, Brown SE, Christian JM et al (2003) Derangements of hippocampal calcium/calmodulin-dependent protein kinase II in a mouse model for Angelman mental retardation syndrome. J Neurosci 23:2634–2644
Weiss LA, Shen Y, Korn JM, Arking DE, Miller DT, Fossdal R, Saemundsen E et al (2008) Association between microdeletion and microduplication at 16p11.2 and autism. N Engl J Med 358(7):667–675
Williams SCP (2011) New mouse models of autism highlight need for standardized tests. Nat Med 17(11):1324. doi:10.1038/nm1111-1324. Nature Publishing Group
Willner P (1984) The validity of animal models of depression. Psychopharmacology (Berl) 83:1–16
Wilson HL, Wong AC, Shaw SR, Tse WY, Stapleton GA, Phelan MC, Hu S, Marshall J, McDermid HE (2003) Molecular characterisation of the 22q13 deletion syndrome supports the role of haploinsufficiency of SHANK3/PROSAP2 in the major neurological symptoms. J Med Genet 40(8):575–584
Won H, Lee H-R, Gee HY, Mah W, Kim J-I, Lee J, Ha S et al (2012) Autistic-like social behaviour in Shank2-mutant mice improved by restoring NMDA receptor function. Nature 486:261–265
Won H, Mah W, Kim E, Maggio N, The Chaim Sheba (2013) Autism spectrum disorder causes , mechanisms , and treatments : focus on neuronal synapses. Front Mol Neurosci 6(August):1–26. doi:10.3389/fnmol.2013.00019
Wong CG-T, III Carter SO (2001) The GABAA receptor: subunit-dependent functions and absence seizures. Epilepsy Curr 1(1):1–5
Yan J, Oliveira G, Coutinho A, Yang C, Feng J, Katz C, Sram J et al (2005) Analysis of the neuroligin 3 and 4 genes in autism and other neuropsychiatric patients. Mol Psychiatry 10:329–332
Yang M, Freeman L, Foley G, Crawley JN (2015a) In tribute to Bob Blanchard: divergent behavioral phenotypes of 16p11.2 deletion mice reared in same-genotype versus mixed-genotype cages. Physiol Behav 146(1):16–27
Yang M, Lewis FC, Sarvi MS, Foley GM, Crawley JN (2015b) 16p11.2 deletion mice display cognitive deficits in touchscreen learning and novelty recognition tasks. Learn Mem 22(12): 622–632
Yang M, Mahrt EJ, Lewis F, Foley G, Portmann T, Dolmetsch RE, Portfors CV, Crawley JN (2015c) 16p11.2 deletion syndrome mice display sensory and ultrasonic vocalization deficits during social interactions. Autism Res 8(5):507–521. doi:10.1002/aur.1465
Yashiro K, Riday TT, Condon KH, Roberts AC, Bernardo DR, Prakash R, Weinberg RJ, Ehlers MD, Philpot BD (2009) Ube3a is required for experience-dependent maturation of the neocortex. Nat Neurosci 12(6):777–783
Yatawara CJ, Einfeld SL, Hickie IB, Davenport TA, Guastella AJ (2016) The effect of oxytocin nasal spray on social interaction deficits observed in young children with autism: a randomized clinical crossover trial. Mol Psychiatry 21(9):1225–31
Yi F, Danko T, Botelho SC, Patzke C, Pak CH, Wernig M, Sudhof TC (2016) Autism-associated SHANK3 haploinsufficiency causes Ih channelopathy in human neurons. Science 352(6286):aaf2669. doi:10.1126/science.aaf2669
Yin HH, Knowlton BJ (2006) The role of the basal ganglia in habit formation. Nat Rev Neurosci 7(6):464–476. doi:10.1038/nrn1919
Yin HH, Knowlton BJ, Balleine BW (2004) Lesions of dorsolateral striatum preserve outcome expectancy but disrupt habit formation in instrumental learning. Eur J Neurosci 19(1):181–189. doi:10.1111/j.1460-9568.2004.03095.x
Yin HH, Knowlton BJ, Balleine BW (2005a) Blockade of NMDA receptors in the dorsomedial striatum prevents action-outcome learning in instrumental conditioning. Eur J Neurosci 22(2):505–512
Yin HH, Ostlund SB, Knowlton BJ, Balleine BW (2005b) The role of the dorsomedial striatum in instrumental conditioning. Eur J Neurosci 22(2):513–523. doi:10.1111/j.1460-9568.2005.04218.x
Yoo H (2015) Genetics of autism spectrum disorder: current status and possible clinical applications. Exp Neurobiol 24(4):257–272

Yuste R (1995) Dendritic spines. Nature 375(6533):682–684. Cambridge, MA: MIT Press
Zhou Y, Kaiser T, Monteiro P, Zhang X, Van der Goes MS, Wang D, Barak B et al (2016) Mice with shank3 mutations associated with ASD and schizophrenia display both shared and distinct defects. Neuron 89(1):147–162
Ziv Y, Burns LD, Cocker ED, Hamel EO, Ghosh KK, Kitch LJ, El Gamal A, Schnitzer MJ (2013) Long-term dynamics of CA1 hippocampal place codes. Nat Neurosci 16(3):264–266
Zoghbi HY (2003) Postnatal neurodevelopmental disorders: meeting at the synapse? Science 302(5646):826–830
Zoghbi HY, Bear MF (2012) Synaptic dysfunction in neurodevelopmental disorders associated with autism and intellectual disabilities. Cold Spring Harb Perspect Biol 4(3):a009886

The Clinical Neuropsychology of ASD

3

Hilde M. Geurts and Anne Geeke Lever

3.1 Clinical Neuropsychology: A Short Introduction

In daily life we are highly dependent on a wide range of cognitive skills, from attention to memory and from the ability to start behavior, to change behavior or to stop behavior, and to the ability to recognize emotions. We often use these skills without even realizing how crucial they are for communicating and interacting with others, for planning all kinds of aspects in your life in order to be able to reach future goals, and when driving a car or when trying to read a book and not letting your mind dwell to the other things you need to do. People with ASD are thought to have difficulties in various cognitive domains underlying the observed challenges they experience in daily life. The main goal of clinical neuropsychology is to use the knowledge regarding the relation between brain and behavior to understand the day-to-day challenges in clinical groups such as ASD. Hence, fundamental research focusing on brain development, brain mechanisms, and specific cognitive processes as well as clinical research focusing on cognitive profiles and the relationship with the observed (disorder specific) symptoms are of importance within the field of clinical neuropsychology. In this chapter, we focus primarily on clinical ASD research. When reading the current chapter, it is, however, good to keep in mind that clinical research and research focusing on neuroscience mutually influence each

H.M. Geurts (✉)
Dutch Autism and ADHD Research Center (d'Arc), Brain and Cognition,
Department of Psychology, University of Amsterdam, Amsterdam, The Netherlands

Dr. Leo Kannerhuis, Mental Health Care Clinic for people with ASD,
Doorwerth, The Netherlands
e-mail: H.M.Geurts@uva.nl

A.G. Lever
Dutch Autism and ADHD Research Center (d'Arc), Brain and Cognition,
Department of Psychology, University of Amsterdam, Amsterdam, The Netherlands

B. Barahona Corrêa, R.-J. van der Gaag (eds.), *Autism Spectrum Disorders in Adults*, DOI 10.1007/978-3-319-42713-3_3

other and are largely intertwined. Some of the theories described below even originated from the observation that patients with specific brain lesions showed similar behaviors as children with ASD (e.g., Damasio and Maurer 1978; Maurer and Damasio 1982). So, even though we will not discuss the functional and structural imaging studies in support of the cognitive constructs related to ASD, the conclusions we draw based on the cognitive behavioral studies are in line with the findings discussed in Chap. 2.

3.2 Cognitive ASD Theories

There are three main cognitive theories of ASD, which are linked to the theoretical constructs of theory of mind, central coherence, and executive functioning (for a review, see Brunsdon and Happé 2014; Happé and Charlton 2012). Below, these three cognitive constructs will be discussed in more detail. However, recently, a number of researchers argued that the ASD-related difficulties in each of these three domains might all be related to a single underlying problem common to all, namely, a problem with predictive coding, which we will also discuss.

3.2.1 Theory of Mind

The first general cognitive explanation of ASD developed around the concept of "theory of mind" (ToM). ToM is the ability to attribute mental states to self and others and is mainly related to the social problems that people with ASD encounter in day-to-day life (e.g., Baron-Cohen et al. 1985). A well-developed ToM is thought to be crucial for making social inferences and guiding social behavior in communicative interactions. Nowadays, ToM is divided into two related systems: an explicit ToM system (i.e., the ability to make cognitive inferences of mental states) and a spontaneous, implicit ToM system (i.e., the ability to explain nonverbal aspects of communication, such as following eye gaze, understanding facial expressions, and interpreting body language). Currently, the global idea is that individuals, and certainly adults, with ASD have difficulties with implicit ToM, but in various occasions, they can compensate by using explicit strategies to draw conclusions regarding the mental states of others. This implies that when there is a sufficient amount of time, individuals with ASD often are able, by using reasoning, to interpret what is going on. However, as social interactions often go rather fast, especially when one is interacting with more than one person at a time, people with ASD might respond too late.

While implicit ToM is typically measured by examining spontaneous eye movements during the presentation of social and emotional videos (e.g., Senju et al. 2009), explicit ToM is, in adults, typically measured with tasks such as the Strange Stories test or the faux pas test. A faux pas is a socially unintended and inappropriate response leading to an awkward social situation (Baron-Cohen et al. 1999), such as criticizing a friend's ugly curtains in his new home without being aware that those curtains were chosen and newly acquired by your friend. The faux pas test contains several stories with and without faux pas situations and related questions, including questions on detection, person identification, content, false belief, explanation, and empathy (Spek et al. 2010; Stone et al. 1998; Zalla et al. 2009). Each of these aspects of ToM is of importance when interacting with others.

More recently it has been argued that people with ASD might differ from people without ASD in social motivation (e.g., Chevallier et al. 2012; Mundy and Neal 2000). The idea is that individuals with ASD assign less importance to social information and relationships and that this lack of social motivation ultimately influences the development of ToM. Put differently, the social motivation theory of ASD (e.g., Chevallier et al. 2012; Mundy and Neal 2000) postulates that deficits in social interactions are due to difficulties in forming reward presentations of social stimuli (hypo-responsivity). However, interestingly, hyperresponsivity has also been hypothesized to be of importance for individuals with ASD but only with respect to specific classes of stimuli such as objects. This might, according to the authors, be an explanation for the observed restricted interests in individuals with ASD (e.g., Cascio et al. 2012; Dichter et al. 2012). Typically, these observed restricted interests and repetitive behaviors have been associated with executive functioning deficits (see later).

3.2.2 Central Coherence (CC)

The second theory is the so-called weak central coherence (WCC) (e.g., Frith and Happé 1994; Frith 1989; Happé 1999; Happé and Frith 2006) or perceptual enhancement (Mottron and Burack 2001) theory. Central coherence is the ability to discern meaning in the surrounding environment and to understand the context when information is processed. The hypothesis is that people with ASD are challenged in this respect. The central coherence theory has been developed not only to explain some weaknesses of individuals with ASD but also to account for some strengths. For example, people with ASD seem to outperform people without ASD in situations where it is beneficial to focus on details, or some may even present certain savant abilities. Depending on one's theoretical standpoint, the WCC theory focuses on atypical perceptual processes which encompass enhanced local processing (Mottron et al. 2006) and/or reduced global processing in people with ASD (e.g., Frith and Happé 1994; Frith 1989; Happé 1999; Happé and Frith 2006). Currently, the idea is that individuals with ASD have a tendency to process information in a fractioned and local way but that they are able to perceive global coherence when instructed to do so (Happé and Frith 2006) or when sufficient time is allowed (Van der Hallen et al. 2015). Atypical perceptual organization has been mainly linked to nonsocial symptoms of ASD, such as insistence on sameness, restricted special interests, or hypersensitivity to sensory stimuli.

Central coherence is often measured with tasks such as the embedded figures test, hierarchical figures or letters, or the Mooney figures (for an overview, see Van der Hallen et al. 2015). For example, in a hierarchical figures test (a well-known example is the Navon test) (Navon 1977), a number of letters composed of smaller letters are shown. These smaller letters can be congruent with the larger figure but can also be incongruent. The tendency to firstly perceive the larger or the smaller letter or the amount of interference occurring when focusing on one of both aspects is indicative of one's proneness to process information globally or locally. A strong focus on details can be beneficial when, for example, reading computer code, checking a contract, or proofreading a text for typographical errors. However, an excessive focus on details is disadvantageous, for example, when watching a romantic movie as every anomaly might distract from the story line or when having a conversation with someone as one might get lost in telling all the details.

3.2.3 Executive Functioning

The third account of ASD postulates a deficit in executive functioning (EF). EF is an umbrella term for those cognitive processes needed to adjust your behavior to the demands of the environment (e.g., inhibition, working memory, cognitive flexibility, generativity, planning). In each of these EF domains, people with ASD seem to encounter problems, such as exerting effortful control when they need to deal with novel, complex, or ambiguous situations in everyday life. In cognitive neuroscience, one often refers to these EF processes as cognitive control. Like EF, cognitive control denotes the ability to maintain task-relevant information in order to suppress inappropriate behaviors and to flexibly adjust behavior according to environmental contingencies (Carter 2005). EF problems are theoretically linked to observed repetitive behavior, and specific interests as repetitive behavior in individuals with ASD might be due to difficulties in suppressing behavior even when the consequences are negative. However, for example, suppression of inappropriate behavior or the literal meaning of words is of course also important in social interactions and communication. So, EF problems might explain some of the observed social difficulties as well.

Typical EF tasks are, for example, the go/no-go task (prepotent response inhibition), the Stroop test (interference control), number-letter sequencing (working memory), the Wisconsin card sorting test (WCST; cognitive flexibility), verbal fluency (generativity), and tower tasks (planning). The common factor in each of these tasks is that there are a lot of degrees of freedom in responding, so it is not immediately evident what the best solution in this new situation is (see also Van Eylen et al. 2011). In a task such as the WCST, one first needs to figure out how to sort information, and suddenly, without a warning, one needs to sort information in a different way. Hence, what is first a correct sorting principle seems unexpectedly wrong, but this is not explicitly told to the participant of this test. So, one needs to respond to unexpected events and flexibly adjust one's behavior to a changing environment. This is exactly what is thought to be hard for people with ASD. As each of the separate EF domains are highly interrelated, it is important to realize that there are no measures that purely measure one domain. For example, also with respect to the WCST, one needs to remember the goal (working memory), and after a change in strategy, one needs to refrain from sorting according to the formerly correct strategy (inhibition).

People with ASD seem to fail most often on EF tasks with implicit instructions as they involve lower degrees of rule constraints (Van Eylen et al. 2011) and higher degrees of open-endedness (Lawson 2003; White et al. 2009). Therefore, some hypothesize that people with ASD experience difficulties in intentional control due to difficulties in the formation of higher-order task intentions rather than to difficulties in implementation of the intentions (Poljac and Bekkering 2012). This means that people with ASD will perform worse on tasks that require them to identify the expected behavior themselves (open systems). Choosing your own goal and your own solutions are more abstract aspects of EF, which are difficult to grasp with most clinical neuropsychological tasks. However, day-to-day observations suggest that also these aspects of EF are especially challenging for individuals with ASD.

3.2.4 Cognition in ASD Summarized

While not everyone with an ASD diagnosis has cognitive problems in each of these three domains and one needs to take developmental changes into account when focusing on cognitive problems (e.g., Hill and Bird 2006; Pellicano 2010; Towgood et al. 2009; Wilson et al. 2014), many individuals with an ASD do encounter cognitive challenges within these domains across the adult life span. Cognitive ASD research is, however, not restricted to the three aforementioned domains.

Moreover, these domains are also interrelated (e.g., Brunsdon and Happé 2014); no cognitive function stands on its own. For example, for many EF tasks, it is crucial that one can use his or her ToM abilities to interpret a task instruction, and for many ToM tasks, it is of importance to keep the goal in mind and to inhibit irrelevant information (i.e., aspects of EF). The development of ToM and EF is strongly related, and there is a lot of debate around which of these cognitive abilities develop first (e.g., Geurts et al. 2010; Pellicano 2010). Also CC has been related to EF and ToM performance. For example, people with WCC seem to perform worse on ToM tasks, and WCC in young children with ASD seem to predict ToM problems later in life (Pellicano 2010), although findings are inconsistent (e.g., Morgan et al. 2003). To circumvent this problem of how these three theories specifically relate to each other, one could assume that there is another cognitive problem that is underlying the observed difficulties with ToM, CC, and EF tasks. Lately, various research groups started to work from a predictive coding framework (Gonzalez-Gadea et al. 2015; Lawson et al. 2014; Palmer et al. 2015; Pellicano and Burr 2012; Van Boxtel and Lu 2013; Van de Cruys et al. 2014), and these researchers are arguing that problems with predictive coding might underlie the observed problems in a wide range of cognitive tasks.

The predictive coding framework is based on the theory that our brains are predictive coding machines. The basic idea is that predictions are used to shape the surrounding environment and that a prediction is compared with the received sensory information. This comparison may lead to errors (i.e., prediction errors) indicating that the current representation of the world is not sufficiently able to explain it (predict it). Once a prediction error is detected, one can attempt to adjust the prediction in order to increase precision, but one also learns how much weight one needs to give to such an error as not every prediction error is equally important. Individuals with ASD might present a deficit in this flexible adjustment (Van de Cruys et al. 2014) or might give too much weight to errors due to violations of the potentially too specific predictions they make (i.e., impaired top-down predictions) (Lawson et al. 2014; Pellicano and Burr 2012). Currently, studies are carried out to test these different perspectives, so the future will teach us whether this indeed is an alternative way of looking at the problems people with ASD encounter in daily life.

In the next sections, we will primarily discuss the cognitive findings in intellectually able adults with ASD with regard to the three dominant cognitive theories, but other related cognitive domains will be also touched upon. We will end with a few specific challenges with respect to older age, gender, and individual differences which are likely to be relevant across each of the cognitive domains.

3.3 Cognition in Young and Middle Adulthood

In general, it seems that the cognitive difficulties in intellectually able adults with ASD are not as profound as in childhood. However, the findings are rather mixed (see, e.g., Altgassen et al. 2012; Hill and Bird 2006; Lai et al. 2011; Sachse et al. 2013; Spek et al. 2009; Spek et al. 2010; Towgood et al. 2009; Wilson et al. 2014). Various studies report hardly any performance differences between those with and without a diagnosis (e.g., Sachse et al. 2013) or show that cognitive problems are only visible in a subgroup of adults with ASD (Hill and Bird 2006; Towgood et al. 2009). Instead of discussing these individual studies in detail, we will discuss various recent informative meta-analyses as these meta-analyses take the wide variety of tests used to test the different cognitive domains into account.

With respect to ToM, it has been shown that in adults (mean age range 20–44 years), there are still considerable ToM problems, as the observed combined effect size was large (Chung et al. 2014). This effect size was based on 17 studies (ToM was measured with the faux pas, Strange Stories, or reading the mind eyes tests) in adults with an ASD (Chung et al. 2014). Indeed, recent individual studies also showed that adults with ASD perform worse on ToM tasks than adults without ASD (see, e.g., Schuwerk et al. 2015; Wilson et al. 2014). During adulthood, age did not seem to have an effect on ToM (Chung et al. 2014). A meta-analysis of ASD studies focusing on emotion recognition (N studies = 48, mean age range 6–41 years) also concluded that age did not have a differential effect on this specific ability (Uljarevic and Hamilton 2013). Hence, individuals with an ASD were challenged when interpreting emotions in both childhood as well as young and middle adulthood. Thus, ToM problems and emotion recognition difficulties are not just present in children.

As we mentioned already, depending on the theoretical standpoint, some will argue that WCC is related to enhanced local processing, while others argue that it related to reduced global processing. A recent meta-analysis was conducted to settle this debate. Based on a wide variety of tasks (N studies = 56, mean age range

6–35 years), it has been shown that there was no enhanced local processing but also no decreased global visual processing in people with ASD (Van der Hallen et al. 2015). Age did not seem to strongly moderate this finding, but the authors suggested that the developmental pace in these processes differs between those with and without ASD, and the performance differences might be stronger among adults (N studies = 16) (Van der Hallen et al. 2015). However, those with ASD seemed to encounter some degree of difficulty, as they were a bit slower in visual processing. Thus, perceptual information seems to be processed differently or at least slower. While this might sometimes be beneficial, it is not the case that this is directly caused by specific strengths or weaknesses in global or local information processing.

All qualitative reviews focusing on all EF domains simultaneously mainly focused on children, although some did also include a few adult studies (e.g., Hill 2004; Kenworthy et al. 2008; Pennington and Ozonoff 1996; Sergeant et al. 2002). Based on these reviews, it seems that across the life span, individuals with ASD do encounter EF problems. Recent meta-analyses that concentrated on specific EF domains included slightly more ASD adult studies from a broader age range. First of all, medium-sized effects were observed in two inhibition meta-analyses (N studies = 41, mean age range 1.5–64 years) (Geurts et al. 2014). While, with respect to prepotent response inhibition (i.e., the ability to stop a response), it seemed that with increasing age, the inhibitory control problems became less profound, age did not exert a different influence on performance of interference control tasks (i.e., the ability to ignore task-irrelevant information) in those with and without ASD. However, only 6 of the 41 studies focused on adults, so the age effect might be largely explained by developmental changes from young childhood to adolescence. Secondly, the findings for working memory (i.e., the ability to keep and manipulate information online) are rather mixed, making it hard to draw strong conclusions (see, for a quantitative review, Boucher et al. 2012). It has been shown, however, that in adolescence spatial working memory and more complex working memory tasks pose a challenge for individuals with ASD (Barendse et al. 2013). These impairments are still observed in adulthood (e.g., Sachse et al. 2013). With respect to the third EF domain, cognitive flexibility (i.e., the ability to change your thoughts and behavior), the effect sizes ranged from small to large, depending on the type of task used to assess cognitive flexibility (N studies = 72, mean age range 5–64 years) (Leung and Zakzanis 2014). For example, flexibility abilities assessed with self-reports yielded the largest discriminative effect, but actually none of the neuropsychological tests reached large effect sizes. Unfortunately, it was not tested whether age of the participants was a relevant factor for explaining the magnitude of the effect even though the age range of the included samples was rather broad. Fourth, regarding generativity (i.e., the ability to generate, create, or produce novel contents, such as words, ideas, or figures), there are no recent reviews or meta-analyses, but most adult studies do report a worse performance on generativity tasks in adults with ASD as compared to adults without ASD (e.g., Ambery et al. 2006; Carmo et al. 2015; Lever and Geurts 2016a; Spek et al. 2009). Finally, recently we (Olde Dubbelink and Geurts 2017) ran a planning meta-analysis (N studies = 50, mean age range 3–64 years) and observed a medium-sized effect size across the broad age span. Age did not seem to be a crucial moderator. Hence, it seems that from childhood to late adulthood, people with ASD encounter EF problems across the different EF domains.

So, also in adulthood there still appear to be difficulties in each of the three cognitive domains that are associated with ASD. However, cognition is not restricted to these domains. There are, for example, various studies reporting that people with ASD process information more slowly (for adult studies, see e.g., Lai et al. 2011; Sachse et al. 2013) and are more variable in responding (N studies = 17, mean age 6–29 years; (Karalunas et al. 2014)) than people without an ASD diagnosis. Processing speed is related to the white matter integrity of the brain (Travers et al. 2014) (see Chap. 2 for details regarding the hypothesis of ASD as a brain connectivity disorder). It is of importance to most cognitive domains and influences performance on almost all neuropsychological tasks used in clinical practice. It is, therefore, key when interpreting neuropsychological results, to take processing speed into account. People with ASD might have another so-called speed accuracy trade-off. This means that they might slow down to make sure that they won't make an error, so they have a more cautious style of responding. In sustained attention (i.e., vigilance), most studies did not report impairments in ASD, but only a very few studies focused on adults (see Sanders et al. 2008, for a review). More recent studies of sustained attention including adults with ASD indicated, however, some difficulties in this domain (Chien et al. 2015; Geurts and Vissers 2012; Murphy et al. 2014). Other aspects of attention such as visual orienting are found to be impaired in ASD. A meta-analysis examining the orienting behavior of people with ASD indicated that the magnitude of the orienting effect is reduced in ASD, but the effect size was small (N studies = 18, mean age 4–29 years) (Landry and Parker 2013). Impairments were most pronounced on so-called arrow cueing tasks and least pronounced on eye-gaze cueing tasks. Impairments increased when trials were rapidly presented and when individuals were older. Nevertheless, the authors raise the question of whether the impairments do not reflect general slowing rather than impaired orienting behavior. Hence, it is not evident whether observed problems in sustained attention and visual orienting are typical for adults with ASD.

For day-to-day life, episodic (declarative) memory is also of importance. It holds contextual information about autobiographical events, such as the when, where, who, what, and why of a certain experience. Episodic memory can be assessed by means of free recall and recognition tasks but also by cued recall tasks. Based on a qualitative review (N studies declarative memory = 39, mean age 4–40 years) (Boucher et al. 2012), it has been concluded that in the majority of studies in intellectually able individuals with ASD, the recognition of verbal and visual nonsocial stimuli is unimpaired or even superior. Less consistent are the findings for social stimuli, as both impaired and unimpaired recognition have been observed. The free recall findings are also mixed. Intact performance is reported on both direct and delayed recall of unrelated stimuli, but with related stimuli, detailed analyses do suggest some impairment regarding specific memory effects (for details see Boucher et al. 2012), while other studies concluded that also in this case, people with ASD are unimpaired. As to recall performance on tasks providing target-related cues, evidence shows that it is generally unimpaired in ASD (Boucher et al. 2012).

In sum, cognition encompasses various different constructs like emotion recognition, theory of mind, perceptual processing, executive functioning, attention, and memory. In each of these domains, adults with ASD might encounter some challenges, even though there are large individual differences (see later).

3.4 Cognition and ASD in Late Adulthood

Given that cognitive deterioration is common in typically aging individuals, it seems plausible that this is also the case in older adults with ASD. However, this group has hardly been studied (Mukaetova-Ladinska et al. 2012). In the section focusing on young and middle adulthood, the highest mean age was 64, but this was often caused by just one or two studies that were included in these meta-analyses. The paucity of studies on adults with ASD in late adulthood does not allow us to draw firm conclusions regarding cognition as this would be rather premature. Therefore, in this section we will solely discuss the few studies that have been conducted on cognitive functioning. The central question we will address here is whether there is evidence for accelerated cognitive aging in older adults with ASD (see also Chap. 6).

A recent epidemiological study (Croen et al. 2015) of 1507 adults with ASD and 15,070 adults without ASD (age range 18–65+) reported a more than four times higher rate of dementia in adults with ASD as compared to the control group. This might suggest that cognitive aging is indeed accelerated, especially as only 9.5 % of the participants were older than 50 years and only 0.4 % older than 65 years. From the dementia literature, we know that the prevalence of dementia is especially high in those older than 65 years of age. Next to dementia, Croen and colleagues also reported whole series of other medical and psychiatric comorbidities that were more prevalent in adults with ASD. Various of these comorbid conditions (i.e., depression, hypertension, diabetes) are considered risk factors for cognitive decline in the general population. Moreover, socio-environmental factors such as high levels of stress, high number of negative life events, low perceived social support, inadequacy of social activity as well as actual low social participation status, and less physical activity are all known risk factors for age-related cognitive decline. Each of these risk factors is thought to be prominent in adults with ASD, which might point toward a risk of accelerated cognitive aging in older adults with ASD. However, the problem with the current literature is that in most studies, the majority of participants had an intellectual disability next to the ASD diagnosis. Therefore, it is hard to determine which findings can be extrapolated to older adults with ASD normal to high IQs.

So far, only three studies actually tested cognitive functioning in older adults with ASD without intellectual disability. In a first small study (*N* ASD = 23; *N* w/o ASD = 23) including individuals aged 51–83 years of age, cognitive problems were observed with respect to sustained attention, working memory, and generativity (Geurts and Vissers 2012). However, older adults with ASD performed equally well as their age-, gender-, and IQ-matched controls on planning and visual and verbal episodic declarative memory tasks. Exploratory analyses also revealed that aging had a smaller impact on generativity in the ASD group but a larger impact on visual memory. In a much larger recent study (*N* ASD = 118; *N* w/o ASD = 118; age range 19–80 years), not all findings were replicated (Lever and Geurts 2016a). Similar to the previous study, group differences were observed in generativity but not in visual and verbal episodic declarative memory tasks. However, the findings of age-related differences were slightly different. Age played a similar role in those with and without ASD with respect to generativity, verbal memory, and ToM but seemed to have a smaller impact on visual memory. Hence, the large impact of age on visual memory performance in the first study was not replicated. In a study solely directed at working memory (*N* ASD = 118; *N* w/o ASD = 167; age range 19–80 years), it was shown that while those with ASD were slower, they did perform equally well on a working memory task (Lever et al. 2015). The impact of age was smaller in the adults with ASD as compared to the adults without ASD. So, as for visual memory, the age-related changes in working memory are smaller in adults with ASD than in typical aging adults. These contradictory findings become even more complex when we focus on the self-report cognitive concerns of the older adults with ASD. While the problems were rather small on the cognitive tests, in day-to-day life, adults with ASD do experience various cognitive challenges (Lever and Geurts 2016a), but these challenges, like in the comparison group, did not augment with increasing age. In sum, in these three cross-sectional cognitive adult studies, no strong indications emerged that there will be accelerated cognitive decline in older adults with ASD. However, to confirm this we desperately need longitudinal studies including even older adults.

3.5 Cognition and Gender Differences

In most cognitive studies, the majority of the participants are males, as ASD is more often diagnosed in males than in females (see Chap. 7). Similar to cognitive aging in ASD, it was only recently that a few studies were published focusing on gender differences in cognitive profiles of people with ASD (Bolte et al. 2011; Carter et al. 2007; Goddard et al. 2014; Lai et al. 2012; Lemon et al. 2011; Memari et al. 2013; Nydén et al. 2010; Schneider et al. 2013), although the findings are rather inconsistent and most studies focus on children (Bolte et al. 2011; Carter et al. 2007; Goddard et al. 2014; Lemon et al. 2011; Nydén et al. 2010). Moreover, in various studies, males and females with ASD are compared with one another, while no attention is paid to whether an observed gender difference is specific for ASD, or whether it is similar to what will be observed when comparing non-ASD males and females with one another. However, a methodological sound study in adults has been performed by Lai et al. (2012). In this study (*N* ASD males/females = 45/38; *N* w/o ASD males/females = 33/35; age range 18–49 years), there were no gender differences with respect to ToM, emotion recognition, and inhibitory control performance, although adults with ASD did perform worse than adults without ASD. There were gender differences with respect to working memory and generativity (females outperformed males), but this was not specific for adults with ASD. With respect to central coherence, there was a marginal differential effect of group by gender which seems to suggest that while males with ASD do have problems on the embedded figures test as compared to males without ASD, females with ASD perform equally well as their female counterparts without ASD. In studies focusing on cognitive aging (Lever and Geurts 2016a; Lever et al. 2015), gender was not taken into account, or no gender-by-group interactions were observed, suggesting that with respect to cognition, there is currently no evidence for different cognitive profiles of males and females with ASD in adulthood. However, while, for example, males and females with ASD did perform similarly in emotion recognition tasks, brain activation differed between the genders (Schneider et al. 2013). Hence, we cannot exclude the possibility that while there are no differences with respect to cognitive performance, the underlying processes necessary to reach the observed performance might actually differ between males and females with ASD.

3.6 Cognition and Individual Differences

All of the aforementioned studies were group studies in which adults with ASD were directly compared with a group of adults without ASD. However, a group difference does not imply that every single individual within this specific group actually has a strength or weakness in the tested cognitive domain. Heterogeneity in symptomatology (Volkmar et al. 2004), comorbidity (Hofvander et al. 2009; Joshi et al. 2013; Lever and Geurts 2016b), genetics (Betancur 2011; Geschwind 2011; Ronald et al. 2006), brain morphology (Lenroot and Yeung 2013), and developmental trajectories (e.g., Magiati et al. 2014) is often described for people with ASD.

Adults with ASD often report that they do encounter cognitive failures in daily life (Lever and Geurts 2016a; van Heijst and Geurts 2014), but the heterogeneity does also exist in the discussed cognitive domains. For example, three studies that each mainly focused on adults with DSM-IV Asperger syndrome (Gonzalez-Gadea et al. 2013; Hill and Bird 2006; Towgood et al. 2009) all report large individual differences. For instance, it was demonstrated that some, but not all, individuals with ASD showed EF impairments ($N = 22$; 16–61 years) on planning, mental flexibility, and generativity (Hill and Bird 2006). On classic EF tests, there were no differences in performance at a group level between adults with ASD and without ASD after controlling for psychomotor speed, even though at an individual level 18 % did show dysfunctions. On certain newer EF tests, especially those involving response initiation and intentionality, 62 % of ASD adults performed within the clinical range with reference to the control group distribution, along observed group differences. In a study ($N = 21$; aged 19–47 years) across a broader range of cognitive domains, including executive functioning, perception, language, and memory, large heterogeneity was observed as well (Towgood et al. 2009). While some (9–28 %) individuals outperformed controls on certain measures, others (5–28 %) underperformed on the same measures. Considerable variation was not only observed between individuals but also within individuals with subnormal and supranormal performance on different measures within an individual. Similarly, this heterogeneous cognitive profile was also found when, next to executive functions (working memory, cognitive flexibility, multitasking), social cognition was measured (*N* = 23, mean age 35 years) (Gonzalez-Gadea et al. 2013). While these interindividual differences were also observed in a large study among adults with all ASDs (*N* = 118, aged 19–80 years), only a few individuals showed impairments on memory, generativity, and ToM measures compared to a group of adults without ASD (Lever and Geurts 2016a). Interestingly, again, the number of adults without ASD and the number of adults performing atypically did not differ. In sum, these studies using multiple case series analysis revealed significant individual differences in cognitive profiles among adults with ASD on all cognitive domains.

Although both subnormal and supranormal performances have been reported, there is preliminary evidence that clinically relevant atypicalities are less pronounced in older than in younger adults with ASD. However, as aforementioned in the current studies to date, old-old adults have hardly been included in cognitive studies, so future research is warranted to determine whether this conclusion will hold.

3.7 Clinical Implications

Most importantly, the given overview of the cognitive literature suggests that, although cognition is of importance when studying ASD, neuropsychological measures are not sufficient to distinguish adults with ASD from adults without ASD. Hence, it has no classification value. Cognitive problems are not universal across all adults with ASD, and not all cognitive domains are similarly impaired. Nevertheless, the large individual differences across individuals indicate that it is of importance to determine individual cognitive profiles. Identifying cognitive strengths and weaknesses can be relevant for treatment purposes as people themselves will know what they can and cannot do, and therapists can take this into account when setting up the intervention plan. While with respect to symptomatology and comorbidity (e.g., see Chap. 7 and Lever and Geurts 2016b) it is of importance to be alert to gender differences, this does not seem to be the case with respect to cognition. However, it is of importance to not just assess someone's cognitive profile only once over the subject's lifetime, as a cognitive profile is not static. Changes in cognitive profiles with increasing age need to be monitored to determine whether or not cognitive age-related deterioration is at hand and to make sure that learned coping strategies are still adequate.

References

Altgassen M, Koban N, Kliegel M (2012) Do adults with autism spectrum disorders compensate in naturalistic prospective memory tasks? J Autism Dev Disord 42(10):2141–2151

Ambery FZ, Russell AJ, Perry K, Morris R, Murphy DGM (2006) Neuropsychological functioning in adults with asperger syndrome. Autism: Int J Res Pract 10(6):551–564

Barendse EM, Hendriks MP, Jansen JF, Backes WH, Hofman PA, Thoonen G et al (2013) Working memory deficits in high-functioning adolescents with autism spectrum disorders:

neuropsychological and neuroimaging correlates. J Neurodev Disord 5(1):14. doi:10.1186/1866-1955-5-14 [doi]

Baron-Cohen S, Leslie AM, Frith U (1985) Does the autistic child have a "theory of mind"? Cognition 21(1):37–46

Baron-Cohen S, O'Riordan M, Stone V, Jones R, Plaisted K (1999) Recognition of faux pas by normally developing children and children with asperger syndrome or high-functioning autism. J Autism Dev Disord 29(5):407–418

Betancur C (2011) Etiological heterogeneity in autism spectrum disorders: more than 100 genetic and genomic disorders and still counting. Brain Res 1380:42–77

Bolte S, Duketis E, Poustka F, Holtmann M (2011) Sex differences in cognitive domains and their clinical correlates in higher-functioning autism spectrum disorders. Autism : Int J Res Pract 15(4):497–511. doi:10.1177/1362361310391116 [doi]

Boucher J, Mayes A, Bigham S (2012) Memory in autistic spectrum disorder. Psychol Bull 138(3):458–496

Brunsdon VE, Happé FGE (2014) Exploring the 'fractionation' of autism at the cognitive level. Autism 18(1):17–30

Carmo JC, Duarte E, Pinho S, Marques JF, Filipe CN (2015) Verbal fluency as a function of time in autism spectrum disorder: an impairment of initiation processes? J Clin Exp Neuropsychol 37(7):710–721

Carter CS (2005) Applying new approaches from cognitive neuroscience to enhance drug development for the treatment of impaired cognition in schizophrenia. Schizophr Bull 31(4):810–815

Carter AS, Black DO, Tewani S, Connolly CE, Kadlec MB, Tager-Flusberg H (2007) Sex differences in toddlers with autism spectrum disorders. J Autism Dev Disord 37(1):86–97

Cascio CJ, Moana-Filho EJ, Guest S, Nebel MB, Weisner J, Baranek GT, Essick GK (2012) Perceptual and neural response to affective tactile texture stimulation in adults with autism spectrum disorders. Autism Res 5(4):231–244

Chevallier C, Kohls G, Troiani V, Brodkin ES, Schultz RT (2012) The social motivation theory of autism. Trends Cogn Sci 16(4):231–239

Chien Y, Gau S, Shang C, Chiu Y, Tsai W, Wu Y (2015) Visual memory and sustained attention impairment in youths with autism spectrum disorders. Psychol Med 45(11):2263–2273

Chung YS, Barch D, Strube M (2014) A meta-analysis of mentalizing impairments in adults with schizophrenia and autism spectrum disorder. Schizophr Bull 40(3):602–616

Croen LA, Zerbo O, Qian Y, Massolo ML, Rich S, Sidney S, Kripke C (2015) The health status of adults on the autism spectrum. Autism : Int J Res Pract 19(7):814–823

Damasio AR, Maurer RG (1978) A neurological model for childhood autism. Arch Neurol 35(12):777–786

Dichter GS, Felder JN, Green SR, Rittenberg AM, Sasson NJ, Bodfish JW (2012) Reward circuitry function in autism spectrum disorders. Soc Cogn Affect Neurosci 7(2):160–172. doi:10.1093/scan/nsq095 [doi]

Frith U (1989) Autism: explaining the enigma. Blackwell, Oxford

Frith U, Happé FGE (1994) Autism: beyond "theory of mind". Cognition 50(1):115–132

Geschwind DH (2011) Genetics of autism spectrum disorders. Trends Cogn Sci 15(9):409–416

Geurts HM, Vissers ME (2012) Elderly with autism: executive functions and memory. J Autism Dev Disord 42(5):665–675

Geurts HM, Broeders M, Nieuwland MS (2010) Thinking outside the executive functions box: theory of mind and pragmatic abilities in attention deficit/hyperactivity disorder. Eur J Dev Pssychol 7(1):135–151

Geurts HM, van den Bergh SFWM, Ruzzano L (2014) Prepotent response inhibition and interference control in autism spectrum disorders: two meta-analyses. Autism Res 7(4):407–420

Goddard L, Dritschel B, Howlin P (2014) A preliminary study of gender differences in autobiographical memory in children with an autism spectrum disorder. J Autism Dev Disord 44(9):2087–2095

Gonzalez-Gadea ML, Baez S, Torralva T, Castellanos FX, Rattazzi A, Bein V et al (2013) Cognitive variability in adults with ADHD and AS: disentangling the roles of executive functions and social cognition. Res Dev Disabil 34(2):817–830

Gonzalez-Gadea ML, Chennu S, Bekinschtein TA, Rattazzi A, Beraudi A, Tripicchio P et al (2015) Predictive coding in autism spectrum disorder and attention deficit hyperactivity disorder. J Neurophysiol 114(5):2625–2636. doi:10.1152/jn.00543.2015 [doi]

Happé FGE (1999) Autism: Cognitive deficit or cognitive style? Trends Cogn Sci 3(6):216–222

Happé FGE, Charlton RA (2012) Aging in autism spectrum disorders: a mini-review. Gerontology 58(1):70–78

Happé FGE, Frith U (2006) The weak coherence account: detail-focused cognitive style in autism spectrum disorders. J Autism Dev Disord 36(1):5–25

Hill EL (2004) Executive dysfunction in autism. Trends Cogn Sci 8(1):26–32

Hill EL, Bird CM (2006) Executive processes in asperger syndrome: patterns of performance in a multiple case series. Neuropsychologia 44(14):2822–2835

Hofvander B, Delorme R, Chaste P, Nydén A, Wentz E, Ståhlberg O et al (2009) Psychiatric and psychosocial problems in adults with normal-intelligence autism spectrum disorders. BMC Psychiatry 9(1):35–44

Joshi G, Wozniak J, Petty C, Martelon MK, Fried R, Bolfek A et al (2013) Psychiatric comorbidity and functioning in a clinically referred population of adults with autism spectrum disorders: a comparative study. J Autism Dev Disord 43(6):1314–1325

Karalunas SL, Geurts HM, Konrad K, Bender S, Nigg JT (2014) Annual research review: reaction time variability in ADHD and autism spectrum disorders: measurement and mechanisms of a proposed trans-diagnostic phenotype. J Child Psychol Psychiatry 55(6):685–710

Kenworthy L, Yerys BE, Anthony LG, Wallace GL (2008) Understanding executive control in autism spectrum disorders in the lab and in the real world. Neuropsychol Rev 18(4):320–338

Lai M, Lombardo MV, Pasco G, Ruigrok A, Wheelwright SJ, Sadek SA et al (2011) A behavioral comparison of male and female adults with high functioning autism spectrum conditions. PLoS One 6(6):e20835

Lai M, Lombardo MV, Ruigrok AN, Chakrabarti B, Wheelwright SJ, Auyeung B et al (2012) Cognition in males and females with autism: similarities and differences. PLoS One 7(10):e47198

Landry O, Parker A (2013) A meta-analysis of visual orienting in autism. Front Hum Neurosci 7:62–73

Lawson J (2003) Depth accessibility difficulties: an alternative conceptualisation of autism spectrum conditions. J Theory Soc Behav 33(2):189–202

Lawson RP, Rees G, Friston KJ (2014) An aberrant precision account of autism. Front Hum Neurosci 8:302. doi:10.3389/fnhum.2014.00302

Lemon JM, Gargaro B, Enticott PG, Rinehart NJ (2011) Brief report: executive functioning in autism spectrum disorders: a gender comparison of response inhibition. J Autism Dev Disord 41(3):352–356

Lenroot RK, Yeung PK (2013) Heterogeneity within autism spectrum disorders: what have we learned from neuroimaging studies? Front Hum Neurosci 7:733. doi:10.3389/fnhum.2013.00733

Leung RC, Zakzanis KK (2014) Brief report: cognitive flexibility in autism spectrum disorders: a quantitative review. J Autism Dev Disord 44(10):2628–2645

Lever AG, Geurts HM (2016a) Age-related differences in cognition across the adult lifespan in autism spectrum disorder. Autism Res 9(6):666–76. doi:10.1002/aur.1545 [pii]

Lever AG, Geurts HM (2016b) Psychiatric co-occurring symptoms and disorders in young, middle-aged, and older adults with autism spectrum disorder. J Autism Dev Disord 46:1916–1930

Lever AG, Werkle-Bergner M, Brandmaier AM, Ridderinkhof KR, Geurts HM (2015) Atypical working memory decline across the adult lifespan in autism spectrum disorder? J Abnorm Psychol 124(4):1014–1026

Magiati I, Tay XW, Howlin P (2014) Cognitive, language, social and behavioural outcomes in adults with autism spectrum disorders: a systematic review of longitudinal follow-up studies in adulthood. Clin Psychol Rev 34(1):73–86

Maurer RG, Damasio AR (1982) Childhood autism from the point of view of behavioral neurology. J Autism Dev Disord 12(2):195–205

Memari AH, Ziaee V, Shayestehfar M, Ghanouni P, Mansournia MA, Moshayedi P (2013) Cognitive flexibility impairments in children with autism spectrum disorders: Links to age, gender and child outcomes. Res Dev Disabil 34(10):3218–3225

Morgan B, Maybery M, Durkin K (2003) Weak central coherence, poor joint attention, and low verbal ability: independent deficits in early autism. Dev Psychol 39(4):646–656
Mottron L, Burack JA (2001) Enhanced perceptual functioning in the development of autism. In: Burack JA, Charman T, Yirmiya N, Zelazo PR (eds) The development of autism: perspectives from theory and research. Lawrence Erlbaum Associates Publishers, Mahwah, pp 131–148
Mottron L, Dawson M, Soulieres I, Hubert B, Burack J (2006) Enhanced perceptual functioning in autism: an update, and eight principles of autistic perception. J Autism Dev Disord 36(1):27–43
Mukaetova-Ladinska EB, Perry E, Baron M, Povey C (2012) Ageing in people with autistic spectrum disorder. Int J Geriatr Psychiatry 27(2):109–118
Mundy P, Neal AR (2000) Neural plasticity, joint attention, and a transactional social-orienting model of autism. Int Rev Res Ment Retard 23:139–168
Murphy CM, Christakou A, Daly EM, Ecker C, Giampietro V, Brammer M et al (2014) Abnormal functional activation and maturation of fronto-striato-temporal and cerebellar regions during sustained attention in autism spectrum disorder. Am J Psychiatry 171(10):1107–1116
Navon D (1977) Forest before trees: the precedence of global features in visual perception. Cogn Psychol 9(3):353–383
Nydén A, Niklasson L, Stahlberg O, Anckarsater H, Wentz E, Rastam M, Gillberg C (2010) Adults with autism spectrum disorders and ADHD neuropsychological aspects. Res Dev Disabil 31(6):1659–1668
Olde Dubbelink, L. M. E, Geurts, H. M. (2017). Planning skills in ASD across the lifespan: a meta-analysis and meta-regression. Jourrnal of Autism and Developmental Disorders
Palmer CJ, Seth AK, Hohwy J (2015) The felt presence of other minds: predictive processing, counterfactual predictions, and mentalising in autism. Conscious Cogn 36:376–389
Pellicano E (2010) Individual differences in executive function and central coherence predict developmental changes in theory of mind in autism. Dev Psychol 46(2):530–544
Pellicano E, Burr D (2012) When the world becomes 'too real': a bayesian explanation of autistic perception. Trends Cogn Sci 16(10):504–510
Pennington BF, Ozonoff S (1996) Executive functions and developmental psychopathology. J Child Psychol Psychiatry 37(1):51–87
Poljac E, Bekkering H (2012) A review of intentional and cognitive control in autism. Front Psych 3:436. doi:10.3389/fpsyg.2012.00436
Ronald A, Happe F, Bolton P, Butcher LM, Price TS, Wheelwright S et al (2006) Genetic heterogeneity between the three components of the autism spectrum: a twin study. J Am Acad Child Adolesc Psychiatry 45(6):691–699
Sachse M, Schlitt S, Hainz D, Ciaramidaro A, Schirman S, Walter H et al (2013) Executive and visuo-motor function in adolescents and adults with autism spectrum disorder. J Autism Dev Disord 43(5):1222–1235
Sanders J, Johnson KA, Garavan H, Gill M, Gallagher L (2008) A review of neuropsychological and neuroimaging research in autistic spectrum disorders: attention, inhibition and cognitive flexibility. Res Autism Spectr Disord 2(1):1–16
Schneider K, Regenbogen C, Pauly KD, Gossen A, Schneider DA, Mevissen L et al (2013) Evidence for gender-specific endophenotypes in high-functioning autism spectrum disorder during empathy. Autism Res 6(6):506–521
Schuwerk T, Vuori M, Sodian B (2015) Implicit and explicit theory of mind reasoning in autism spectrum disorders: The impact of experience. Autism : Int J Res Pract 19(4):459–468. doi:10.1177/1362361314526004 [doi]
Senju A, Southgate V, White S, Frith U (2009) Mindblind eyes: an absence of spontaneous theory of mind in asperger syndrome. Science (New York, NY) 325(5942):883–885. doi:10.1126/science.1176170 [doi]
Sergeant JA, Geurts H, Oosterlaan J (2002) How specific is a deficit of executive functioning for attention-deficit/hyperactivity disorder? Behav Brain Res 130(1):3–28
Spek AA, Schatorjé T, Scholte E, van Berckelaer-Onnes I (2009) Verbal fluency in adults with high functioning autism or asperger syndrome. Neuropsychologia 47(3):652–656
Spek AA, Scholte EM, Van Berckelaer-Onnes IA (2010) Theory of mind in adults with HFA and asperger syndrome. J Autism Dev Disord 40(3):280–289

Stone VE, Baron-Cohen S, Knight RT (1998) Frontal lobe contributions to theory of mind. J Cogn Neurosci 10(5):640–656

Towgood KJ, Meuwese JDI, Gilbert SJ, Turner MS, Burgess PW (2009) Advantages of the multiple case series approach to the study of cognitive deficits in autism spectrum disorder. Neuropsychologia 47(13):2981–2988

Travers BG, Bigler ED, Tromp DPM, Adluru N, Froehlich AL, Ennis C et al (2014) Longitudinal processing speed impairments in males with autism and the effects of white matter microstructure. Neuropsychologia 53:137–145

Uljarevic M, Hamilton A (2013) Recognition of emotions in autism: a formal meta-analysis. J Autism Dev Disord 43(7):1517–1526

Van Boxtel JJ, Lu H (2013) A predictive coding perspective on autism spectrum disorders. Front Psych 4:19. doi:10.3389/fpsyg.2013.00019

Van de Cruys S, Evers K, Van der Hallen R, Van Eylen L, Boets B, de-Wit L, Wagemans J (2014) Precise minds in uncertain worlds: predictive coding in autism. Psychol Rev 121(4):649–675

Van der Hallen R, Evers K, Brewaeys K, Van den Noortgate W, Wagemans J (2015) Global processing takes time: a meta-analysis on local–global visual processing in ASD. Psychol Bull 141(3):549–573

Van Eylen L, Boets B, Steyaert J, Evers K, Wagemans J, Noens I (2011) Cognitive flexibility in autism spectrum disorder: explaining the inconsistencies? Res Autism Spectr Disord 5(4):1390–1401

van Heijst BFC, Geurts HM (2014) Quality of life in autism across the lifespan: a meta-analysis. Autism 19(2):158–167

Volkmar FR, Lord C, Bailey A, Schultz RT, Klin A (2004) Autism and pervasive developmental disorders. J Child Psychol Psychiatry 45(1):135–170

White SJ, Burgess PW, Hill EL (2009) Impairments on "open-ended" executive function tests in autism. Autism Res 2(3):138–147

Wilson CE, Happé FGE, Wheelwright SJ, Ecker C, Lombardo MV, Johnston P et al (2014) The neuropsychology of male adults with high-functioning autism or asperger syndrome. Autism Res 7(5):568–581

Zalla T, Sav A, Stopin A, Ahade S, Leboyer M (2009) Faux pas detection and intentional action in asperger syndrome. A replication on a french sample. J Autism Dev Disord 39(2):373–382

Outcomes for Adults with Autism Spectrum Disorder and Intellectual Disability

4

Lisa Underwood, Jane McCarthy, and Eddie Chaplin

4.1 Introduction

Research on adults with ASD began in the late 1960s when those children who were among the first to be diagnosed with autism reached adulthood. Studies were mainly descriptive but found indications that adult outcome, in terms of social functioning, for most of those with ASD was poor and appeared to be related to IQ and verbal skills (Lockyer and Rutter 1969; Lotter 1974; Rutter et al. 1967). Kanner (1971) explored the 'destinies' of the original sample that he used to define the clinical criteria for autism and surmised that those who were not admitted to hospital and lived in a supportive environment had a better outcome. Lotter (1974) commented that '...it remains easier to predict a poor outcome than a good outcome' (pp. 273).

Research that followed largely confirmed these earlier findings (Kanne et al. 2011) and, in general, continued to use vague outcome criteria rather than standardised measures (Henninger and Taylor 2013). Howlin's (2000) review of adult life for those with high-functioning ASD identified just six studies. Results were 'extremely variable'; however, most studies reported low rates of employment (maximum 44 %) and

L. Underwood (✉)
Centre for Longitudinal Research, Faculty of Medical and Health Sciences, University of Auckland, Auckland, New Zealand

Forensic and Neurodevelopmental Science, Institute of Psychiatry, Psychology and Neuroscience at King's College London, London, UK
e-mail: l.underwood@auckland.ac.nz

J. McCarthy
Forensic and Neurodevelopmental Science, Institute of Psychiatry, Psychology and Neuroscience at King's College London, London, UK

E. Chaplin
Mental Health and Learning Disabilities, School of Health and Social Care, London South Bank University, London, UK

B. Barahona Corrêa, R.-J. van der Gaag (eds.), *Autism Spectrum Disorders in Adults*, DOI 10.1007/978-3-319-42713-3_4

independent living (maximum 50 %). Those with a 'good outcome' were in the minority (maximum 44 %). The review also found there was a suggestion of increased mortality among people with ASD (further increased for those with low IQ) (Howlin 2000). The subsequent literature on life for adults with ASD and intellectual disabilities has continued to rely on these earlier studies to provide evidence that this group has the poorest outcomes (Van Dooren et al. 2016). However, (on the surface at least) much has changed in recent years with the introduction of ASD-specific legislation in some countries including the United Kingdom and the United States (Autism Act 2009; Congress 2006) plus a roll-out of strategy documents and guidelines (Department of Health 2010; National Audit Office 2009; NICE 2012). These developments were designed to improve the lives of all those on the autism spectrum including those with intellectual disability (Mccarthy et al. 2015).

This chapter re-evaluates the evidence on life outcomes for adults with ASD and intellectual disability with a focus on studies published since 2000. Literature searches carried out for this review revealed that adult outcomes for those with the full spectrum of ASD have still not been systematically studied (Levy and Perry 2011; Van Dooren et al. 2016). This is problematic because it is not clear whether poor outcomes for those with 'low-functioning' ASD are related to the impact of ASD itself, intellectual disability (also known to be associated with poor outcomes in adult life) or a combined effect of having both conditions. An ideal study would compare, over time from childhood to adulthood, outcomes for comparative groups (with respect to gender, age and socio-economic status) of individuals with (1) ASD without intellectual disability, (2) ASD and intellectual disability, (3) intellectual disability without ASD and (4) neither ASD nor intellectual disability. To date, as Section 4.4 shows, research involving comparison groups has been rare and thus limits our ability to understand the epidemiology of observed poor outcomes in adults with ASD and intellectual disability. In the next section, we discuss some of the reasons that research evidence on adults with ASD and intellectual disability is so limited.

4.2 Researching Adult Outcome in ASD and Intellectual Disability

Research on adults with ASD and intellectual disability is in its infancy (relatively speaking; compared with research on children with ASD or on adults with other neuropsychiatric conditions). This is in part because of the challenges of carrying out research with this complex group. A lack of earlier research makes designing studies difficult; there is little evidence on which to base decisions about eligibility criteria, sample size, measures and analyses.

There are a number of practical challenges that face researchers when including participants with complex needs. People with ASD and/or intellectual disability are a heterogeneous group and vary greatly in terms of their characteristics and also their ability to understand research, engage with others, make decisions and express their views. This section explores some of the considerations that should be taken into account when conducting research on adults with ASD and intellectual disability. Sources of data and recruitment issues are briefly discussed.

4.2.1 Sources of Data

We know that using a range of the best available sources and collecting data in a systematic way can increase confidence in the findings of research and reduce measurement bias (Prince 2003). Information about participants can be assembled from existing records (e.g. medical notes), the persons themselves or someone who knows them personally or in a professional capacity. The more structured and standardised the method of data collection, the easier it is to compare individuals or groups of participants. Where available, it is preferable to use existing measures that have been methodically developed and tested (Prince 2003).

Assessment tools for adults with ASD and intellectual disability may be participant-, informant- or observation-based. Participants can be asked to self-rate items on a questionnaire or they can be interviewed face-to-face by a researcher. However, this can be difficult for people with ASD and/or intellectual disability who may not be able to describe their feelings and experiences or may be unaware of the impact their behaviour has on others (Underwood et al. 2011). They may also have difficulty understanding the questions being asked of them. Many people with ASD and/or intellectual disability have limited verbal skills, and some are unable to speak at all. In these situations it may be appropriate to ask someone who knows the person well to act as their 'informant' and answer questions on their behalf. Though largely accepted, this method of data collection is not without its biases (Stewart 2003). An informant will often be asked to make judgements about an individual's thoughts, feelings and behaviour. In some situations, informants may have reason to under- or overplay a person's difficulties, perhaps if they feel they are being judged as a carer or if they hope to improve their access to services. Informants may be so accustomed to an individual's problems that they no longer consider them challenging or unusual. Additionally, researchers might use standardised tools to record and code their observations of a person's behaviour during structured or unstructured activities with others or with the researcher. In all of these cases, the data collected might be qualitative or quantitative.

4.2.2 Recruitment Issues

Adults with ASD and/or intellectual disability are often socially excluded and may also have limited access to health, social or educational services. This can make it difficult to identify potential participants and also causes problems when approaching people to take part in research. Individuals may rely on other people to open and read their mail, be unable to access a telephone and have limited direct contact with service providers/practitioners. Their approachability is often dependent on the willingness of others to facilitate their involvement (such as family or paid support workers). This can introduce an element of sampling bias if individuals who agree to take part differ from those who refuse or are not approached to take part; e.g. they are more independent or have fewer problems.

A further barrier for research is the relatively small proportion of the general population who have both ASD and intellectual disability (estimated to be around

0.05 %), impeding the ability of single-site studies to recruit sufficient sample sizes. Having a small number of potential participants is likely to make random sampling unfeasible or even unnecessary since it may be more practical to approach and attempt to recruit as many people as possible from a sample population. Researchers and clinicians have strived to rise above these challenges to ensure that research about adults with ASD and/or intellectual disability takes place and is methodologically sound. A key remaining issue is how best to determine whether a person with ASD and intellectual disability has a 'good outcome' and how best to measure this objectively and, if possible, quantitatively.

4.3 Measuring Outcome in Adults with ASD and Intellectual Disability

Common measures of outcome for people with intellectual disability are life expectancy, physical and mental health, adaptive functioning, service contact, independent living, employment and relationships (Henninger and Taylor 2013; O'Brien 2001). Research on adults with ASD has also used a wide range of methods to define and measure 'outcome' (Henninger and Taylor 2013). In Howlin's (2000) review of adult outcome for people with ASD, seven types of measure were identified: '(1) IQ, academic skills and adaptive behaviours; (2) language ability; (3) behavioural problems; (4) education and employment history; (5) independence and social relationships; (6) psychiatric history; and (7) stability of IQ over time and variables related to outcome' (pp. 67).

It is now clear that adults with ASD are more likely to have intellectual disability/cognitive deficits and language difficulties and experience physical, behavioural and mental health problems than those without ASD (Findon et al. 2016; Taylor 2016; Underwood et al. 2010). However, evidence on social outcomes such as education, employment, independence and relationships remains relatively lacking. Some of the measures used in research on adult life for people with ASD are summarised in Table 4.1. The most common themes have been employment, education and independence. It is often standard practice for studies to use a composite scale based on information from a range of instruments rather than any direct data collection or use of an existing measure of social functioning. Many measures have been based on criteria developed by Howlin et al. (2004) or Lotter (1974).

There are some limitations to these measures particularly for adults with ASD and intellectual disability. For example, Lotter's definition of poor outcome included 'obvious severe handicap'; therefore, those with intellectual disability were more likely to fall into these categories. Most adults with intellectual disability would score poor or very poor on these criteria because of their low IQ or adaptive functioning (Levy and Perry 2011). This is problematic because it takes a somewhat narrow view of what constitutes a positive outcome. It does not take into account the individual's views nor does it contrast their current situation with the highest level of outcome that they could be expected to achieve given their level of functioning (Henninger and Taylor 2013).

Table 4.1 Measures of adult outcome in ASD and intellectual disability

(**Howlin et al.** 2000; **Mawhood et al.** 2000) Four composite measures: language, friendship, independence and autistic-type stereotyped behaviours Each rated 0 (normal/near-normal), 1 (moderate/fair) or 2 (poor/very poor) Composite score (sum of above) comprising 3 levels: 0–1 = near-normal functioning 2–4 = moderate difficulties 5–8 = considerable levels of difficulty
Language: Good (uses sentences with mature grammar, understands 2-/3-step instructions, talks with others so that conversation flows, is able to build on other person's dialogue) = 0 Fair (scores positively on 2 of the above) = 1 Poor (scores on only 1) = 2 Very poor (scores on none) = 2
Friendships: Good (normal relationship) = 0 Fair (some limited friendships) = 1 Poor (no friends; has acquaintances who are met in a group situation, such as work or a club) = 2 Very poor (no friendships involving selectivity and sharing) = 2
Independence: Full (able to cope with all self-care activities, travel independently and manage own finances without help) = 0 Moderate (requires some help in these areas) = 1 Little (significant help required) = 2
Autistic behaviours: ADI scores for unusual preoccupations; rituals/compulsions, resistance to change and unusual attachments to objects Total score of 0/1 (none/minimal problems) = 0 Total score of 2–5 (moderate problems) = 1 Total score of 6 (severe problems) = 2
Also measured was education (university = 0, mainstream college = 1, special college = 2, no further education = 3) and occupation (regular paid work = 0, voluntary/special job arrangements = 1, day or residential centre = 2, no daytime placement = 3)
(**Howlin et al.** 2004; **Eaves and Ho** 2007; **Farley et al.** 2009) Three composite measures: occupation, friendships and independent living. Each rated 0, 1 or 2
Composite score (sum of above) comprising five levels: 0–2 = Very Good (achieving a high level of independence) 3–4 = Good (generally in work but requiring some degree of support in daily living) 5–7 = Fair (some degree of independence, although requires support, and supervision does not need specialist residential provision) 8–10 = Poor (requiring special residential provision/high level of support) 11 = Very Poor (needing high-level hospital care)
Occupation: employed or self-employed = 0, voluntary work/job training or low-pay scheme = 1, supported/sheltered employment = 2, in special centre/no occupation = 3 Friendships: range of scores from >1 close friendships involving sharing and exchange of confidences and range of different activities together = 0 to no friends, no joint activities = 3
Living independently = 0, in semi-sheltered accommodation (or still at home) but with high degree of autonomy = 1, living with parents, some limited autonomy = 2, in residential accommodation with some limited autonomy = 3, specialist autistic or other residential accommodation with little or no autonomy = 4, in hospital care or at home because nowhere else would accept the individual = 5
Support required: see Engstrom et al. (2003)

(continued)

Table 4.1 (continued)

(Marriage et al. 2009) Five composite measures: education, vocation, independence, friendships and intimate relationships. Each rated 1 (poor functioning) to 5 (age-appropriate attainment) Composite score (sum of above)
Education: did not graduate from high school = 1; graduated from an adapted programme in high school = 2; graduated from regular high school = 3; attended college/university (if < 25 years, in college = 5; if > 25 years, attending college = 4); graduated from college/university = 5
Employment: Disability pension, never employed, not in educational programme = 1; employed briefly, unemployed now = 2; series of jobs, briefly in or out of work now, or in school part-time, no job = 3; stable employment or in school full-time, if >25 years = 4; employed at potential or, if <25 and in school full-time = 5
Living arrangements/independence: lives with parents, needs support in activities of daily living and routine = 1; lives with parents, needs some support to manage in community = 2; lives with parents, self-sufficient managing life otherwise, if >25 years = 3; lives independently, needs some support to manage finances, etc. = 4; living independently, manages affairs alone, or, < 25, lives with parents, manages affairs alone = 5
Social relationships (outside the family): isolated, lives in own world, no friends = 1; somewhat isolated, has some acquaintances, not necessarily any shared interests = 2; some acquaintances around shared interests = 3; has one or more friendships only short term = 4; has one or more close and enduring friendships = 5
Intimate relationships: No partner ever, no interest = 1; some attempt at finding partner, brief relationships, unsatisfactory to subject = 2; relationships of a few months or more = 3; one or more long-term (>6/12) relationships or divorced = 4; married/living common-law, satisfactory to both partners = 5
(Billstedt et al. 2005**; Engstrom et al.** 2003**; Lotter** 1974) Composite score comprising five levels: Good outcome: (a) employed or in education or training plus (b) living independently (for those aged 23 and over) or >2 friends or steady relationship (for those aged under 23)
Fair outcome: (a) or (b)
Restricted outcome: neither (a) nor (b) + no mental health problem
Poor outcome: obvious severe handicap, no independent social progress, some clear verbal or non-verbal communicative skills
Very poor outcome: obvious very severe handicap, unable to lead any kind of independent existence, no clear verbal or non-verbal communication
(Engstrom et al. 2003) **Criteria for level of support** Public: none (no public support); low (advice and support from habilitation, regular home-help service); moderate (continuous home support, sheltered job, job assistant, regular support from psychiatry and/or habilitation; high (supported living, group home or institution, daycentre, personal assistant)
Private: none (no contact with family); low (normal or near-normal contact with parents, siblings and other relatives; support and practical assistance from time to time); moderate (regular practical assistance at home; daily contact by phone or physically; help with local authorities); high (extensive help with social contacts and employment sites; total control of economic affairs; lives with relatives from time to time)

There could also be problems applying the two criteria developed by Howlin to people with ASD *and* intellectual disability. For example, in the earlier criteria (Howlin et al. 2000), the composite score included measures of autistic behaviours and language; therefore, those with ASD would be more likely to score higher and appear to have poorer social functioning if compared to a group without ASD. To date there is little evidence on the psychometric properties of these measures (Billstedt et al. 2005; Levy and Perry 2011). Marriage et al. (2009) acknowledged that such methods 'should be considered more qualitative than quantitative' (pp. 327). In addition to social functioning measures, studies have used quality-of-life measures. Quality-of-life domains have been identified as social inclusion, physical well-being, interpersonal relationships, material well-being, emotional well-being, self-determination, personal development and rights (Schalock et al. 2002).

The measures described in this chapter have all been designed by clinicians and researchers. On the whole, previous research has not been based on measures developed by asking adults with ASD and intellectual disability what they think is important or optimum. The challenges of assessing outcomes for adults with ASD and intellectual disability and the limitations of commonly used measures should be taken into account when evaluating the evidence described in the rest of this chapter. It is clear that further work that includes the voices of adults with ASD and/or intellectual disability is needed before we can accurately describe what life is like for this complex group of individuals.

4.4 Evidence on Outcomes for Adults with ASD and Intellectual Disability

4.4.1 ASD Functional Outcome

Since the review by Howlin (2000), described in the introduction to this chapter, there has been an increasing interest in adult outcomes for people with ASD, and a number of further studies have been published (Henninger and Taylor 2013). Among these studies, rates of unemployment for those with ASD ranged from 24 to 98 %; many participants left school without qualifications, and only 8–20 % were living independently (Barnard et al. 2001; Billstedt et al. 2011; Cederlund et al. 2008; Engstrom et al. 2003; Eaves and Ho 2007; Esbensen et al. 2010; Farley et al. 2009; Howlin 2000; Howlin et al. 2004; Mawhood et al. 2000; Renty and Roeyers 2006; Saldana et al. 2009). One study found that 24 % of all those with ASD were not engaging in any meaningful activity and 31 % were not involved in any social activities (Barnard et al. 2001). Green et al. (2000) reported that even those with ASD who have 'normal' cognitive ability struggle with practical day-to-day functioning.

A significant number of studies that concentrated on people with high-functioning ASD (Howlin et al. 2013; Howlin et al. 2014) did not make clear how many of their participants had additional intellectual disability (Kirby 2016) or used non-standardised measures of intellectual functioning (Gillespie-Lynch et al. 2012; Gotham et al. 2015). Many looked at the impact of IQ on social functioning, but few focused on those with intellectual disability to explore outcome among those with low IQ (particularly below 50) (Magiati et al. 2014). In addition, many studies did not include a comparison group so it is not clear whether these individuals with ASD and intellectual disability had poorer social functioning compared to those without any other disorder or with intellectual disability alone. Other studies have included comparison groups of participants with a different disorder or different types of ASD (Billstedt et al. 2005; Cederlund et al. 2008; Green et al. 2000; Howlin 2000).

Some studies have explored associations between intellectual and social functioning for adults with ASD. In Eaves and Ho's study (Eaves and Ho 2007), verbal IQ in childhood was the best predictor of social functioning score which also correlated with performance IQ. Another study found that low IQ and low verbal skills in childhood predicted social functioning (Billstedt et al. 2005). However, it should be noted that *poor* and *very poor* social functioning definitions included these items. In a study of 19-year-olds who had been diagnosed with ASD at age 2–3, Anderson et al. (2014) found that those with a verbal IQ <70 had significantly lower adaptive skills than those with a verbal IQ ≥70 but commented: 'adaptive skills were a relative strength for this [low verbal IQ] group, beyond what their IQ scores would suggest'.

A selection of studies on outcomes for adults with ASD and intellectual disability are summarised in Table 4.2. The methods used by these studies vary widely, as do their findings. However, research continues to consistently report that individuals with ASD and intellectual disability fare less well in adulthood than those with 'high-functioning' ASD. For example, in a study that compared adult males with autism to those with Asperger syndrome (AS), most participants in both groups had poor social functioning (Cederlund et al. 2008). Those with AS had significantly better social functioning compared to those with autism; none of whom had good social functioning, 5 % had fair social functioning and only 8 % of those over 23 lived independently. The majority of those in the autism group had intellectual disability. Participants with autism had significantly lower Global Assessment of Functioning (GAF) scores than those with AS; GAF score was significantly associated with IQ.

By contrast, in Howlin et al.'s study (Howlin et al. 2004), there was not a significant correlation between IQ and social functioning. But in a sub-analysis comparing participants with an IQ of 50–69 and those with IQ > 70, those in the lower IQ group scored significantly higher (indicating a poorer social functioning) on residential status, educational level, level of work and total rating of social functioning. Marriage et al. (2009) compared adults diagnosed with ASD in childhood and those who were diagnosed after 18 years of age. Of those diagnosed as children, participants with intellectual disability scored lower than those without intellectual disability on all measures of outcome except for intimate relationships.

Similarly, research indicates differences between those who have intellectual disability with and without ASD. For example, a series of studies from Wales explored the mental health and social functioning of adults with intellectual disability. Sub-analyses of those with ASD (as assessed using items on the Disability Assessment Schedule (DAS) (Holmes et al. 1982) relating to the ASD triad of

Table 4.2 Studies on the social functioning of adults with ASD and intellectual disability

Study	Participants	Comparison group	Measure(s)	Source of data	Results
Saldana et al. (2009)	74 adults with 'autism' (n = 48), Asperger syndrome (n = 8) and ASD/PDD (n = 18) (clinical diagnoses). Unclear how many had ID	None	Quality of life, employment, health, social network	Parent interview, comprehensive quality-of-life questionnaire, social/language DAS items, CARS, ICAP	Poor quality of social interaction, low levels of structured activity (16 %) and independence
Barnard et al. (2001)	450 adults with ASD (according to parent-reported diagnoses which were not assessed). Unclear how many had ID	None	Employment, activities, type of residence	Parent interview	Low levels of employment, activities and independence
Howlin et al. (2004)	68 adults with ASD (confirmed in adulthood by ADI-R) and IQ>50 (23 with IQ of 50–69)	None	Education, employment, friendships, type of residence. Composite score of social functioning[a]	ADI-R, parent interview, case records	Mostly poor social functioning (58 %). Significantly poorer for those with IQ of 50–69
Eaves and Ho (2007)	48 young adults with ASD (according to Rutter criteria) (38 with ID)	None	Quality of life, employment, type of residence, friendship, independence, satisfaction with services (Howlin et al. 2004 criteria[a])	Parent interview	Fair to very good social functioning for majority (54 %), none with very poor
Marriage et al. (2009)	45 adults diagnosed with ASD (according to DSM-IV) in childhood (12 had ID)	35 adults diagnosed with ASD after age of 18 (1 had ID)	Education, vocation, independence, social, intimate relationships	Case note review, Australian Scale for Asperger's Disorder, AQ, Child Symptom Inventory. ADI-R and ADOS	Poorer social functioning for those with ASD and ID compared with ID alone

(continued)

Table 4.2 (continued)

Study	Participants	Comparison group	Measure(s)	Source of data	Results
Billstedt et al. (2005)	78 adults with autism (DSM-IV criteria and DISCO) (62 with ID)	42 adults with atypical autism (36 with ID)	Type of residence, relationships, Lotter's criteria of outcome[a]	Parent interview, DISCO, Global Assessment of Functioning (GAF)	Poor social functioning for majority (89 %), no difference between groups
Cederlund et al. (2008)	70 adult males with autism or atypical autism (according to DSM-III and DISCO) (67 had ID)	70 adult males with Asperger syndrome (IQ>70)	Type of residence, outcome rating based on Lotter's criteria[a]	DISCO, GAF, Vineland Adaptive Behavior Scales	Poor social functioning for majority. Better for those with AS
Esbensen et al. (2010)	79 adults with ASD and ID (confirmed by ADI-R)	70 adults with Down syndrome (matched on age)	Type of residence, social contact with friends, employment, health, functioning (Howlin et al. 2004 criteria[a])	Parent interview, revised Barthel Index, Vineland Screener Scale, Scales of Independent Behavior-Revised	Group with ASD had low levels of independence and contact with friends. Poorer social functioning among those with ASD
Totsika et al. (2010)	Adults with ID and ASD aged 50 years and over (DAS triad of impairments) (65 with matched adaptive behaviour skills)	Adults with ID aged over 50 years (65 in matched group)	Domestic, social and community activities	Index of Community and Index of Participation in Domestic Life, ABC, PIMRA or PAS-ADD	Lower levels of activity for those with ASD but no differences between matched groups
Felce et al. (2011)	158 adults with ID and ASD (triad of impairments on DAS) in staffed community housing	269 adults with ID in staffed community housing	Challenging behaviour, independence variety/ frequency of social and community activities, constructive activities	ABC, AAMR ABS, DAS	No difference in social functioning between those with and without ASD

Beadle-Brown et al. (2009)	51 adults with severe ID and ASD (according to ICD-10 criteria)	21 adults with severe ID	Life satisfaction, community satisfaction, recreation satisfaction, job satisfaction, challenging behaviour	Lifestyle Satisfaction Scale, Schedule of Handicaps Behaviours and Skills, AAMR ABS, Leiter International Performance Scales, QoLQ, Reynell Language Development Scales	ASD was not a significant predictor of quality of life once challenging behaviour and IQ were accounted for
Matson et al. (2009)	65 adults with ASD and 104 with PDD-NOS (diagnosed using checklist with the combined ASD criteria from DSM-IV and ICD-10) and severe ID	65 adults with severe ID	Daily living skill functioning	Adaptive behaviour task analysis checklist	Those with ASD or PDD-NOS had lower scores for dressing, grooming and hygiene domains but no significant differences for bathing, housekeeping or meal preparation
Anderson et al. (2014)	53 'less cognitively able' (verbal IQ <70) adults with ASD (diagnosed at age 2 using ADI-R and ADOS)	32 'more cognitively able' (verbal IQ ≥70) adults with ASD (diagnosed at age 2 using ADI-R and ADOS)	Adaptive skills, ASD core features, behaviour problems, psychotropic medication	Vineland-II scales, ABC, CDRS-R	Less cognitively able group had significantly lower adaptive skills, higher levels of hyperactivity and more likely to be on psychotropic medication

[a]See Table 4.1. *AAMR ABS* American Association on Mental Retardation Adaptive Behavior Scale, *ABC* Aberrant Behavior Checklist, *ADI* Autism Diagnostic Interview, *ADOS* Autism Diagnostic Observation Schedule, *CDRS-R* Childhood Depression Rating Scale, *DAS* Disability Assessment Schedule, *DISCO* Diagnostic Interview for Social & Communication disorders, *ICAP* Inventory for Client & Agency Planning, *ID* intellectual disability, *PAS-ADD* Psychiatric Assessment Schedule for Adults with Developmental Disorders, *PIMRA* Psychopathology Instrument for Mental Retarded Adults, *QoLQ* Quality of Life Questionnaire

impairments) have been carried out. Totsika et al. (2010) compared quality of life for older adults with and without ASD. Participants with ASD were involved in a significantly lower number of domestic, social and community activities than those without ASD. They also spent a lower proportion of their time engaged in any activity (39 % vs. 59 %). Those with ASD had significantly more behaviour problems (a higher mean score on the Aberrant Behavior Checklist (Aman et al. 1985) than those without ASD. However, in a sub-analysis of those with matching adaptive skills, there were no significant differences between those with and without ASD on any quality-of-life measure or problem behaviours (Totsika et al. 2010).

A more recent study from this series looked at adults with intellectual disability who lived in staffed community housing (Felce et al. 2011). Participants with ASD were more likely to have severe challenging behaviour (36 % vs. 15 %) and had higher levels of problem behaviour and lower levels of adaptive behaviour than those without ASD. When participants were matched on adaptive behaviour, there remained significant differences in levels of problem behaviour and prevalence of challenging behaviour. Other measures included variety/frequency of social and community activities, household independence and engagement in constructive activities; this time there were no significant differences between those with and without ASD. However, the authors of these studies acknowledge limitations with regard to the way participants were categorised into those with and without ASD (Felce et al. 2011; Totsika et al. 2010).

The 'Camberwell Cohort' was a total population sample of children with severe ASD and/or intellectual disability in South London; this group was followed up as adults to explore their life satisfaction (Beadle-Brown et al. 2009). Participants with ASD had lower levels of community satisfaction than those without ASD, but there was no difference on any other measure. The only childhood predictor of quality of life among the whole sample was independent living skills. Of the measures taken when participants were adults, the most important factors associated with quality of life were challenging behaviour and IQ.

Esbensen et al. (2010) compared individuals with ASD and intellectual disability to those with Down syndrome. Few participants had high or very high levels of independence. Most of those with ASD had low or very low levels of independence, whereas those with Down syndrome tended to be classed as having moderate or low levels. Predictors of social functioning for those with and without ASD were total functional abilities and service receipt. Severity of intellectual disability and maladaptive behaviours were not significant predictors of social functioning. This study found that those accessing mental health services had poorer social functioning and concluded that 'It will be important for future researchers to examine the best ways to assess psychological and psychiatric needs among adults with autism spectrum disorders so that appropriate interventions can be put in place' (Esbensen et al. 2010) pp. 287.

It is clear that the social functioning of people with ASD and intellectual disability varies greatly over time, geographical areas and between individuals. Evidence on which factors are significantly associated with outcomes is weak. This is because the few good quality studies in this area have included diverse populations and used a range of methods to define/diagnose ASD, collect data and measure outcomes

(Levy and Perry 2011). However, there is some consistent evidence on the characteristics that appear to be related to outcomes for people with ASD and intellectual disability.

The following factors have been found to have a positive relationship with outcomes: IQ, expressive communication, early language skills, adaptive functioning and level of perceived informal support. Severity of ASD/ASD symptoms and level of unmet formal support needs have been found to have a negative relationship with social functioning. It is important that studies examining differences in the social functioning of adults who have intellectual disability with and without ASD explore the effect of these variables, that is, whether they are better predictors of social functioning than ASD itself or effect moderators that have a different impact on individuals with and without ASD.

4.4.2 ASD Symptom Outcome

In addition to research on social functioning, a number of studies have investigated changes in ASD symptomatology and diagnostic outcome – that is, whether adults who were diagnosed with ASD as children continue to meet criteria as adults (Anderson et al. 2014; Fein et al. 2013). There appears to be some evidence that a small minority of children diagnosed with 'high-functioning' ASD do not meet diagnostic criteria as adults. However, this may indicate that they were initially misdiagnosed (Fein et al. 2013). Other research reports that for some individuals, the severity of their ASD symptoms decreases as they age (Howlin et al. 2015). Evidence on the extent to which children with intellectual disability who are diagnosed with ASD in childhood improve over time is lacking, and there is some evidence that ASD symptoms in those with severe intellectual disability worsen over time (Magiati et al. 2014).

4.5 Research and Clinical Implications

Few studies of adults with intellectual disability report the number of participants with ASD or investigate whether presence of ASD has any impact on their findings. The situation is similar for research on adults with ASD which does not always take intellectual disability into account unless it is specifically on those with low-functioning ASD. However, research indicates that those with ASD form a distinct group among adults with intellectual disability and that adults with ASD and intellectual disability have different patterns of mental health, problem behaviour and social functioning outcomes compared to those without ASD (Bradley et al. 2014; Underwood et al. 2012).

Future research should be prospective, longitudinal and population-based, although given the difficulties carrying out these types of studies, clinic-based, cross-sectional studies could provide a valuable snapshot of individuals' lives (Elison et al. 2010; Engstrom et al. 2003). An improved understanding of the characteristics that predict social functioning and the course of adult outcomes would aid the provision of services and interventions for adults with ASD and intellectual disability.

It is vital that services for adults with ASD and intellectual disability better understand their users. This includes recognising the importance of characteristics that group individuals together and impact on their needs and outcomes. Once recognised and better understood, these characteristics (either at a group or individual level) should inform the delineation of assessment and care pathways; the identification of people that services should be prioritising for improved access to assessment, services and monitoring; and choice of evidence-based intervention. Individuals with intellectual disability may require specialist assessment to determine whether they meet the criteria for ASD. Unfortunately, standardised tools for this group are currently lacking (Sappok et al. 2015). Adults with ASD should receive comprehensive neuropsychological assessment to identify their cognitive strengths and limitations and determine their level of intellectual functioning. It is also important that adaptive functioning is assessed in those with ASD and/or intellectual disability as this may not match expected levels given an individual's cognitive functioning.

The following suggested policy and practice strategies may lead to better outcomes for adults with ASD and intellectual disability:

- Efforts to identify groups and individuals who are not effectively accessing services and increase equity of access, particularly among those with high needs
- Better assessment and monitoring of individuals' needs using standardised methods plus proactive intervention to meet or eliminate specific needs
- Improved assessment and monitoring of outcomes, ensuring that action is taken when outcomes do not improve
- Proactive identification of factors that may be limiting an individual's opportunity for a better outcome
- Improved awareness and understanding of ASD (among support staff and carers but also health and social care staff and the general public)
- Improved assessment, for ASD among those with intellectual disability and of intellectual functioning among those with ASD, in order to better understand an individual's presentation
- Improved assessment for mental and physical health problems to better inform treatment and care decisions
- Less fragmented assessment of need and implementation of care packages across the range of services used by adults with ASD and intellectual disability

Conclusion

In early studies, adults with ASD appeared to have generally poor life outcomes (Howlin et al. 2004) (Henninger and Taylor 2013). More recent research found that, as a group, their social functioning was better than expected and has improved over time, particularly now that more people with ASD are living in the community. IQ and verbal skills appear to be the most significant predictors of outcome, and there is evidence that those with intellectual disability or more severe ASD do less well in adult life (Cederlund et al. 2008; Marriage et al. 2009). More research is needed that bridges the gap between childhood and adulthood to explore the period of transition between these two life stages (Kirby 2016). Similarly, few studies have looked at life outcomes for older adults with ASD (Howlin et al. 2015).

The literature offers few recommendations on what might be done to improve outcomes for adults with ASD and intellectual disability. Howlin (2000) suggested that although life for people with ASD appears to have improved over time, it is likely this is due to less institutionalisation and more opportunities, stating: '…there is no evidence to suggest that long-term outcome can be dramatically improved following the implementation of any particular intervention programme' (pp. 78). Emerging evidence suggests that adults with ASD respond well to interventions designed to increase social participation and functioning and that these can lead to increased quality of life (Tobin et al. 2014). However, again there is a lack of research on the effectiveness of these interventions for adults with ASD and intellectual disability.

Many of the characteristics associated with poorer social functioning among those with ASD and intellectual disability are factors that tend not to change such as IQ and severity of ASD symptoms. However, it is possible that early recognition and intervention could improve individuals' adaptive functioning and skills and that this could in turn lead to better life outcomes. Certainly, better recognition and effective treatment should improve quality of life for those with ASD and intellectual disability who experience co-occurring mental health, behavioural and physical health problems.

References

Aman MG, Singh NN, Stewart AW, Field CJ (1985) The aberrant behavior checklist: a behavior rating scale for the assessment of treatment effects. Am J Ment Defic 89:485–491

Anderson DK, Liang JW, Lord C (2014) Predicting young adult outcome among more and less cognitively able individuals with autism spectrum disorders. J Child Psychol Psychiatry 55:485–494

Autism Act 2009. Autism Act UK. In: Hm Government (ed).

Barnard, J., Harvey, V., Potter, D. & Prior, A. 2001. Ignored or ineligible? The reality for adults with autism spectrum disorders. The National Autistic Society, London

Beadle-Brown J, Murphy G, Diterlizzi M (2009) Quality of life for the Camberwell Cohort. J Appl Res Intellect Disabil 22:380–390

Billstedt E, Gillberg C, Gillberg C (2005) Autism after adolescence: population-based 13- to 22-year follow-up study of 120 individuals with autism diagnosed in childhood. J Autism Dev Disord 35:351–360

Billstedt E, Gillberg IC, Gillberg C (2011) Aspects of quality of life in adults diagnosed with autism in childhood: a population-based study. Autism 15:7–20

Bradley E, Caldwell P, Underwood L (2014) Autism Spectrum Disorder. In: Mccarthy J, Tsakanikos E (eds) Handbook of psychopathology in intellectual disability. Springer, New York

Cederlund M, Hagberg B, Billstedt E, Gillberg IC, Gillberg C (2008) Asperger syndrome and autism: a comparative longitudinal follow-up study more than 5 years after original diagnosis. J Autism Dev Disord 38:72–85

Congress, U.S. (2006) Combating Autism Act Pub. Law No. 109–416. In: Congress, U.S. (ed)

Department of Health (2010) 'Fulfilling and rewarding lives' The strategy for adults with autism in England (2010). Department of Health, London

Eaves LC, Ho HH (2007) Young adult outcome of autism spectrum disorders. J Autism Dev Disord 38:739–747

Elison S, Stinton C, Howlin P (2010) Health and social outcomes in adults with Williams syndrome: findings from cross-sectional and longitudinal cohorts. Res Dev Disabil 31:587–599

Engstrom I, Ekstrom L, Emilsson B (2003) Psychosocial Functioning in a Group of Swedish Adults with Asperger Syndrome or High- Functioning Autism. Autism 7:99–110

Esbensen AJ, Bishop S, Seltzer MM, Greenberg JS, Taylor JL (2010) Comparisons between individuals with autism spectrum disorders and individuals with Down Syndrome in adulthood. Am J Intellect Dev Disabil 115:277

Farley MA, Mcmahon WM, Fombonne E, Jenson WR, Miller J, Gardner M, Block H, Pingree CB, Ritvo ER, Ritvo RA, Coon H (2009) Twenty-year outcome for individuals with autism and average or near-average cognitive abilities. Autism Res 2:109–118

Fein D, Barton M, Eigsti IM, Kelley E, Naigles L, Schultz RT, Stevens M, Helt M, Orinstein A, Rosenthal M, Troyb E, Tyson K (2013) Optimal outcome in individuals with a history of autism. J Child Psychol Psychiatry 54:195–205

Felce D, Perry J, Lowe K, Jones E (2011) The impact of autism or severe challenging behaviour on lifestyle outcome in community housing. J Appl Res Intellect Disabil 24:95–104

Findon J, Cadman T, Stewart CS, Woodhouse E, Eklund H, Hayward H, De Le Harpe Golden D, Chaplin E, Glaser K, Simonoff E, Murphy D, Bolton PF, Mcewen FS (2016) Screening for co-occurring conditions in adults with autism spectrum disorder using the strengths and difficulties questionnaire: a pilot study. Autism Res 9:1353–1363

Gillespie-Lynch K, Sepeta L, Wang Y, Marshall S, Gomez L, Sigman M, Hutman T (2012) Early childhood predictors of the social competence of adults with autism. J Autism Dev Disord 42:161–174

Gotham K, Marvin AR, Taylor JL, Warren Z, Anderson CM, Law PA, Law JK, Lipkin PH (2015) Characterizing the daily life, needs, and priorities of adults with autism spectrum disorder from Interactive Autism Network data. Autism 19:794–804

Green J, Gilchrist A, Burton D, Cox A (2000) Social and psychiatric functioning in adolescents with Asperger syndrome compared with conduct disorder. J Autism Dev Disord 30:279–293

Henninger NA, Taylor JL (2013) Outcomes in adults with autism spectrum disorders: a historical perspective. Autism 17:103–116

Holmes N, Shah A, Wing L (1982) The Disability Assessment Schedule: a brief screening device for use with the mentally retarded. Psychol Med 12:879–890

Howlin P (2000) Outcome in Adult Life for more Able Individuals with Autism or Asperger Syndrome. Autism 4:63–83

Howlin P, Mawhood L, Rutter M (2000) Autism and developmental receptive language disorder - follow-up comparison in early adult life. II: social, behavioural, and psychiatric outcomes. Journal of Child Psychology and Psychiatry 41:561–578

Howlin P, Goode S, Hutton J, Rutter M (2004) Adult outcome for children with autism. Journal of Child Psychology and Psychiatry 45:212–229

Howlin P, Moss P, Savage S, Rutter M (2013) Social outcomes in mid- to later adulthood among individuals diagnosed with autism and average nonverbal IQ as children. J Am Acad Child Adolesc Psychiatry 52:572–581 e1

Howlin P, Savage S, Moss P, Tempier A, Rutter M (2014) Cognitive and language skills in adults with autism: a 40-year follow-up. J Child Psychol Psychiatry 55:49–58

Howlin P, Arciuli J, Begeer S, Brock J, Clarke K, Costley D, Di Rita P, Falkmer T, Glozier N, Gray K, Guastella A, Horstead S, Rice L, Stancliffe RJ, West S, Yam C, Einfeld S (2015) Research on adults with autism spectrum disorder: Roundtable report. J Intellect Dev Disabil 40:388–393

Kanne SM, Gerber AJ, Quirmbach LM, Sparrow SS, Cicchetti DV, Saulnier CA (2011) The role of adaptive behavior in autism spectrum disorders: implications for functional outcome. J Autism Dev Disord 41:1007–1018

Kanner L (1971) Follow-up study of eleven autistic children originally reported in 1943. J Autism Child Schizophr 1:119–145

Kirby AV (2016) Parent expectations mediate outcomes for young adults with autism spectrum disorder. J Autism Dev Disord 46:1643–1655

Levy A, Perry A (2011) Outcomes in adolescents and adults with autism: a review of the literature. Research in Autism Spectrum Disorders 5:1271–1282

Lockyer L, Rutter M (1969) A five- to fifteen-year follow-up study of infantile psychosis. Br J Psychiatry 115:865–882

Lotter V (1974) Factors related to outcome in autistic children. J Autism Child Schizophr 4:263–277

Magiati I, Tay XW, Howlin P (2014) Cognitive, language, social and behavioural outcomes in adults with autism spectrum disorders: a systematic review of longitudinal follow-up studies in adulthood. Clin Psychol Rev 34:73–86

Marriage S, Wolverton A, Marriage K (2009) Autism Spectrum Disorder grown up: a chart review of adult functioning. J Can Acad Child Adolesc Psychiatry 18:322–328

Matson JL, Dempsey T, Fodstad JC (2009) The effect of Autism Spectrum Disorders on adaptive independent living skills in adults with severe intellectual disability. Res Dev Disabil 30:1203–1211

Mawhood L, Howlin P, Rutter M (2000) Autism and developmental receptive language disorder – a comparative follow-up in early adult life I: cognitive and language outcomes. J Child Psychol Psychiatry 41:547–559

Mccarthy J, Chaplin E, Underwood L (2015) An English perspective on policy for adults with autism. Advances in Autism 1:61–65

National Audit Office 2009. Supporting people with autism through adulthood. Report by the Comptroller and Auditor General. HC 556 Session 2008–2009. National Audit Office, London

NICE (2012) Autism: recognition, referral, diagnosis and management of adults on the autism spectrum, National Institute for Health and Clinical Excellence, London

O'Brien G (2001) Adult outcome of childhood learning disability. Dev Med Child Neurol 43:634–638

Prince M (2003) Measurement in psychiatry. In: Prince M, Stewart S, Ford T, Hotopf M (eds) Practical psychiatric epidemiology. Oxford University Press, Oxford

Renty JO, Roeyers H (2006) Quality of life in high-functioning adults with autism spectrum disorder: the predictive value of disability and support characteristics. Autism 10:511–524

Rutter M, Greenfeld D, Lockyer L (1967) A five to fifteen year follow-up study of infantile psychosis. Br J Psychiatry 113:1183–1199

Saldana D, Alvarez RM, Lobaton S, Lopez AM, Moreno M, Rojano M (2009) Objective and subjective quality of life in adults with autism spectrum disorders in southern Spain. Autism 13:303–316

Sappok T, Heinrich M, Underwood L (2015) Screening tools for autism spectrum disorders. Adv Autism 1:12–29

Schalock RL, Brown I, Brown R, Cummins RA, Felce D, Matikka L, Keith KD, Parmenter T (2002) Conceptualization, measurement, and application of quality of life for persons with intellectual disabilities: report of an international panel of experts. Ment Retard 40: 457–470

Stewart R (2003) Inference 1: chance, bias, and confounding. In: Prince M, Stewart S, Ford T, Hotopf M (eds) Practical psychiatric epidemiology. Oxford University Press, Oxford

Taylor LJ (2016) Psychopharmacologic intervention for adults with autism spectrum disorder: a systematic literature review. Res Autism Spectr Disord 25:58–75

Tobin MC, Drager KDR, Richardson LF (2014) A systematic review of social participation for adults with autism spectrum disorders: support, social functioning, and quality of life. RASD 8:214–229

Totsika V, Felce D, Kerr M, Hastings RP (2010) Behavior problems, psychiatric symptoms, and quality of life for older adults with intellectual disability with and without autism. J Autism Dev Disord 40:1171–1178

Underwood L, Mccarthy J, Tsakanikos E, Howlin P, Bouras N, Craig TJ (2012) Health and social functioning of adults with intellectual disability and autism. J Policy Pract Intellect Disabil 9:147–150

Underwood L, McCarthy J, Tsakanikos E (2010) Mental health of adults with autism spectrum disorders and intellectual disability. Current Opinion in Psychiatry 23(5):421–426

Underwood L, McCarthy J, Tsakanikos E (2011) Assessment of Co-morbid Psychopathology. In: Matson JLL, Sturmey P, eds. International Handbook of Autism and Pervasive Developmental Disorders. New York: Springer 287–293

Van Dooren K, Mcpherson L, Lennox N (2016) Mapping the needs of adults with autism and co-morbid intellectual disability. Curr Dev Disord Rep 3:82–89

5 The High-Functioning Group: High-Functioning Autism and Asperger Syndrome in Adults

Bernardo Barahona-Corrêa

5.1 Introduction

As a young resident in psychiatry, I once expressed my surprise to a senior colleague at the fact that we never got to see any patients with autism or Asperger syndrome in adult psychiatry. What happened to them when they grew up? Where were they, and where were they being treated or followed up? "Oh, they all become schizophrenic…" was the swift, patronizing answer of the experienced older clinician. Looking back today it seems hardly believable that an experienced and competent clinician should say and, worse still, believe such a nonsensical idea, and yet it eloquently reflects the huge gap in expert training of psychiatrists in the field of autism and autism-related disorders in adults. This is all the more worrying as current evidence shows that the prevalence of autism spectrum disorders in adults is at least equal to (and possibly twice) that of psychosis (Brugha et al. 2011). Moreover, this personal anecdote encloses the three fundamental questions that remain, still today, partly unanswered by adult psychiatry regarding its role in diagnosing and treating adults with an autism spectrum disorder (ASD), namely, what are the medical, psychiatric, and social needs for care of individuals with an autism spectrum disorder who reach adult age? Where, and by whom, should these needs be addressed? What leads these patients to seek help and how do they present clinically? In the case of high-functioning autism spectrum disorders (HFA), these questions materialize in one of two practical scenarios: (1) adults who receive a first-time

B. Barahona-Corrêa, MD, PhD
CADIN – Neurodevelopment, Champalimaud Foundation Clinical Centre, Champalimaud Centre for the Unknown, Nova Medical School – NOVA University of Lisbon, Lisbon, Portugal

Department of Psychiatry and Mental Health, Hospital Egas Moniz, Lisbon, Portugal
e-mail: barahona.correa@nms.unl.pt

B. Barahona Corrêa, R.-J. van der Gaag (eds.), *Autism Spectrum Disorders in Adults*, DOI 10.1007/978-3-319-42713-3_5

diagnosis of an autism spectrum disorder and (2) adults with an autism spectrum disorder that has been known and treated since an early age and who presently go on seeking professional help for one reason or another.

5.2 Adults with Undiagnosed Autism Spectrum Disorders

Surprising as it may be for a disorder that affects sufferers from such an early age and with such devastating results, a significant number of individuals with a high-functioning ASD reach adult age without ever having been correctly diagnosed. In the only population-based epidemiologic survey on adult ASD published to date, Brugha et al. (2011) found that none of the subjects who met diagnostic criteria for an ASD had been diagnosed before. Moreover, these subjects had no more contact with mental health services than the general population (Brugha et al. 2011). The three questions that immediately arise are as follows: (1) What are their autistic clinical features? (2) What explains that they have remained without a diagnosis up to adulthood, i.e., how do they differ from their counterparts diagnosed in infancy? (3) What leads them to seek help from a mental health professional at this point in their lives?

5.2.1 Clinical Features of Adults with a First-Time Diagnosis of ASD

Adults with previously undiagnosed ASD remain a relatively understudied subgroup within the field of adult autism. The overwhelming majority presents an HFA/ Asperger syndrome phenotype (Lehnhardt et al. 2012; Brugha et al. 2011). The epidemiologic survey by Brugha et al. (2011) found that these undiagnosed subjects were mostly males, single, with low educational qualifications, and living in publicly supported housing (Brugha et al. 2011). Those who spontaneously present to specialized clinics for assessment and treatment are of course likely to differ somewhat from these community-dwelling individuals. Several explanations have been put forward to explain why ASD remains undiagnosed until adulthood in a subset of patients. An important explanation resides in the fact that diagnostic criteria for ASD were much more stringent two or three decades ago, in a time when ASD diagnoses, and their compatibility with a wide range of intelligence levels, were also not broadly known (Geurts and Jansen 2011). Additionally, psychiatric comorbidity will often overshadow the underlying ASD and distract clinicians, for the most part unfamiliar with ASD diagnoses, from the underlying developmental disorder (Nylander and Gillberg 2001). Another popular hypothesis is that ASD subjects who remained undiagnosed until adult age must have learned to somehow compensate for their autistic deficits through imitative learning (Lehnhardt et al. 2012). It is suggested that during growth, these subjects have gradually assimilated, in a formal, explicit way, the implicit rules that govern social interactions, allowing them to adequately deal with social situations as long as they unfold in a predictable and conventional way (Lai and Baron-Cohen 2015; Tobin et al. 2014). In accordance with this, in qualitative studies on how adults with ASD dealt with their disorder and with their ASD diagnosis, subjects often report that over time, they learned to consciously hide their symptoms and characteristics, developing a sort of effortful false self to be presented to others in social contexts (Griffith et al. 2012; Punshon et al. 2009). This more or less implies that these individuals have to possess the necessary cognitive ability to achieve such learning, a prediction that seems to be corroborated by evidence showing that subjects with an autism spectrum disorder first diagnosed in adult age characteristically have normal to above-average intelligence (Lehnhardt et al. 2011; Marriage et al. 2009; Cederlund and Gillberg 2004; Hofvander et al. 2009; Engstrom et al. 2003), in contrast to most adults with a childhood diagnosis of ASD (Howlin 2000, 2003; Seltzer et al. 2004). It goes without saying that, in addition to a normal or high intelligence, these subjects must have developed good linguistic skills and must have had access to a supporting psychosocial network, two factors that are well known to influence the prognosis of autism spectrum disorders (Joshi et al. 2013; Howlin and Moss 2012). The problem with this explanation is that it has not yet been confirmed by evidence from studies directly comparing early diagnosed and late-diagnosed individuals. Additionally, IQ measures in autism are, as a rule, difficult to interpret, as in most cases full-scale IQ measures conceal huge heterogeneities in performance across the different domains (Spek et al. 2008; Chiang et al. 2014). Moreover, even autism spectrum disorder subjects with good linguistic skills and high intelligence are often highly impaired in terms of psychosocial functioning (Marriage et al. 2009; Lehnhardt et al. 2012; Magiati et al. 2014). So, even though good linguistic and cognitive abilities and an available supporting social network are probably necessary elements for an ASD to go undiagnosed until adult life, they are in all likelihood not sufficient. It is likely that these patients simply have a less severe phenotype both in terms of the core symptoms of autism and in terms of psychiatric comorbidities, therefore being able to function adaptively until environmental demands exceed their coping abilities (Lugnegård et al. 2011). This is particularly likely to happen upon entering university, the first job, or conjugal life (Lehnhardt et al. 2012; Marriage et al. 2009). In accordance with this hypothesis, samples of patients with late-diagnosed ASD have high proportions (roughly 40–80 %) of individuals who have a university degree, who are professionally successful, who are living independently, or who report having a meaningful intimate relation (Spek et al. 2008; Hofvander et al. 2009; Marriage et al. 2009), in contrast with 25 % or less in adults who were diagnosed in infancy or youth (Howlin 2000, 2003; Cederlund and Gillberg 2004; Billstedt et al. 2005; Seltzer et al. 2004). There are no studies directly comparing the severity of core autistic symptoms in early and late-diagnosed ASD. However, when compared with IQ- and age-matched healthy adults, patients with ASD diagnosed in adulthood do have a significantly worse performance on social cognition tasks, pragmatic language, and executive function tasks (Lehnhardt et al. 2011). In an often cited paper, Tantam (2000) remarks that parental retrospective reports on the childhood behavior of their offspring with late-diagnosed ASD do not differ from the reports of parents of patients diagnosed in childhood (Tantam 2000). However, they tend to report less social inadequacy and less interpersonal tension when describing their children's early behavioral problems, which suggests that parental attitude to the child's autistic traits is probably another determining factor as to whether or not they will remain undiagnosed until adulthood. Marriage et al. (2009) compared adaptive functioning and psychiatric comorbidity in a group of ASD patients diagnosed in adulthood and a group of adults with ASD diagnosed in infancy, all with full-scale IQ above 70 (Marriage et al. 2009). They found that subjects who had been diagnosed as adults had higher scores of adaptive functioning in all domains (education, independent living, employment, social and intimate relationships). They also found similar rates of psychiatric comorbidity in ASD adults with intellectual disability, ASD adults diagnosed in infancy, and ASD adults diagnosed as adults, except for a higher prevalence of depression in the latter (Marriage et al. 2009). This high prevalence of major depression in late-diagnosed individuals with HFA has also been noted by Hofvander et al. (2009) and Lehnhardt et al. (2012) and is in line with the observation that a high IQ and being professionally integrated are vulnerability factors for the development of depression in ASD adults generally, probably reflecting greater exposure to social pressures and challenges, and a deeper awareness, by patients, of their own shortcomings (Tantam 2000; Howlin 2003; Hofvander et al. 2009; Lehnhardt et al. 2012; Tobin et al. 2014). Alternatively, it may simply reflect a greater ability of subjects who are verbally more apt to effectively express internalizing symptoms (Buck et al. 2014). Notwithstanding the higher scores in adaptive behavior, only 25 % of the late-diagnosed subjects were considered to have good adaptive functioning (Marriage et al. 2009).

What brings these patients to seek help at this particular stage in their life course? As mentioned, many patients seek help at times of major changes in their lives (transition to university, entering the labor market, leaving the parental home) that face them with new psychosocial and executive demands and challenges that overwhelm their previously sufficient coping abilities (Tantam 2000; Marriage et al. 2009; Lehn et al. 2012). The loss of employment – often as a consequence of workplace conflicts, loss of a supporting parent, or inability to find a new placement once an employer closes down – is another frequent trigger of the decision to seek help (Holwerda et al. 2012). It is, in this respect, revealing that psychotropic medication use increases sharply in ASD after age 20 (Esbensen et al. 2009). Furthermore, Hutton et al. (2008) noted that onset of new psychiatric disorders often occurs in the early to mid-twenties (Hutton et al. 2008). In their descriptive study of 105 adults aged between 18 and 64 who had just received their first-time ASD diagnosis, Geurts and Jansen (2011) found that 37 % were referred for specialized mental health assessment due to mood- or anxiety-related complaints, with a further 26 % referred due to socialization difficulties (Geurts and Jansen 2011). However, other, more subtle and deeply rooted factors may be at play here. For one thing, Lehnhardt et al. (2012) reported that many of their adult subjects with a first-time diagnosis of ASD described feelings of strangeness and "otherness" beginning by late adolescence that made them uncomfortable and insecure with respect to their ability to engage in meaningful intimate relationships (Lehnhardt et al. 2012). Marriage et al. (2009) reported that part of their sample of adults with late-diagnosed HFA had tried to engage in a sexual relationship and had failed, leading them to develop an asexual attitude in adult life, or even, in a minority, to question their gender identity (Marriage et al. 2009). Other authors report that adults with an ASD tend to regard their social and relational disability as a form of failure or personal inferiority (Howlin et al. 2004; Billstedt et al. 2005). Moreover, there is evidence that social-cognitive adaptation efforts lose momentum beyond late adolescence or early adulthood, which is exactly the opposite of what happens with environmental demands for social-cognitive conforming (Griffith et al. 2012; Taylor and Seltzer 2010). In their survey on how adult subjects with an ASD had experienced their diagnosis, Jones et al. (2014) noticed that for many participants, the trigger that had led them to seek a diagnosis had been a critical negative event such as loss of employment or the breaking up of a significant relationship (Jones et al. 2014). Moreover, the specific complaints that most often led adults in this and other studies to seek help from a mental health professional were awareness of his/her own difficulties with social interactions and relationships, depressive and anxiety symptoms, and prominent ritualistic or obsessive-compulsive-like behaviors (Jones et al. 2014; Geurts and Jansen 2011). Descriptive reports on adults with an ASD attending formal support groups reveal that many subjects describe becoming more aware of their isolation and their differences from their age peers as they grow older, an experience that is invariably reported as being hurtful and a source of anxiety and depressive feelings and thoughts about the self and the future (Tobin et al. 2014). Friendships tend to be perceived by most as superficial and more akin to acquaintances than real friendships, with ASD subjects often describing a sense of impotence with respect to transforming them into more deep and close relationships (Tobin et al. 2014).

5.2.2 Reasons for self-referral to Mental Health services

As we already saw, more often than not, adults with an undiagnosed ASD will seek professional help due to problems that are collateral to their core condition, frequently in times of major changes in their lives that bring to surface the patient's adaptive and interpersonal vulnerabilities and, consequently, impinge on the sufferer's mental health. At other times, patients will seek help due to conditions that, without being a direct cause of the ASD, are well known to co-occur frequently with ASD across the life span.

Much has been written about the emotional consequences of having an ASD (Tantam 2000). High trait anxiety, a low self-esteem, and a life course punctuated by peer rejection, bullying, failure in close relations, and often family tension or breakdown will often result in an adult who is suspicious of others, reluctant to accept the responsibilities of adult life or who simply has withdrawn into the isolated world of his idiosyncratic and restricted interests (Tantam 2000; Lai and Baron-Cohen 2015). As Tantam points out, as adolescents with an ASD grow, they become increasingly more aware of their condition and, consequently, increasingly distressed by it, even though the resulting disability may tend to improve with age. Even for the relatively well-adapted and good-functioning adolescent or young adult with an ASD, progressing through adulthood often proves to be an unanticipated ordeal, as failures in professional, social, and intimate life accumulate and social and family networks that supported him or her during infancy and adolescence gradually disappear (parents die, peer groups from school or high school disintegrate, etc.). In other cases, the breaking up of a long-established or occasionally even marital relationship may prove a catastrophic event and will often be the occasion when professional help is sought. Unsurprisingly, and similarly to what has been reported in adults with an ASD diagnosed in infancy, depression and anxiety disorders are not only the two most frequent mental health problems in adults with a first-time diagnosis of ASD but also the most frequent reason for referral to specialized assessment (Joshi et al. 2013; Takara and Kondo 2014a). Hofvander et al. (2009), in a sample of 122 adults with a first-time diagnosis of ASD, found a lifetime prevalence of mood disorder of 53 %. This was independent of gender or ASD subgroup (i.e., Asperger syndrome, autistic disorder, or pervasive developmental disorder not otherwise specified). Interestingly, only a minority of patients had ever been treated with an antidepressant, which suggests that, although overrepresented, depression tends to be underdiagnosed and undertreated in ASD (Hofvander et al. 2009). Marriage et al. (2009), in their sample of 34 adults with a first-time diagnosis of ASD, likewise found major depression to be the most prevalent mental disorder (44 %) (Marriage et al. 2009). Lehnhardt et al. (2012) found that 50 % of their adult patients newly diagnosed with ASD either had been treated for depression in the past or were being currently treated for it. Moreover, they found that 30 % of their patients had significant depressive symptoms at the time of assessment (Lehnhardt et al. 2012). Joshi et al. (2013), in their sample of 63 adults with a first-time diagnosis of ASD, found a lifetime prevalence of major depression as high as 77 % and a prevalence of current major depression of 31 % (Joshi et al. 2013). Importantly, the former figure was significantly higher than the lifetime prevalence of a control group of non-ASD adults referred to the same clinic. In an alternative approach, Takara and Kondo (2014a, b) showed that up to 16 % of first-visit adult patients with major depression visiting a psychiatric outpatient clinic met formal criteria for an ASD (Takara and Kondo 2014a). In their descriptive study of 54 adult subjects with Asperger syndrome, of which 28 were diagnosed as adults, Lugnegård et al. (2011) found a lifetime prevalence for depression of 69 % (Lugnegård et al. 2011).

Anxiety disorders are the second most frequent comorbid psychiatric condition in adult-diagnosed ASD. Hofvander et al. (2009) reports the highest prevalence, with 50 % of their sample having a current or past history of at least one anxiety disorder (other than obsessive-compulsive disorder (OCD), which at the time of the study was classified within the group of anxiety disorders) (Hofvander et al. 2009). Again there were no gender differences regarding prevalence of this group of disorders, nor were there differences between the several ASD syndromes. Lugnegård et al. report similar prevalence rates of 54 % in their mixed sample of adult- and childhood-diagnosed Asperger syndrome cases (Lugnegård et al. 2011). Marriage et al. (2009) and Lehnhardt et al. (2012) report much lower lifetime prevalences of 23 % and 16 %, respectively, again excluding OCD (Marriage et al. 2009; Lehnhardt et al. 2012). Joshi et al. (2013) found that 59 % of their sample of adult-diagnosed ASD cases had at least two comorbid anxiety disorders, including OCD (Joshi et al. 2013). Among these, social phobia was the most prevalent disorder, both lifetime and at the time of assessment at 56 % and 40 %, respectively. This is a much higher figure than has been reported in children with ASD (Joshi et al. 2010) or in adults with childhood-diagnosed ASD (Mouridsen et al. 2008; Buck et al. 2014). It is possible that this again reflects the fact that adults who are being diagnosed with ASD for the first time are usually functioning at a comparatively high level and are consequently exposed to much more frequent and complex social challenges than the typical ASD subject. These are ASD adults who are aware of their difficulty managing social relationships and the need to overcome them if they are to be fully integrated and successful. Their failure to do so inoculates their attempts with growing social anxiety and ultimately phobic social avoidance (Joshi et al. 2013). Interestingly, all cases of social phobia in the sample described by Joshi et al. (2013) had an IQ above 70, and two thirds met diagnostic criteria for at least a second comorbid anxiety disorder (including OCD in 31 %). In line with these findings, and even though their lifetime prevalence figures were much lower (9 %), Lehnhardt et al. (2012) also found social phobia to be the most frequent anxiety disorder in their sample (Lehnhardt et al. 2012).

Obsessive-compulsive disorder seems to be overrepresented in adults with a first-time diagnosis of ASD in some series, but not in others. The issue is certainly complicated by the obvious difficulty in operationalizing the complex differential diagnosis between the two disorders. Hofvander et al. (2009) found an OCD diagnosis in 24 % of their patients, equally distributed between males and females and across the three ASD diagnostic categories (Hofvander et al. 2009). Their figure is strikingly similar to the lifetime prevalence of 24 % reported by Joshi et al. (2013), who also found a current diagnosis of OCD in 16 % of their sample, both figures significantly higher than those found in the control non-ASD clinical sample (Joshi et al. 2013). Lugnegård et al. found 12 % of their sample meeting criteria for an OCD diagnosis (Lugnegård et al. 2011). In sharp contrast to these two studies, Lehnhardt et al. found an OCD diagnosis in only 3.4 % of their group of adults with a first-time diagnosis of ASD (Lehnhardt et al. 2012). In an often cited study, Ailsa Russel et al. (2005) explored OCD psychopathology in a sample of 40 adults with high-functioning ASD. They found that one quarter met formal ICD-10 criteria for OCD and that subsyndromic obsessions and compulsions were extremely prevalent in the ASD group (Russell et al. 2005). Apart from subtle differences in terms of obsessive thought contents, they did not find relevant differences in OCD symptoms when they compared the ASD group with a second group of adults with OCD and no ASD. Importantly, these results contrast with what has been found in ASD patients with low IQ and speech delay, who tend to manifest predominantly repetitive behaviors like touching, tapping, self-injuring, or hoarding, rather than the more typical cleaning or checking compulsions that predominate in OCD patients (Russell et al. 2005).

Although bipolar disorder is often claimed to occur more frequently in ASD than in the general population or clinical non-ASD populations, the evidence base supporting this in ASD patients diagnosed in adulthood is contradictory. Joshi et al. (2013) found a lifetime prevalence of bipolar disorder of 25 % in their sample, against a mere 13 % in the control clinical population (Joshi et al. 2013). However, other groups report much lower prevalence figures varying between 3 and 8 % (Stahlberg et al. 2004; Hofvander et al. 2009; Rydén and Bejerot 2008; Lugnegård et al. 2011). Regardless of the true prevalence, there is evidence that few of these patients are medicated with a mood stabilizer (Hofvander et al. 2009). This should be a cause of concern for all those involved in assessing and treating this special group of individuals with ASD, as bipolar disorder is a highly disabling, albeit, treatable disorder. Stahlberg et al. noted, in their study, that the prevalence of bipolar disorder or psychosis was not higher in the relatives of ASD probands with any of these two diagnoses than it was in relatives of ASD probands without bipolar disorder or psychosis, which could reflect an unspecific vulnerability for these two major disorders in ASD, rather than the action of specific genetic factors (Stahlberg et al. 2004).

Even though it is never too much to insist that ASD is not a form of early onset psychosis, and notwithstanding the caveat that many of the manifestations of ASD, especially in adults, may easily be mistaken for psychotic symptoms, the truth is that psychosis does occur in ASD and is particularly likely to be seen in late adolescence and early adulthood, similar to what occurs in non-ASD individuals (Stahlberg et al. 2004). Reported prevalence numbers for non-affective psychosis in adults with a first-time diagnosis of ASD vary between 5 and 8 % (Stahlberg et al. 2004; Ghaziuddin and Zafar 2008; Marriage et al. 2009; Lehnhardt et al. 2012) and 12–13 % (Hofvander et al. 2009; Joshi et al. 2013). The higher figures were reported by groups who used the Structured Clinical Interview for DSM to screen for comorbid diagnoses (Stahlberg et al. 2004; Hofvander et al. 2009; Joshi et al. 2013), while the lower numbers mostly come from studies that resourced to chart reviews or unstructured psychiatric assessments (Ghaziuddin and Zafar 2008; Marriage et al. 2009; Lehnhardt et al. 2012). It is noteworthy that Stahlberg et al. (2004), when comparing their sample of adults with late-diagnosed ASD with a group of adults with late-diagnosed attention deficit/hyperactivity disorder, found a similar prevalence, in both groups, of bipolar disorder, but a higher prevalence of psychosis, including schizophrenia, in the ASD group (Stahlberg et al. 2004). Again, there is a risk of simultaneous over- and underdiagnosis of psychosis in ASD, and while many ASD patients with psychosis remain untreated, previous treatment with antipsychotics is relatively prevalent in ASD, including in adults with a first-time diagnosis (Hofvander et al. 2009; Esbensen et al. 2009).

In spite of the fact that DSM-IV and DSM-IV TR precluded a diagnosis of ADHD in the presence of an ASD, many studies in children found an association between the two disorders in a substantial proportion of children with an ASD (Joshi et al. 2010; Gillberg et al. 2015). Studies in adults have been much more rare, and particularly so in adults with a first-time diagnosis of ASD. Hofvander et al. (2009) found enough criteria for a diagnosis of ADHD in 43 % of their sample, with a predominance of the inattentive and combined subtypes (17 % and 19 %, respectively) (Hofvander et al. 2009). Joshi et al. (2013) likewise found that 42 % of their late-diagnosed adult ASD patients qualified for a diagnosis of ADHD at the time of assessment, with a much higher lifetime prevalence of ADHD in this group, of around 68 % (Joshi et al. 2013). Lugnegård et al. report a prevalence of current ADHD of 31 % in their sample of Asperger syndrome cases (Lugnegård et al. 2011). In spite of these impressive figures, ADHD had rarely been diagnosed and adequately treated before in most cases when patients finally looked for expert advice. Moreover, both ASD and ADHD are severely underdiagnosed in adults by general psychiatrists without expertise in the field, adding to the unlikelihood of a timely and correct diagnosis outside a specialized clinical setting. Again, this is regrettable as ADHD is easily treated with success, and untreated ADHD is likely to aggravate the many executive and psychosocial difficulties already faced by most ASD subjects. Stahlberg et al. (2004), studying a mixed clinical sample of adults with a first-time diagnosis of ASD and adults with a first-time diagnosis of ADHD, found that 38 % of those with a primary diagnosis of ASD also fulfilled criteria for ADHD, while 30 % of those with a primary diagnosis of ADHD also had an ASD (Stahlberg et al. 2004). Ghaziuddin and Zafar (2008) found a somewhat lower rate (18 %), possibly because they did not use a structured interview for diagnosis (Ghaziuddin and Zafar 2008). Rydén and Bejerot (2008) found a diagnosis of ADHD in 37 % of their sample and, importantly, found that late-diagnosed ASD adults with comorbid ADHD were significantly less prone to develop repetitive and stereotyped routines and were therefore more likely to go undiagnosed (i.e., in the presence of a diagnosis of ADHD, the ASD diagnosis is more likely to be missed) (Ryden et al. 2008).

Disorders related to the use of alcohol or drugs are not rare in late-diagnosed adults with an ASD. Marriage et al. found that 4 (11 %) of their 34 cases had a present or past history of substance abuse, and Hofvander et al. report a lifetime prevalence of 16 % for substance use-related disorders in their sample of 122 adults, close to the 19 % reported by Lugnegård et al. (2011) (Hofvander et al. 2009; Marriage et al. 2009). Joshi et al. (2013) found a lifetime prevalence of 33 % for substance use disorders in their sample. Most cases were related to alcohol abuse or dependence (29 % and 13 %, respectively), although drug abuse and drug dependence also occur in a minority of patients (14 % and 5 % lifetime prevalence, respectively) (Joshi et al. 2013). Cannabis is by far the most frequently abused drug among adults with ASD, although other drugs like hallucinogens, benzodiazepines, and cocaine are also relatively common among those with a history of drug use (Joshi et al. 2013). It is not clear what makes late-diagnosed ASD adults in particular so vulnerable to alcohol abuse or dependence, but it probably reflects the fact that these patients, being relatively more exposed to social conformity pressures from their peers (age-peer groups at school, work colleagues, etc.), resource to alcohol to "fit in" with behavior patterns that are prevalent in these social contexts. Moreover, it is likely that many patients gradually learn to use alcohol to control social anxiety and to overcome behavioral inhibition in social situations perceived as intimidating. In the long run, however, this poses them at risk of a worse psychosocial outcome. In their study of 70 ASD adults who had been referred to one of two specialized centers for the diagnosis of ASD in adults, Sizoo et al. (2010) found a prevalence of substance use disorders of 30 %, which, the authors claim, is similar to the prevalence of comorbid substance use disorders in psychiatric disorders in general (Sizoo et al. 2010). These subjects had a worst psychosocial functioning than counterparts with no history of substance use disorders. Risk factors associated with the odds of developing a substance use disorder were the same as in subjects with no ASD: a family history of substance use disorders, a disturbed early family environment, and early onset of smoking (Sizoo et al. 2010).

Eating disorders have rarely been studied in adults with ASD, and even less so in adults with a first-time diagnosis of an ASD (Råstam 2008). Lehnhardt et al. (2012) found a diagnosis of eating disorder in 9 % of their sample, and Hofvander et al. (2009), using the SCID, diagnosed an eating disorder in 5 % of their sample (Hofvander et al. 2009; Lehnhardt et al. 2012). Neither of these authors specifies any further which subtype of eating disorder was found in their patients. Given that eating disorders, and specially anorexia nervosa, may have extremely adverse outcomes and have very specific treatment needs, this is clearly an area where more research is warranted. In a systematic review of published literature on eating disorders and ASD, Rastam (2008) found that eating problems (from food refusal to pica, overeating, and other forms of abnormal eating behavior) have been frequently reported in ASD patients of all ages and are present in up to 90 % of cases in childhood (Råstam 2008). Patients of all ages will often limit their choice of foods to just a few varieties and will often reject certain colors, textures, or smells (Gillberg 2002; Attwood 2007; Leekam et al. 2007). This is particularly frequent in patients with prominent perceptual abnormalities like texture hypersensitivity. Interestingly, the opposite may also be a problem, with low sensitivity to taste leading to exaggerated use of salt or other seasonings. Ritualized eating may also be problematic and socially conspicuous, e.g., eating all the potatoes first, separating all the ingredients in the plate, or grouping foods by color or some other criterion. Interest restriction may also be reflected in eating behaviors in this group, and there is some evidence that vegetarianism, orthorexia nervosa (an obsessive concern with eating supposedly healthy foods), and other forms of excessive concern over the composition of meals may be quite frequent in adults with ASD (Råstam 2008). Other patients may develop odd beliefs about what is healthy or not or about what sort of nutrients their bodies need. The end result of all these dyspragmatic concerns about food is often an extremely unbalanced and unhealthy diet and a host of somatic problems from gastrointestinal problems to vitamin and mineral deficiencies. Regarding anorexia nervosa specifically, there is evidence that it may be more common in the extended families of patients with ASD than in the general population, and women with anorexia nervosa often disclose a history of autistic-like traits in childhood, with few peer relations, perfectionism, obsessive adherence to routines, emotional restraint, and deficits in the expression of empathy (Zucker et al. 2007). Moreover, excessive focusing on details to the detriment of a coherent perception of relevant information as a whole, i.e., weak central coherence, seems to be a cognitive feature of both ASD and anorexia nervosa (Carina Gillberg et al. 2007). In summary, there is a fair amount of evidence that anorexia nervosa and ASD may share vulnerability and etiologic factors. Furthermore, there seems to be a gender bias by which ASD tends to be underdiagnosed in girls with anorexia nervosa, and anorexia nervosa tends to be underdiagnosed in low weight boys with ASD.

Most adults with an ASD also meet diagnostic criteria for at least one personality disorder, and it is not infrequent, when these patients first seek help from specialized clinicians, that a prior diagnosis of personality disorder has been formulated (Hofvander et al. 2009). Indeed, differential diagnosis is often difficult between ASD and certain personality disorders such as schizoid personality disorder or anankastic personality disorder (Lehnhardt et al. 2012). Moreover, social clumsiness and lack of empathic skills may lead adult subjects to behave in ways that are perceived and described by others as aggressive, provocative, or plainly antisocial, often prompting an inappropriate diagnosis of cluster B personality disorder. Unsurprisingly, many, if not most, adults with a first-time diagnosis of ASD meet formal diagnostic criteria for at least one and often two or more personality disorders. Hofvander et al. (2009), for instance, found that 62 % of their 117 adults with late-diagnosed ASD met criteria for one personality disorder, while 35 % met criteria for two, and 17 % met criteria for at least three different personality disorders (Hofvander et al. 2009). Paranoid, schizoid, schizotypal, avoidant, and anankastic personality disorder were the most frequently diagnosed personality disorders (Hofvander et al. 2009). Rydén and Bejerot (2008) found that their sample of late-diagnosed ASD adults had a median of four personality disorders as diagnosed by the Structured Clinical Interview for DSM Axis II Disorders (SCID-II), the most frequently diagnosed disorders being avoidant, borderline, and anankastic personality disorder, closely followed by schizoid and schizotypal personality disorder (Rydén and Bejerot 2008). Joshi et al. (2013) found 8 % of their adult patients meeting the criteria for antisocial personality disorder, while Lehnhardt et al. report much lower prevalence figures for personality disorder, with a predominance of schizoid and borderline personality disorder (Lehnhardt et al. 2012; Joshi et al. 2013). Such disparity in numbers, and the fact that such a high proportion of patients meet criteria for more than one personality disorder, clearly show the limited utility of this construct to describe and classify the symptoms, problems, and disabilities of adults with ASD. In contrast, a dimensional characterization of the predominant personality traits present in late-diagnosed ASD adults does seem to provide a useful profile. Rydén and Bejerot, using the Swedish Universities Scales of Personality, a self-assessment questionnaire, found that ASD adults in this particular subgroup predominantly describe themselves as avoidant and withdrawn, highly susceptible to stress, insecure, and unable to be self-assertive in social situations while at the same time being prone to feelings of envy and blaming toward others (Rydén and Bejerot 2008). This important observation clearly shows that, far from naïve, self-centered or indifferent to others and to their own social ineptness, ASD adults are painfully aware of their disabilities, tending to see themselves as inferior to others and to resent their exclusion from normal, successful social intercourse. In another study, Rydén et al. (2008) set out to study the prevalence of ASD in a sample of successive adult women with a diagnosis of borderline personality disorder. They concluded that 15 % of these patients, a substantial proportion, also met the criteria for ASD and found that this particular subgroup had not only a much worse outcome with respect to living autonomously, having a partner or being employed, but also had a much higher number of previous suicide attempts, in comparison with women with borderline personality disorder without ASD (Ryden et al. 2008). It is not fully clear what to make out of these surprising results. Are these truly comorbid cases or do they simply reflect the fact that a young female adult with marked difficulties managing interpersonal relationships, impaired social and occupational functioning, and unpredictable, often disturbing or self-injuring behavior is much more likely to receive a diagnosis of borderline personality disorder than one of ASD, even in cases in whom the latter diagnosis would much more aptly capture the constellation of her problems and disabilities? It also probably reflects the fact that women with ASD are much more likely to remain undiagnosed until adulthood regardless of their level of functioning, in contrast with male late-diagnosed ASD subjects, who tend to be high functioning. Rydén et al. (2008) therefore recommend that in women with a working diagnosis of borderline personality, an additional (or possibly alternative) diagnosis of ASD should be contemplated and investigated if there is no history of substance abuse or in the presence of frequent suicidal ideation or suicide attempts that are unrelated to separation fears or devoid of any obvious manipulative motivation, and when the patient manifests a pronounced and relentlessly negative self-image (Ryden et al. 2008). The distinction is, evidently, of paramount importance, as it is doubtful if interventions for borderline personality disorder would be any good for young women with ASD.

Suicide remains flagrantly understudied in adults with ASD, and even more so in the case of adults with and undiagnosed ASD. This is all the more surprising as the few data that have been published suggest that suicide attempts may actually be a frequent event in this particularly vulnerable subgroup, and possibly more frequent than in other vulnerable groups such as patients with psychosis or multiple physical illnesses (Cassidy et al. 2014). Rydén and Bejerot (2008), for instance, found that 17 % of the subjects in their sample had made at least one suicide attempt in the past (Rydén and Bejerot 2008). Lehnhardt, in a similar sample, also found a history of suicide attempts in 11 % of their ASD cases (Lehnhardt et al. 2012). On the other hand, Kato et al. (2013), in a study of 587 adults consecutively admitted to a general hospital's critical care unit following severe nonfatal suicide attempts, found that 7.3 % had an ASD (Kato et al. 2013). Moreover, this important study also found that ASD adults who attempted suicide were much more likely than non-ASD suicide attempters to choose high-lethality self-harm methods such as carbon monoxide poisoning or self-cutting/self-stabbing (Kato et al. 2013). Unlike non-ASD suicide attempters, most (81 %) ASD subjects in this clinical sample were males, and suicide attempts were apparently not related to events in the last 24 h, suggesting that they were less impulsive and more closely planned than those of non-ASD suicide attempters. In line with these findings, Takara and Kondo (2014a, b) found that among depressed adults attending a psychiatric outpatient clinic, previously undiagnosed ASD features figured as one of three factors that were significantly associated with suicide attempts, the others being agitation and a past history of suicide attempts (Takara and Kondo 2014b). Again, ASD subjects were more likely to attempt suicide by violent methods (hanging, in 44 % of cases), in contrast with non-ASD patients, who more often resourced to drug overdose (Takara and Kondo 2014b). Social isolation, lack of a confident, and awareness of the discrepancy between demands for social adjustment and true social and interpersonal abilities have all been cited as factors contributing to the high risk of attempted or completed suicide in ASD adults. A further, seldom mentioned factor is the lack of access to appropriate mental health care, mostly due to underdiagnosis of both the ASD and related comorbidities. This is supported by the fact that in the study by Kato et al. (2013), the overwhelming majority of ASD suicide attempters had no previous contacts with mental health services or a previous history of psychiatric treatment (Kato et al. 2013).

It must be stressed that all these figures refer to convenience clinical samples and not to population-based samples and are therefore in all likelihood overestimations. Nonetheless, on the whole, it is clear that adults with undiagnosed ASD are particularly vulnerable to comorbid psychiatric disorders in general. It is difficult to disentangle to what extent this clinically apparent comorbidity reflects shared biological factors, overlapping phenomenological features between ASD and certain disorders (e.g., social phobia), or an increased vulnerability of ASD adults to the multiple factors that influence the risk of developing a psychiatric disorder in the non-ASD general population. An important study by Kreiser and White found, in a sample of university students, that the load of previously undiagnosed ASD traits correlates with the likelihood of meeting diagnostic criteria for comorbid psychiatric disorders, particularly mood disorders (including bipolar disorder), anxiety disorders, and substance use disorders (Kreiser and White 2015). This suggests that, regardless of the role almost certainly played by other factors, ASD constitute in themselves a source of vulnerability to the development of other mental disorders in affected adults.

5.2.3 Differential Diagnosis Issues in Adults with a First-Time Diagnosis of Autism Spectrum Disorder

As we saw in the previous section, psychiatric comorbidity in adults with a first-time diagnosis of ASD is the rule rather than the exception. This faces the managing clinician or therapist with a double diagnostic challenge. The first difficulty is that of diagnosing an ASD in the presence of a major psychiatric comorbidity that may modify or masquerade the ASD. The second difficulty has to do with the fact that common mental disorders such as major depression or anxiety disorders often manifest in a totally atypical way in adults with ASD (or for that matter, in any adults with a developmental disorder), which is often misleading for the inexperienced health professional and may lead to unnecessary, un-indicated, or even plainly harmful treatments and interventions. This is particularly likely to happen when symptoms of ASD are attributed to another mental disorder characterized by impairments in social interaction, social isolation, atypical communication style, or stereotyped behavior (Takara and Kondo 2014a; Lai and Baron-Cohen 2015). The few studies that have looked at previous non-ASD diagnoses in adults with a first-time diagnosis of ASD have indeed found that a substantial proportion of cases had been in contact with mental health services before, often for a significant number of years, and had received alternative diagnoses. The most frequently diagnosed disorders in these undiagnosed ASD adults were depressive (10–12 %) and anxiety disorders (10–15 %), although, worryingly, psychosis had also been diagnosed in between 10 and 25 % of these subjects (Geurts and Jansen 2011; Nylander and Gillberg 2001).

The most problematic differential diagnosis dilemma, even for the experienced clinician, is probably the distinction between ASD and disorders in the schizoid spectrum, particularly schizoid personality disorder, schizotypal disorder, and certain presentations of schizophrenia, such as simple schizophrenia or hebephrenic schizophrenia. Mouridsen et al. (2008), in a study of 89 adults who had been diagnosed with an ASD in childhood, found that roughly 35 % had received a diagnosis of a schizophrenia spectrum disorder at least once in their lifetime, clearly illustrating the tendency to overdiagnose this disorder in ASD adults and adolescents (Mouridsen et al. 2008). Every clinician with experience in diagnosing and treating adults with ASD will have met several cases that had previously been misdiagnosed (and consequently mistreated) as schizophrenia or atypical psychosis, a risk that is probably higher in those cases that are higher functioning (Fitzgerald 2012; Underwood et al. 2015). The potentially catastrophic consequences of such a misdiagnosis are self-evident: unnecessary treatment with antipsychotics, unnecessary hospitalizations, and inadequate rehabilitation settings, to name a few. For the clinician with no experience in the field, the often eccentric, or even frankly odd interests; the rigid, stereotyped, or apparently emotionless expression and avoidant gaze; the overly pedantic, often incessant speech; the original though many times bewilderingly literal or concrete ideas; or the atypical mimic and motor stereotypies all concur to a comprehensible confusion with the idiosyncrasies of delusional, formally disordered thought processes, emotional inadequacy, and paranoid rapport that are typical of schizophrenia or severe psychosis (Lai and Baron-Cohen 2015). Reduced body language and facial expression, monotonous prosody, laconic speech, lack of initiative, social withdrawal, vague, overelaborate or disorganized thought processes are other characteristics that are common to both schizophrenia and ASD. Unsurprisingly, adult subjects with schizophrenia tend to score high on the Autism Diagnostic Observation Schedule, and their score on this instrument correlates positively with their score on negative symptom scales (Bastiaansen et al. 2011). Moreover, ASD adults are prone to engage in self-talk and to invent new words, something that may be easily misinterpreted by the observing clinician as evidence of auditory hallucinations and neologisms. Things are made worse by the potential for reciprocal misunderstanding between clinician and ASD patient in the course of a standard psychiatric interview (Buck et al. 2014). Closed questions regarding certain psychotic symptoms will be interpreted and answered literally, the typical example being the patient who answers affirmatively when asked if he hears voices because he is indeed hearing voices: his own, the clinician's, and those of people sitting next room or passing by the door (Fitzgerald 2012; Lai and Baron-Cohen 2015). Unusual perceptual experiences often described by ASD individuals, especially those involving smell, will invariably be taken as further evidence of hallucinatory phenomena, and the abrupt, clumsy way in which ASD patients often will force their favorite subjects into the conversation as evidence of formal thought disorder. Things are made even more confusing by the fact that both patients with schizophrenia and subjects with ASD manifest difficulties negotiating theory of mind challenges. It must be said, however, that, tantalizing as they may be, these overwhelming similarities are no more than superficial and will succumb to an attentive and detailed semiological investigation. It is helpful to think about the differentiation of the two disorders in terms of both cross-sectional differences and longitudinal differences. For one thing, it is of fundamental importance to keep in mind that bizarre is not necessarily, and as a matter of fact is not even usually, synonymous with psychotic. The Jasperian concept of incomprehensibility as the central defining characteristic of psychotic life experiences is immensely useful here. The ASD patient, unlike the psychotic patient, will not provide a delusional justification for his unusual perceptual experiences. Neologisms, rather than the idiosyncratic, undecipherable words whose meaning is accessible exclusively to the subject, as typically found in schizophrenia, are unusual but meaningful in ASD, frequently resulting from fusing two or more words, two idioms, or from turning nouns into verbs or vice versa, in what often amounts to a playful if pedantic display of verbal agility. Unusual thoughts and beliefs likewise prove nonpsychotic when subject to a careful inquiry into their genesis: rather than the product of primarily paranoid phenomena such as delusional perceptions or delusional intuitions, they typically result, in the ASD patient, from over-literal, concrete, often even naïve ways of assimilating and reproducing complex information that has been heard from others, or read in the Internet or in books, and misinterpreted (Buck et al. 2014). These are thoughts and beliefs that are comprehensible (in the Jasperian sense of the word) in light of the difficulty of the ASD individual to read between the lines and capture implicit and metaphoric meanings, to understand humor, or to decipher irony. Moreover, when compared to adults with schizophrenia, adults with an ASD tend, in spite of quantitative overlaps in total ADOS[1] scores, to show higher scores in the items related to stereotyped language, lack of reciprocal social communication, qualitatively poor social responses, and overall rapport quality (Bastiaansen et al. 2011). Longitudinally, the most obvious difference is that ASD core signs and symptoms are present from birth and tend to improve with age, while schizophrenia develops much later and deficits tend to worsen with age. In ASD the first years of life are invariably marked by atypical psychomotor development. Even HFA patients often spoke their first words late or walked later than usual. Moreover, poor eye contact, passivity, lack of interest for physical contact, lack of anticipatory approach behavior, and fascination with parts of objects or spinning objects, in short, the whole myriad of typical early autistic signs, are of course absent from the developmental history of patients with schizophrenia (Tantam 2000; Fitzgerald 2012). Certain features, such as savant skills, when present, argue vehemently in favor of an ASD diagnosis (Fitzgerald 2012). Moreover, even if attenuated in adolescence and adulthood, the typical autistic phenotype is semiologically stable in the long term, unlike schizophrenia, which frequently alternates crises with remissions. Needless to say, an exhaustive and careful anamnesis of early development and childhood is the decisive element here (Lai and Baron-Cohen 2015).

In the case of schizoid personality disorder, the sexual indifference and social aloofness, as well as the apparent emotional coldness and the lack of initiative that characterize so many young adults with ASD certainly make this a tempting

[1] Autism Diagnostic Observation Schedule; see (Lord et al. 2000)

alternative diagnosis. However, unlike ASD subjects, individuals with a schizoid personality have impaired social functioning as a result of their detached, avoidant style of rapport, rather than as a consequence of impairments in communication abilities (Tantam 2000). As for schizotypal personality disorder, current definitions make the distinction easier as they tend to overemphasize the disorder's quasi-psychotic features and its proximity to the positive features of other disorders of the schizoid spectrum such as schizophrenia (American Psychiatric Association (institution) 2013). Furthermore, restriction of interests and activities is not typically seen in schizoid or schizotypal disorder (Lai and Baron-Cohen 2015).

Anankastic personality disorder is another disorder where many ASD-like behaviors and symptoms occur that may make differential diagnosis more difficult, mostly due to the fact that in both disorders patients may develop excessively ritualized behaviors and routines, social isolation, poor expression of emotions, limited, rigid body language and high levels of trait anxiety (Tantam 2000). It is interesting to note here that ASD adults, when responding to self-rating questionnaires, tend to report as OCD symptoms behaviors that are reported by their parents as being part of the ASD core symptoms and as having been present from childhood (Moss et al. 2015). This highlights the difficulty of reliably assessing psychiatric comorbidity in ASD adults using screening instruments that were designed for the general population. Things are made more complicated by the fact that obsessive-compulsive disorder (OCD) seems to be more prevalent in ASD patients than in the general population (Russell et al. 2005). The phenomenology of repetitive behaviors is, again, decisive for differential diagnosis. Obsessions in OCD are experienced by the subject as intrusive, unwanted, and disturbing thoughts that the subject feels as incongruent with his view of himself and of the world around him (i.e., obsessions in OCD are by definition egodystonic). As such, they arouse severe and often incapacitating anxiety in the subject, who tries to suppress them from consciousness, typically by way of compulsive rituals. In contrast, the repetitive behaviors of ASD are usually a reflection of the subject's restricted, over-invested interests and are not seen as intrusive or disturbing to the patient, who will usually take great pleasure and satisfaction from their performance (Miguel et al. 2001; Lai and Baron-Cohen 2015). Additionally, the manifestations of ASD typically present from a very early age, while OCD typically develops at school age or later (Bernardo Barahona-Corrêa et al. 2015).

Antisocial and narcissistic personality disorder may also occasionally be diagnosed in adults with an ASD, given their self-centeredness, lack of emotional reciprocity and empathy, and apparent emotional coldness. However, adults with antisocial or narcissistic personality disorder are clearly distinguishable from adults with an ASD by having intact theory of mind abilities and normal or above-average deception ability but reduced ability to respond with the appropriate emotion to another person's emotional state. In contrast, ASD subjects typically may fail to recognize signs of emotional distress in others but will respond with concern and the appropriate emotion when explicitly alerted to them (Lai and Baron-Cohen 2015).

Social phobia and avoidant personality disorder are another two disorders that manifest from late adolescence onward and may easily be mistaken for, or diagnosed in place of, an ASD. Cross-sectional comparisons show considerable symptom overlap between ASD and social anxiety, and both socially phobic and avoidant individuals may display abnormal nonverbal communication skills and avoidant gaze when socially uncomfortable or when they feel scrutinized by others (Cath et al. 2008; Tyson and Cruess 2012). Interestingly, in spite of these phenomenological similarities, their initial face-scanning pattern is actually similar to that of neurotypical subjects, unlike that of ASD adults (Tyson and Cruess 2012). In situations of social scrutiny, adults with social phobia may even manifest socially clumsy reactions to approaches from others, stereotyped, restricted mimic, and inappropriately laconic speech, which are all features typically found in the young adult with an ASD (Tyson and Cruess 2012; Lehnhardt et al. 2013). In addition to the absent history of abnormalities in social interaction and communication since childhood, a diagnosis of social phobia or avoidant personality should be favored if the affected subject only shows abnormal social behavior when faced with unfamiliar social situations where he or she fears negative judgment by others (Lai and Baron-Cohen 2015). Finally, socially phobic and avoidant individuals do not exhibit the intensely pursued, restricted interests and activities typical of ASD (Tantam 2000).

5.2.4 Diagnosing Psychiatric Comorbidity in Adults with an Autism Spectrum Disorder

One of the great challenges for the psychiatrist dealing with adults with an ASD is that of deciphering the extremely atypical clinical presentation of other mental disorders in this population, especially as the most unusual manifestations will tend to be those of common mental disorders, i.e., major depression or generalized anxiety are more likely to manifest with highly atypical and unexpected changes in behavior that will often divert clinical reasoning away from the correct diagnosis, while rare, severe mental disorders will manifest with symptoms and signs that are closer to those found in the non-ASD population (Underwood et al. 2015). This means that the clinician has to constantly bear in mind the relative frequency of possible comorbid mental disorders when assessing an individual case, rather than any specific, telltale symptoms. Moreover, the old medical precept that we are more likely to meet unusual presentations of common disorders than to meet common presentations of rare disorders cannot be overemphasized in the context of mental disorders in subjects with a neurodevelopmental disorder.

As we saw, major depression is by far the most common mental disorder in adults with an ASD and also holds the distinction of being the single mental illness that is most likely to be both over and underdiagnosed in this population (Ghaziuddin et al. 2002; Ghaziuddin and Zafar 2008; Takara and Kondo 2014a). Indeed, the monotonous prosody, the poverty of body language and mimic, or the apparently emotionless attitude of many adults with ASD will easily be mistaken for depressive symptoms (Ghaziuddin et al. 2002; Takara and Kondo 2014a), more so as adolescents and young adults with ASD often use powerful or disturbing idiomatic expressions, often including terms such as death, suicide, or even psychopathological jargon to convey trivial messages. One patient, for example, complained that watching football matches on the TV with his high school mates was such an ordeal to him that he might as well kill himself. Another patient said that life was a walk through the shadow of the valley of death, but what he actually meant by this was that his almost complete devotion to the Internet was a perfect substitute for real life with real people and real places. Identification of depressive symptoms in adults with an ASD is often difficult due to the fact that patients have great difficulty recognizing and describing their own emotional states and affective symptoms (Ghaziuddin et al. 2002; Underwood et al. 2015). Moreover, the often poor baseline emotional expressivity of ASD patients renders depressive signs much harder to detect by the clinical observer. Other, more indirect signs and symptoms are therefore much more important and should be watched for by those caring for this particular group of patients, namely, changes in appetite and energy, sudden unexpected crying spells, an aggravation of social withdrawal with much more time spent in bed than usual, or loss of interest for usual activities, including previously highly rewarding repetitive or stereotyped activities linked to the subject's idiosyncratic, restricted interests (Ghaziuddin et al. 2002; Stewart et al. 2006). Autistic preoccupations may suffer a subtle change in character or content, and obsessions and typical obsessive-compulsive behaviors such as hand-washing may become aggravated or may appear de novo (Ghaziuddin et al. 2002). In other patients, especially those who have a lower level of functioning, there may be an aggravation of certain autistic manifestations, such as hand flapping, echolalia, or ritualistic behavior (Stewart et al. 2006). Increased or unusual physical complaints are another frequent presentation of depression in ASD adults, as are changes in sleep or sleep quality. Finally, it is always important to watch out for significant changes of behavior from a previous habitual baseline and to bear in mind that, similarly to non-ASD subjects, ASD adults often develop major depressive episodes following stressful life events (Ghaziuddin et al. 2002; Lai and Baron-Cohen 2015; Underwood et al. 2015).

Similar to depressive symptoms, signs and symptoms of anxiety may also be difficult to identify in an adult with an ASD. Patients' inability to identify and describe inner states again means that anxiety manifests more clearly in terms of physical and behavioral signs, often better described by those who know the patient well, such as spouses or work colleagues, than as subjective complaints (Davis et al. 2008; Underwood et al. 2015). Examples of such signs are increased intensity of stereotyped behaviors, sleep disturbance, an increase in motor stereotypies, gross agitation with hand flapping and other motor or vocal stereotyped behaviors, and, evidently, signs of autonomic activation (Ghaziuddin et al. 2002; Rodgers et al. 2012). The latter occasionally may lead the patient to seek medical help out of fear of having a cardiovascular disorder. Again, it is important and revealing to explore the antecedents of symptoms, as anxiety typically develops or aggravates in ASD adults in situations that are unpredictable or that imply significant changes to the subject's established routines (Davis et al. 2008; Lai and Baron-Cohen 2015).

Assessing psychiatric morbidity in high-functioning adults with an ASD is challenging and requires time, repeated observation over several occasions, and experience. The recognition of common psychopathology is made difficult not only, as we mentioned already, by patients' difficulty in recognizing their own inner states and emotions but also by their deficits in social communication and nonverbal language. It is important to bear in mind that patients with higher scores of ASD core symptoms tend to be less able to report on their own psychopathology, regardless of cognitive and verbal ability (Moss et al. 2015). The examiner should use a simple and straightforward language, avoiding abstract terms and metaphorical expressions that are likely to be taken literally or will not be understood at all. Time must be given for the patient to fully process questions and answers, and the examiner must constantly make sure that the patient understands what is being asked. Moreover, obtaining complementary anamnestic data from a second informant is of paramount importance, the ideal being persons who have frequent regular contact with the patient and the patient's routines. It is nevertheless worthwhile remembering that self-ratings and ratings by parents on psychopathology screening instruments are only modestly correlated, with the patients tending to score much higher on certain dimensions such as depression, anxiety, or OCD than their parents (Buck et al. 2014; Moss et al. 2015). Access to previous clinical reports and a good description of previous mental health episodes, and how they were treated, is another important complement to the assessment of present psychopathology. Screening instruments and structured interviews to assess psychopathology in high-functioning ASD adults specifically have yet to be developed. A review by Underwood et al. found only two instruments for the assessment of psychopathology in ASD adults with intellectual disability, and none for high-functioning ASD adults (Underwood et al. 2011), a situation that has since known little change (Moss et al. 2015). Psychiatric diagnoses will therefore have to be formulated based on standard DSM-5 and ICD-10 criteria for the latter group of patients.

5.3 Psychosocial Functioning of Adults with a Newly Diagnosed Autism Spectrum Disorder

The few studies on adults with a first-time diagnosis of ASD report psychosocial functioning patterns that seem to be similar or only slightly better than those found in HFA subjects diagnosed in childhood or adolescence. Although the psychosocial functioning of this particular subgroup is almost unanimously described as fair, a more detailed look at the available evidence quickly shows that the term fair is a misleading oversimplification. Indeed, most studies actually show that ASD patients diagnosed in adulthood receive extensive support from their families, are seldom fully employed in regular paid jobs, and are mostly living alone and without close partner relationships.

5.3.1 Work

Findings vary greatly across studies with respect to the occupational status of adults with newly diagnosed ASD, similarly to follow-up studies of ASD children into adult age (Engstrom et al. 2003; Stahlberg et al. 2004; Rydén and Bejerot 2008; Hofvander et al. 2009; Marriage et al. 2009; Lehnhardt et al. 2012; Joshi et al. 2013). This variation naturally reflects the inevitable differences, across studies, in recruitment and sampling methods, as well as regional and national specificities and macroeconomic changes over the years. Notwithstanding this, the available evidence shows that adults with newly diagnosed ASD, like those whose disorder has been diagnosed in a more typical age, tend to be underemployed, i.e., working in sheltered jobs, with relatives, or in occupations that are below their academic level of achievement. A substantial proportion of these subjects have either completed a university degree or are studying at university level, with at least one author (Lehnhardt et al. 2012) reporting a predominance of technical and scientific areas such as mathematics, computer science, or mechanics (Hofvander et al. 2009; Lehnhardt et al. 2012; Joshi et al. 2013). A history of grade repetition or special personalized support needs during schooling is a relatively frequent finding, possibly in as much as a half to two thirds of subjects in this special subgroup (Joshi et al. 2013). Compared to subjects diagnosed at younger ages, late-diagnosed adults with ASD do achieve higher rates of university or college-level education and employment (Marriage et al. 2009), but they have higher rates of unemployment when compared with adults with other neurodevelopmental disorders such as ADHD, which shows that finding and keeping a job is a particular problem in ASD (Rydén and Bejerot 2008). For instance, in their study of adults with Asperger syndrome, Lugnegård et al. found that 42 % had finished high school, and 15 % were attending university or had completed a university degree, yet only 4 % had a regular employment, and 62 % were living on a disability pension (Lugnegård et al. 2011). It is unclear which – if any – factors influence the probability of being and remaining fully employed in this group of ASD subjects (or, for that matter, in adults with a high-functioning ASD generally). Communication difficulties, socially inappropriate behaviors, difficulties in adapting to unpredictable changes, poor hygiene, poor coping with multiple tasks, and low productivity are recurrent problems identified in ASD workers by their neurotypical work colleagues, and probably decrease the probability that a worker with an ASD will be able to keep his job in a non-sheltered setting, regardless of his or her level of ability and competence (Howlin et al. 2005). Although it is logical to presume that having an university degree, higher intellect, or a milder phenotype have a positive impact on opportunities, this has not been proved, and the available evidence actually shows that even more able individuals with an university degree often lapse into inactivity after or shortly after they complete their formal training (Taylor and Seltzer 2011; Holwerda et al. 2012). Access to effective formal support in this domain, in the form of sheltered employment, in-job coaching, or other resources and support modalities, is probably more determinant for the occupational outcome of adults with an ASD than the individual's symptom profile or cognitive ability (Howlin and Moss 2012; Holwerda et al. 2012; Howlin et al. 2005). However, adults with a first-time diagnosis of ASD in adult age are unlikely to have any access to these forms of support prior to their diagnosis. For those who do manage to enter the competitive work market and remain employed for significant periods of time, the experience often proves overwhelming and a source of stress and anxiety. Interviews of adults diagnosed with ASD in adulthood have shown that many of those who had been employed earlier eventually surrendered to their difficulties and gave up from trying to remain employed (Griffith et al. 2012).

5.3.2 Family and Partnership

Although most adults with a high-functioning ASD, including those diagnosed late in their life course, are either living alone or with their families of origin (usually their parents), a significant proportion of the latter group are either married or living with a partner at the time of diagnosis (16 % according to Hofvander et al. 2009; the same figure is reported by Joshi et al. (2013); 17 % in the study by Rydén and Bejerot 2008) (Hofvander et al. 2009; Joshi et al. 2013), and many have children (Stahlberg et al. 2004; Rydén and Bejerot 2008; Lehnhardt et al. 2012). Lehnhardt et al. (2012) found that 58 % of their sample had a current or previous partnership or conjugal relationship, including 27 % who were either married or divorced and 16 % who had children (Lehnhardt et al. 2012). In the sample of 84 subjects described by Rydén and Bejerot, 7 (8.4 %) had children (Rydén and Bejerot 2008). In their comparison of ASD adults diagnosed before and after 18 years of age, Marriage et al. (2009) found that those diagnosed as adults had higher scores of adaptive functioning in the "intimate relations" domain, but the difference was not statistically significant, possibly due to the very low number of subjects in the early diagnosis group (Marriage et al. 2009).

5.3.3 Autonomous Living

Independent living is probably one of the domains of psychosocial functioning where late-diagnosed ASD adults differ the most from their counterparts diagnosed in infancy (Marriage et al. 2009). Engström et al. (2003) found up to 56 % of their late-diagnosed ASD patients living in their own houses, although with varying levels of support from their families or public entities (Engstrom et al. 2003). Hofvander et al. (2009) likewise found that half of the subjects above 23 years of age in their sample had independent living arrangements, and Lehnhardt et al. (2012) report that 39 % of their newly diagnosed ASD adults were living completely alone, and a further 29 % were living with a partner (or wife/husband) or with a partner and children (Hofvander et al. 2009; Lehnhardt et al. 2012). Rydén and Bejerot rather less optimistically report that only 27 % of their sample could be considered to have a good level of functioning, defined as having a job or an IQ-appropriate level of education, and living independently (Rydén and Bejerot 2008).

5.4 Diagnosing Autism Spectrum Disorders in High-Functioning Adults

5.4.1 Assessing ASD Symptoms and Signs

Diagnosing an ASD in an adult subject is a difficult clinical challenge even for the experienced clinician (Bastiaansen et al. 2011; Lai and Baron-Cohen 2015). Notwithstanding the growing literature calling attention to the need for more and better training in ASD-related issues for general psychiatrists and psychologists and even for primary care physicians, it is evidently unrealistic to expect that the necessary skills, experience, and training for accurately diagnosing and assessing ASD in adults will ever be widespread across all levels of care. A service organization perspective is therefore inescapable when addressing this issue, the objective being to cost-effectively identify and evaluate individuals in the general service-using population who may have a previously unidentified ASD and, within a reasonable time interval and with the highest possible accuracy, refer those with special needs to the adequate level of specialized care. Unfortunately, literature on how this diagnostic evaluation in an outpatient setting should proceed is scarce. In recent years a relatively consensual view has been developing that proposes a two or three-level pathway to diagnosis and care, epitomized in the recent guidelines issued in the United Kingdom by the National Institute for Health and Care Excellence (National Institute for Health and Care Excellence 2012). The rate-limiting step in the process clearly resides in the ability to identify those subjects whose clinical features mark them as being probable ASD cases, a task made more difficult by the fact that most cases that go undiagnosed until adult age probably correspond to what was formerly defined as Asperger syndrome, with normal language and intellectual development and subtle, difficult to elicit autistic spectrum core symptoms (Nylander and Gillberg 2001; Pilling et al. 2012; Lehnhardt et al. 2013; Lai and Baron-Cohen 2015). Furthermore, comorbidity is the rule rather than the exception, calling for an additional differential diagnostic effort (Lai and Baron-Cohen 2015). More often than not, adult patients with an undiagnosed ASD will seek help from mental health services due to co-occurring, common mental health problems such as anxiety or depression, whose presence can easily mask the underlying neurodevelopmental disorder – which, anyway, is unlikely to be considered by most professionals unfamiliar with this group of disorders in the first place (Nylander and Gillberg 2001; Geurts and Jansen 2011). The presence of a limited number of clues or "red flag" signs that every primary care physician, or general psychiatrist or psychologist should be able to identify, should prompt a more detailed screening for ASD core symptoms when associated with persistent, lifelong difficulties in initiating or maintaining friendships, persistent difficulties in academic achievement, vocational training or sustaining employment, a lifelong history of contact with mental health or learning disability services, or a known history of any neurodevelopmental condition (Nylander and Gillberg 2001; National Institute for Health and Care Excellence 2012; Pilling et al. 2012):

Social isolation since childhood
Inconvenient or un-empathic social behavior
Inappropriate self-centeredness
Poor, absent, or inappropriate (e.g., excessively fixed) eye contact
Poor facial mimic and limited use of expressive gesticulation during conversation
Atypical or stereotyped and monotonous prosody
Difficulty deciphering implicit social rules, second meanings, metaphors, or irony
Overinvestment in circumscribed areas of interest, lonesome passionate collecting
Inordinate accumulation of factual knowledge on restricted, unusual themes with little or no practical application
Rigid insistence on sameness in terms of habits and routines

All these red flag signs fall into one of the three core ASD phenomenological dimensions of disturbances of social interaction, impaired communication, and restricted interests and repetitive behavior patterns, which in DSM-5 have been grouped into a dyadic construct of disturbances in communication and social interaction and restricted interests and repetitive behaviors (Barahona-Corrêa and Filipe 2016). Interestingly, in a recent cluster analytic study of ASD core features in a large general adult population sample, Palmer et al. (2014) found that subclinical ASD features tend to occur in two distinct profiles: social difficulties with weak detail-oriented attention and good social skills with strongly detail-oriented attention (Palmer et al. 2014). This means that adult individuals being considered for a diagnosis of ASD should best be rated along these two independent dimensions of social difficulties (comprising a mixture of sociability deficits and theory of mind skills) and detail orientation (comprising features like being fascinated with numbers or dates, excessive collection of factual information, or fascination with patterns) (Palmer et al. 2014). Other clues that may be suggestive of an ASD diagnosis are a history of motor clumsiness or atypical reactivity to sensory stimuli (e.g., aversion to particular textures, smells or sounds, or indifference to painful stimuli) (Lehnhardt et al. 2013). If any of these clues are present and associated with relevant consequences in terms of psychosocial functioning, then it is appropriate to apply a screening instrument for ASD in adults. There are various screening instruments available that may be used to explore ASD signs and symptoms in adult subjects. Most have not been adequately validated and are in all likelihood not available in most idioms. Some screen ASD generically as a syndrome, while others specifically explore symptoms of Asperger syndrome (Matson and Boisjoli 2008; Lehnhardt et al. 2013; Lai and Baron-Cohen 2015). Even though the predictive value of many of these instruments is suboptimal or even frankly limited, their greatest usefulness resides in the fact that they offer the inexperienced clinician a score for systematically exploring and eliciting the core symptoms of ASD. The most unanimously recommended are the Autism Spectrum Quotient, the Social Responsiveness Scale-Adult version, and the Ritvo Autism Asperger Diagnostic Scale-Revised. All three of them are self-assessment questionnaires, and all have been shown to have good sensitivity and specificity for identifying adults with ASD in isolated studies (Lai and Baron-Cohen 2015). NICE guidelines specifically advise the use of the short version of the Autism Spectrum Quotient, commonly known as AQ-10 (National Institute for Health and Care Excellence 2012). This is a 10-item self-assessment questionnaire that includes only the most informative items of the larger version. A positive answer in six or more of the ten items is indicative of a probable ASD. It should be noted here that most screening instruments have a reasonable negative predictive value, but that a positive result by no means guarantees that an ASD is present, as subjects with other unrelated disorders such as schizophrenia or affective psychosis may also score highly in most instruments and scales (Lehnhardt et al. 2013; Lai and Baron-Cohen 2015). A word of caution is warranted with respect to diagnosing ASD in adult high-functioning women. There is ample evidence that high-functioning females with an ASD tend not only to be diagnosed at a later age than males, but also tend to be misdiagnosed with social phobia, borderline personality disorder, or avoidant personality disorder (Attwood 2007; Lugnegård et al. 2011; Van Wijngaarden-Cremers et al. 2014). In terms of symptom profile, there is evidence that females show less interest restriction and repetitive and stereotyped behaviors than males, with several authors claiming that ASD diagnostic criteria are based exclusively, or at least predominantly, on the male ASD behavioral phenotype (Van Wijngaarden-Cremers et al. 2014). This means that diagnosis in adult high-functioning females may be easily missed. It is therefore important for the clinician considering an ASD diagnosis in a young adult woman to bear in mind that ASD girls tend to have better imaginative play than boys, are socially more engaged, and tend to cultivate more socially acceptable special interests such as horses or popstars (Gillberg 2002; Attwood 2007; Van Wijngaarden-Cremers et al. 2014). In a head-to-head comparison of age and IQ-matched adult females and males with an ASD, Lai et al. (2011) found that women had better sociabilization and communication abilities and higher scores of lifetime sensory symptoms (Lai et al. 2011). Moreover, the same group noted that, unlike their adult male counterparts, adult ASD women with a history of delayed language development had lower cognitive ability than ASD females with normal language development history.

Once a diagnosis of ASD is suspected, a more formal investigation of the core symptoms of ASD should take place, preferentially by a mental health-care specialist with training and experience in diagnosing ASD in adults. This is a lengthy process that ideally involves a multidisciplinary approach and several sources of information as well as structured and nonstructured assessments (Lai and Baron-Cohen 2015). The fundamental goal is to ascertain the presence of a lifelong, pervasive history of impairment in social interaction, impaired communication abilities, and restricted interests and repetitive behaviors. The importance of the terms "lifelong" and "pervasive" cannot be overemphasized. Symptoms, as well as signs of impairment, should be present since early childhood, and although most high-functioning patients will have been aware of their impairments since as early as they can remember, an interview with the patient's parents, childhood caregivers, an older sibling, a neighbor, or friend of the family is, whenever possible, a decisive source of valuable information (Lai and Baron-Cohen 2015). This must include a detailed developmental history – it is not rare to find peculiarities in this area, such as late walking, early speech development, sudden late appearance of fully developed speech, or early use of sophisticated and pedantic vocabulary. It is important to bear in mind here that severe early affective and social deprivation may also lead to autistic-like manifestations and syndromes and should therefore be actively explored if suspected, namely, in those cases that have been through early institutionalization or have a history of foster care (Rutter et al. 2007). Clumsiness, communication impairment, interest restriction, and social isolation must be explicitly asked for and must be further investigated using more open or tangential questions, such as (to cite a few examples) (Lai and Baron-Cohen 2015) did the patient ever learn to ride a bike (motor skills)? What was the patient's favorite playing activity (interest restriction)? How did the patient compare to his/her siblings? When did the parents first become concerned that something might be wrong? Did the patient enjoy playing football or other team sports (motor skills, theory of mind skills, social skills)? Did the patient ever bring his school friends to the house or would he usually be invited by peers to go to theirs (social skills, reciprocal relationship deficits)? Changes and major transitions help informants to frame relevant time windows and are invariably a period of great, sometimes overwhelming stress to an ASD subject, therefore meriting careful exploration. In adolescence many of the core autistic features become more evident as the patient comes under peer pressure to conform to group norms and identity-forming age-typical stereotypes. Bullying is a particularly frequent occurrence at this time of life and should be explicitly investigated. In a study of adults with major depression and undiagnosed ASD, a past history of bullying was found to be one of the significant indicators that discriminated ASD patients from non-ASD subjects (Takara and Kondo 2014a). Other significant discriminators identified in the same study were a past history of school absenteeism, of quasi-psychotic experiences in childhood and adolescence, and of repeated interpersonal problems at work or school. Though unspecific in isolation, in the context of other clues, the presence of these factors is very supportive of an ASD diagnosis and should prompt a careful anamnestic exploration. It is important to note here that although adult patients with an ASD will evidently be able to provide accurate data on most of their developmental trajectory, it is not rare for young ASD adults to omit or distort relevant facts in an attempt to present a more favorable image to the clinician, at least in the first encounters. Tangential questioning about habits, preferences, friends and girl-/boyfriends, living situation, and other aspects of the patient's everyday life is again useful here, perhaps more useful than direct formal questioning about abstract ASD symptoms (Lehnhardt et al. 2013). Parent or sibling information is again decisive, as are other indirect sources of information such as end-of-period reports from teachers, photographs, and home videos (Lehnhardt et al. 2013; Lai and Baron-Cohen 2015). It is important to repeatedly confirm that impairments persisted continuously during the patient's life course and that they were evident in all areas of functioning, i.e., school, family life, occupational life or peer relations, among others. The retrospective assessment of these pervasive impairments is occasionally made more difficult by cross-generational differences with respect to views on what is normal or not, differences in educational practices, and the relative weight given to specific impairments and specific symptoms and signs (Lai and Baron-Cohen 2015; Attwood 2007). Structured assessment of core ASD symptoms and signs at this stage should ideally include the gold standards of diagnostic assessment of ASD, namely, the Autism Disorder Observation Schedule (ADOS) (Lord et al. 2000) for direct patient assessment and the Autism Diagnostic Interview-Revised (ADI-R) to interview caregivers (Lord et al. 1994; Matson and Goldin 2014). Possible alternatives to the latter, though much less studied and validated, might be the Adult Asperger Assessment (AAA) (Baron-Cohen et al. 2005), the Asperger Syndrome Diagnostic (and high-functioning autism) Interview (Gillberg et al. 2001), or the Diagnostic Interview for Social and Communication Disorders (Wing et al. 2002; Billstedt et al. 2007; Lai and Baron-Cohen 2015; Matson and Wilkins 2008). The AAA instrument has the advantage of allowing a simultaneous interview with the patient and the informant and additionally includes questions on peculiarities of communication not usually covered by other instruments, like pedantic speech or social inopportunity and lack of tact (Baron-Cohen et al. 2005; Lai and Baron-Cohen 2015).

Box 5.1
The ADI-R is a semi-structured clinical interview for caregivers of children and adults for whom a diagnosis of an ASD is being contemplated. The revised version follows a diagnostic algorithm that produces ASD diagnoses according to ICD-10 and DSM-IV criteria. The interview comprises 93 items organized into five sections: opening questions, early and current communication and language, early and current quality of social interactions, early and current repetitive and restricted behaviors (including unusual preoccupations, motor stereotypies, or perceptual abnormalities), and an additional number of questions assessing general behavior problems that might provide relevant complementary information or additional treatment needs, such as savant skills or self-injury (Lord et al. 1994). Each item is scored by the examiner based on the caregiver's responses and specific descriptions of the examinee's current and early behavior. The ADI-R was recently shown to have good sensitivity (88 %) and specificity (80 %) for diagnosing ASD in adults with an intellectual disability (Sappok et al. 2013). There is also evidence that the instrument has robust validity, sensitivity, and specificity, regardless of age and cognitive ability, except for very young age groups (below 5 years of age) (Tsuchiya et al. 2013). Notwithstanding these findings, the instrument's results must be interpreted with care when applied to adult subjects with elderly childhood caregivers as informers.

5.4.2 Cognitive Profile and Adaptive Functioning

Additionally, other structured assessments may be indicated, namely, IQ and IQ profile assessment, social cognition assessments, adaptive functioning assessments, or even neurological (e.g., electroencephalogram, neuroimaging, polysomnography) or genetic tests. It is important not to underestimate the importance of assessing adaptive behavior, a concept that encompasses the ability to function at age-appropriate levels of proficiency in areas that are critical to independent living, such as dressing and grooming, using money or public transportation, or being able to ask for a direction (Klin et al. 2007). Adaptive behavior is usually measured in three domains: socialization, communication, and daily living. ASD subjects, regardless of age, typically show deficits in all of these areas of adaptive functioning, with socialization being the most impaired domain. There is inconsistent evidence that severity of ASD symptoms correlates with adaptive behavior scores in these domains, especially with deficits in the socialization domain of adaptive behavior (Klin et al. 2007). The most important point, however, is that neither ASD severity nor IQ are good predictors of adaptive functioning (Klin et al. 2007; Kenworthy et al. 2010; Matthews et al. 2015). Indeed, in clinical practice it is not rare to meet adult patients with an apparently mild to moderate ASD phenotype and above-average IQ who have severe impairments in terms of independent living and adaptive functioning in general. This wide gap between cognitive ability and adaptive functioning has been empirically demonstrated by Matthews et al. (2015) in a study that assessed adaptive functioning in 75 ASD subjects aged between 16 and 58 years (Matthews et al. 2015). The two most studied and most commonly used instruments for assessing adaptive behavior in ASD are the Adaptive Behavior Assessment System (ABAS) (Harrison and Oakland 2003) and the Vineland Adaptive Behavior Scales (VABS) (Sparrow et al. 2005). Both have been extensively used for research purposes in samples of adults with ASD without intellectual impairment, and both have reasonable psychometric properties. Importantly, scores on the ABAS assessment instrument have been shown to correlate with real-world executive function measures, particularly with cognitive flexibility and planning and organization abilities in adults with high-functioning ASD (Wallace et al. 2015).

Box 5.2

The Autism Diagnostic Observation Schedule (ADOS) is a semi-structured assessment of communication, social interaction, and imagination used to diagnose ASD in all age groups. The ADOS interview comprises four modules specifically designed for different age groups and developmental and linguistic levels. Module four is used to assess adolescents and adults with fluent speech. The ADOS consists of standardized activities that offer the examiner the opportunity to observe the patient's social behavior and communication ability over 30–45 min and in a standardized context. The great advantage of this instrument, the gold standard of semi-structured ASD diagnosis, is that it provides the examiner with an opportunity for direct observation of the core behavioral and communicational manifestations of ASD in patients with a suspected diagnosis. This circumvents the fact that ASD adults, even those with good linguistic abilities and mild symptoms, have poor self-referential cognition that limits the validity of self-report measures of autistic symptoms (Bastiaansen et al. 2011). The revised version of the instrument's algorithm incorporates the DSM-5 position that condenses social interaction and communication deficits into a single dimension of social affect (Hus and Lord 2014; Pugliese et al. 2015). The instrument's total score incorporates scores in this dimension and scores in a second restricted and repetitive behaviors dimension. The total score is able to accurately discriminate between adults with ASD and both neurotypical subjects and subjects with antisocial personality disorder (psychopathy) and has good inter-rater reliability and internal consistency (Bastiaansen et al. 2011). However, there is a large overlap between the scores of ASD subjects and patients with schizophrenia, mostly those with prominent negative symptoms. Moreover, sensitivity for higher-functioning individuals with mild ASD phenotypes is limited (Bastiaansen et al. 2011). In their validation study of the revised 2014 algorithm first proposed by Hus and Lord (2014); Pugliese et al. (2015) showed that both sensitivity and specificity are lowest in individuals with a verbal IQ between 85 and 115 (specificity may be as low as 65 % in this particular group), but they also confirmed that the instrument has a good performance in subjects aged 16–20 and subjects above 20 (Pugliese et al. 2015). The limited sensitivity of the ADOS interview means that, in clinical settings, where sensitivity is more important than specificity, a less stringent cutoff of eight should be adopted, while a less inclusive cutoff of ten will probably be more appropriate in a research context where false positives are to be avoided (Pugliese et al. 2015). In a clinical setting, and especially when dealing with high-functioning adults with no intellectual disability, ADOS scores should always be complemented with careful exploration of early development and current daily functioning, as well as careful in-depth exploration of suspected schizophrenia-like phenomenology (Bastiaansen et al. 2011). In the absence of any evidence of psychosis, a positive score on the ADOS means that there is a very high probability that the examinee has indeed an ASD. Finally, it must be borne in mind, when interpreting ADOS scores, that in high-functioning adolescents and adults, the core symptom profile tends to be dominated by impairments in nonverbal communication and social reciprocity, rather than deficits in verbal communication and interest restriction/stereotyped behaviors (Seltzer et al. 2003; Shattuck et al. 2007). The 2014 revision also includes a severity assessment scale (the calibrated severity metric), but doubts have been raised regarding how it should be interpreted and how it relates to other measures of ASD severity, measures of functional impairment, or measures of cognitive ability (Pugliese et al. 2015).

Cognitive ability and cognitive profile are ideally assessed using the Wechsler Adult Intelligence Scale. The classical profile is one of huge disparities in performance across the various subtests of the instrument, frequently with a significant difference between verbal and performance IQ that invalidates the use of full-scale scores as reliable measures of cognitive ability (Gillberg 2002; Spek et al. 2008; Chiang et al. 2014). In spite of this, research in high-functioning adults with an ASD has shown that IQ profiles vary wildly across subjects, and mean differences between verbal and performance IQ are not statistically significant at the group level (Spek et al. 2008). In summary, while there is no pathognomonic IQ profile in adult ASD, a heterogeneous profile does add some weight to a hypothetical diagnosis of ASD in the presence of other signs and symptoms. Other classical cognitive measures are probably of little practical clinical value in ASD adults without cognitive impairment. In contrast, assessing the so-called real-world executive functions may prove a valuable contribute to understanding patients' disabilities in an ecologically valid manner (Wallace et al. 2015).

Box 5.3
The Vineland Adaptive Behavior Scales (VABS) is a standardized, structured caregiver interview that assesses adaptive skills at all ages between birth and 90 years and 11 months and has been shown to have a robust reliability and validity. It produces a score (the Adaptive Behavior Composite) comprised by standard scores in the three domains of communication, daily Living, and socialization (Sparrow et al. 2005).

The Adaptive Behavior Assessment System (ABAS), Second Edition, is a questionnaire that measures adaptive functioning, both at home and in community settings, at all ages between birth and 89 years and 11 months. Several forms are available for application to parents of children of different ages, teachers, or adults. The overall General Adaptive Composite score comprises a conceptual domain (communication, functional academics, self-direction), a social domain, and a practical domain (self-care, home living, community use, health and safety). The instrument has reasonable psychometric properties and has been used as an alternative to the VABS (Harrison and Oakland 2003).

5.4.3 Coping with the Diagnosis of ASD

Little has been written on how adult subjects react to and cope with a novel diagnosis of ASD. Clearly, importing psychological models of reaction to physical disease into the field of ASD is inadequate. The classical stage theories based on Kubler-Ross's stages of bereavement are clearly more useful to understand individual reactions to acute, catastrophic health events that impinge on the subject's lifeline and drastically change the subject's future, self-image, and self-esteem (Punshon et al. 2009). Adults with an undiagnosed ASD invariably have spent their lives coping with their symptoms and their difficulties, and in most instances are probably functioning better and are more aware of their inabilities at the time of the first diagnosis than they were as children, i.e., to a certain extent their illness tended to improve rather than the opposite. In this respect, adults facing a first-time diagnosis of ASD may be more readily compared to subjects with a chronic physical disorder who have experienced symptoms of their illness for some time and have therefore grown increasingly aware that there is something wrong with their health (Punshon et al. 2009). Every psychiatrist who has diagnosed ASD in adults will confirm that subjects often react with a mixture of relief and surprise to their diagnosis and often perceive it as something that finally allows them to make sense of their lifelong difficulties. Relief from lifelong feelings of guilt and reproach by the self and others is often conveyed by this revelation that chronic difficulties "fitting in" are not a manifestation of personal failure or inferiority but a clinical problem with a scientific label, even though there is no straightforward cure (Punshon et al. 2009; Griffith et al. 2012). For a proportion of those receiving a diagnosis of Asperger syndrome, the label may even be felt to represent a mark of distinction or subtle cognitive superiority over "non-ASD commons," as well as a liberation from the self-imposed duty to try to conform with the constraints of neurotypical thinking processes (Punshon et al. 2009; Griffith et al. 2012; Kite et al. 2013; Spillers et al. 2014).

The relatively positive experience of receiving a diagnosis for the first time is, for many adults with a previously undiagnosed ASD, tempered by the perception that society as a whole – and health services in particular – are totally unprepared to deal appropriately with individuals with an ASD. Studies that have looked at how ASD adults and their supporters describe their experience of health-care services and professionals have found that the most recurrently mentioned theme is providers' lack of knowledge about ASD, their general attitude toward the disorder, and their skill in dealing with ASD subjects, namely, in facilitating communication and tolerating deviations from standard practice such as allowing the patient to put his or her complaints and questions in writing or allowing a parent or spouse to accompany the patient during each consultation (Nicolaidis et al. 2011; Griffith et al. 2012; Jones et al. 2014). In one study, subjects expressed their mistrust of health services due to having previously been wrongly diagnosed with other mental disorders (Punshon et al. 2009), and in another study interviewed subjects explained that their lack of trust in health-care providers was aggravated further by the prescription of mainstream therapeutic interventions that patients perceived as unhelpful (in this particular case, cognitive behavioral therapy) (Griffith et al. 2012). Studies that have looked at health-care providers' knowledge and beliefs about ASD have widely corroborated this negative perception of services by patients. Although there are, in all likelihood, national specificities, data show that most health-care providers, not only at the primary care level but also in mental health services, consider themselves unprepared to deal with adults with an ASD (Bruder et al. 2012). There seems to be a lack of both theoretical knowledge and practical skills, linked with stereotyped misconceptions like the belief that ASD are only present in children or that ASD adults never engage in drug or alcohol use or do not have a sexual life (Zerbo et al. 2015). The latter misconception is particularly worrisome as it means that adult women with an ASD are probably not receiving all the medical care that they should, including preventive and screening interventions that are routinely offered to adult women with active sexual lives (Bruder et al. 2012). Most professionals identify the improvement of skills for communicating effectively with ASD patients as one of the most pressing training needs and see difficulties in communicating with ASD patients as the main barrier for working effectively with this special group of service users (Zerbo et al. 2015).

Employers' and work colleagues' lack of information about ASD is also often reported as a source of problems in the workplace and may even contribute to chronic unemployment as subjects perceive their difficulties in dealing with the communication and socializing challenges in the workplace as an overwhelming source of stress and anxiety (Griffith et al. 2012). Finally, though by no means less important, adults with newly diagnosed ASD will often find themselves, once diagnosed, in contact with support services that are not in the least adequate to their needs and to their level of functioning (Griffith et al. 2012). Indeed, although there are probably national and regional variations in this regard, most adults with high-functioning ASD, regardless of when in their life course they were first diagnosed, find themselves referred to support services that have originally been designed and planned to address the needs of much lower-functioning populations such as individuals with chronic psychosis or physical or intellectual disabilities (Jones et al. 2014). High-functioning ASD subjects, especially those who have only recently been diagnosed, often find this shocking and unacceptable. This sort of rehabilitation services do not usually offer the flexible, intermittent low-level, individually tailored support that most adults with high-functioning ASD need or wish for (Griffith et al. 2012). For those who have been newly diagnosed with an ASD, adequate information on the meaning of the diagnosis and offer of adequate post-diagnostic support, possibly the mere opportunity for post-diagnostic follow-up appointments, are often cited in the literature as unmet needs for care identified by patients themselves (Punshon et al. 2009; Jones et al. 2014). Punshon et al. (2009) pertinently comment in this respect that adapting to a novel diagnosis of ASD is not a single episodic event, but rather a complex and gradual process that may drag for months or years as the subject comes to terms with the new meaning the diagnosis gives to their lifelong difficulties and negative self-appraisals (Punshon et al. 2009).

5.5 Adult Outcome of High-Functioning Autism Spectrum Disorders Diagnosed in Childhood

Specialists and researchers working with autism have always been intrigued by the long-term prognosis of ASD, not only in pragmatic terms such as psychosocial functioning and treatment needs but also in terms of symptom profile. What happens to autistic subjects when they reach adult age? Do they improve in terms of autonomy? Is there a recovery from ASD? Do symptoms change with aging or do patients, especially those who are more cognitively able, simply learn to live with their symptoms and characteristics and learn to compensate for them or to "disguise" them from the ruthless eyes of a competitive, meritocratic society? Surprising as it may be, answering these questions is, in terms of research methodology, far from straightforward. The ideal research approach to these questions would be to follow-up cases diagnosed in infancy all the way to adult age. This is not only a formidable endeavor, given the very long follow-up periods required, but is also further complicated by the fact that diagnostic criteria for autism and related disorder have changed so much since the disorder made its first appearance in DSM-III. Indeed, since the inclusiveness of autism's definitions has varied so much over the years, it is not always clear whether patients have outgrown the disorder or whether diagnostic criteria have outgrown the patients. For instance, while earlier definitions were clearly more exclusive and earlier cohorts were consequently composed of more severe, lower-functioning cases, many higher-functioning patients with Asperger syndrome or pervasive developmental disorder not otherwise specified diagnosed in the 1990s now fail to qualify for ASD under DSM-5 (Barahona-Corrêa and Filipe 2016). Consequently, cohorts diagnosed in the 1990s will display an apparently better evolution over the years, in terms of autonomy and symptom evolution, than earlier diagnosed cohorts. Notwithstanding these difficulties, several long-term longitudinal studies have looked at the adult outcome of ASD. These studies may roughly be divided into two groups: those studies that looked at adult outcome proper in terms of psychosocial functioning, autonomy, employment, or psychiatric comorbidity, among other indicators and studies that have looked at the longitudinal evolution of the core symptoms of autism as patients grow older. In both types of studies, results have not always been consistent, mainly due to the methodological issues already mentioned.

5.5.1 Psychosocial Functioning

In terms of psychosocial functioning, studies mostly show that adult outcomes are modest for the majority of patients (Magiati et al. 2014). The earliest studies on adult outcome of children with HFA appeared in the 1970s and 1980s and were for the most part based on very small samples (Lord and Venter 1992; Howlin and Moss 2012). Very few of these studies were population based. In all follow-up studies of ASD children, regardless of their level of functioning, adult outcome was invariably found to be poor or very poor in terms of social adjustment in as much as 60–75 % of subjects. A good outcome was found only in 5–15 % of subjects (Nordin and Gillberg 1998; Howlin and Moss 2012). In general, evidence from these studies suggested that adult outcome in terms of academic achievement and adaptive behavior is to some degree correlated with full-scale IQ and particularly with verbal IQ or with performance on executive tasks highly correlated with verbal IQ (Howlin and Moss 2012). Subjects with an IQ of 50 or less by age 6 were almost universally found to have a poor outcome as adults, with a high proportion eventually being placed in long-term institutions (Lord and Venter 1992; Nordin and Gillberg 1998). Speech was also repeatedly found to be a potentially relevant prognostic factor, with good speech at age 5 predicting, to some degree, a better outcome in adult age (Howlin and Moss 2012). Individual variability, however, was found to be huge, with these group predictors proving totally unreliable when it came to predict individual outcomes (Nordin and Gillberg 1998; Magiati et al. 2014). Surprisingly, the predictive value of the severity of core ASD symptoms in childhood has been omitted from most studies. The available evidence is again inconsistent: while severity of ASD core symptoms as a whole seems to be an unreliable predictor of psychosocial outcome in adult age, severity of stereotyped and repetitive behaviors, or, alternatively, the severity of social impairments, especially in reciprocal social interactions, has been shown to predict a worse adult outcome, particularly in terms of gainful employment and ability to develop and sustain close relationships (Howlin and Moss 2012; Howlin et al. 2013).

In the specific case of high-functioning individuals, IQ and early speech development seem to be much less reliably predictive of adult outcome, with a significant gap between cognitive ability and adaptive functioning that widens with increasing IQ scores (Rumsey et al. 1985; Szatmari et al. 1989; Venter et al. 1992; Lord and

Venter 1992; Nordin and Gillberg 1998). From among these earlier studies, the group of patients described by Szatmari et al. (1989) achieved the best outcomes in all areas. Almost half of the 16 patients were university graduates, six had remunerated jobs, and four had stable intimate affective relationships (Szatmari et al. 1989). Notwithstanding this, about two thirds had limited nonverbal communication skills or excessively formal speech and almost one half were described as socially clumsy. The samples described in the two other studies had much worse outcomes, despite having normal IQs (Rumsey et al. 1985; Venter et al. 1992). Only a minority was competitively employed, and the overwhelming majority of those subjects who were employed had either low-level jobs or were in sheltered employment programs. Furthermore, the majority was still living with relatives or with some form of supervision, and none had affective relationships (Rumsey et al. 1985; Venter et al. 1992). In a 2000 paper that reviewed earlier studies on the adult outcome of subjects with high-functioning autism, Howlin observed that results up to that point had been extremely heterogeneous, despite the fact that the studied groups – almost invariably small samples varying in size between 9 and 43 subjects – were reasonably homogeneous in terms of composition. Employment rates varied between 5 and 44 %, the proportion of adult subjects living independently varied between 16 and 50 %, outcomes rated as good were observed in 16–44 % of subjects followed up to adulthood, and psychiatric comorbidity was reported in 11–67 % of cases (Howlin 2000). In general, the studies described in this review concluded that IQ remained reasonably stable over time, especially performance IQ scores (there was some evidence for a modest improvement in verbal IQ in a proportion of subjects). Again, in most studies IQ correlated with adult outcome and with adult Vineland scores, in spite of the recurrent mention of a gap between cognitive ability and adaptive functioning. Finally, childhood verbal ability was a robust predictor of adult linguistic and social functioning (Howlin 2000). In almost all the studies, adult subjects remained significantly handicapped in terms of social functioning, even if a substantial minority were able to live with a partner or even get married. In a follow-up study of 68 patients with ASD and a performance IQ of 50 or higher, Howlin et al. (2004) generally confirmed the conclusions of earlier smaller studies. Upon reaching adult age, most subjects in this sample (78 %) did not have any formal school qualifications, and only 10 out of the 68 had been educated in mainstream schools (Howlin et al. 2004). Only 34 % of these subjects were working as adults, and of these, only 35 % (i.e., 12 % of the total sample) were working independently, the rest being in some form of sheltered or supported work. Most of the jobs were of low level anyway and had mostly been obtained through parental contacts. More than half (56 %) had no friends or acquaintances whatsoever. Half of the group were living in supported residential accommodation, and close to a third were still living at home with their parents. Again, there was an association between higher adult IQ and higher adult verbal IQ and better social outcome measures. Moreover, IQ scores remained remarkably stable over time, with a significant correlation between childhood and adult IQ scores (both verbal and performance), particularly in those who had scores above 70–74 from the outset (Howlin et al. 2004). Childhood performance IQ was shown in this sample to correlate with adult outcome not only in terms of social functioning but also in terms of academic achievement and, to a lesser extent, language competence, severity of ASD symptoms, and frequency of ritualistic behaviors. An important further observation in this study, and one that replicated previous observations from smaller studies, was that outcome in terms of adaptive behavior is generally worse in women, despite equivalent cognitive and linguistic abilities.

In a large cohort of 120 children diagnosed with autism in the 1980s Billstedt, Gillberg and Gillberg found that 78 % of the included subjects had very poor or poor outcome as adults, none having what the authors defined as a good outcome and only 8 % showing fair outcome (Billstedt et al. 2005). Only four subjects were fully independent. Importantly, most subjects in this sample had either severe or moderately severe intellectual disability, 40 % had a present or past history of epilepsy, and 49 % had a major medical or neurological problem requiring regular medical care (Billstedt et al. 2005). Nevertheless, the authors found that normal IQ score before age 10 and the presence of some communicative phrase speech at age 6 were predictive of a better outcome in adult age. Because this sample included a substantial proportion of low-functioning ASD individuals, conclusions are not necessarily valid for high-functioning individuals.

In an important study specifically focused on high-functioning ASD, Cederlund et al. (2008) followed up a group of 70 Asperger syndrome patients for 5 years after initial assessment, into late adolescence or early young adulthood (Cederlund et al. 2008). This was a sample with above-average cognitive ability. All but eight of the individuals continued to meet diagnostic criteria for Asperger syndrome or an ASD. Again, the authors were surprised to find that adult outcome was, in terms of global functioning, independent living, or occupational status, way below what could be expected given the group's cognitive ability. Only 27 % of the subjects had a good outcome, and, again, higher full-scale IQ scores were associated with better outcomes. Only seven subjects had full-time paid jobs, and 17 % had no occupation whatsoever. A substantial proportion of all individuals were living alone, but all depended financially from parental support. Only three subjects had long-term affective relationships. Importantly, full-scale IQ scores remained essentially stable over time, with a significant decrease of the initial gap between verbal IQ and performance IQ over time, mainly due to an increase in performance IQ. Interestingly, the only patients who showed a decrease in IQ scores were the three subjects who developed psychosis during the follow-up (Cederlund et al. 2008).

In another study that compared adaptive functioning of ASD subjects diagnosed in infancy and ASD subjects diagnosed as adults, Marriage et al. (2009) reported the follow-up until adulthood of the former group, comprising 45 individuals, 33 of whom had a normal IQ (Marriage et al. 2009). Adult psychosocial functioning outcome was extremely variable, ranging from dependence on a disability pension to a successful family and professional life. Very few of these high-functioning ASD subjects diagnosed in childhood had ever benefited from specific therapeutic interventions for ASD, and only 15 % of the whole sample achieved what the authors considered a good level of adaptive behavior (Marriage et al. 2009).

A further study of high-functioning ASD subjects by Farley et al. (2009) assessed the adult outcome of a group of 41 subjects with autism diagnosed in childhood and a performance or full-scale IQ of at least 70 (Farley et al. 2009). Fifty-six percent of these subjects had attended special education public school programs, and 39 % had received post-secondary education. Half of the subjects were working in independent, paid jobs, and a further 7 % were working in supported employment positions. Fourteen percent were either married or engaged in a long-term relationship, half of them with offspring. Twelve percent lived independently, but 56 % were still living with their parents. In terms of caregiver support, 27 % of the subjects required a moderate level of help in their daily lives, and 46 % required high-level assistance, meaning, for example, that they needed someone to control their finances or to help them with social contacts. In terms of overall social outcome, the study authors considered that 48 % of the subjects had either good or very god outcome, while 17 % had a poor outcome. In terms of the need for support from social services, 29 % of the subjects had no need for formal support; 20 % required moderate support in the form of continuous home support, sheltered job, or regular support from mental health or rehabilitation services; and a further 32 % needed a high level of support including, for example, supported living, a group home, or a personal assistant (Farley et al. 2009). In terms of adaptive behavior, subjects generally showed significantly higher functioning in terms of daily living skills than they did in the communication and socialization domains. Current performance IQ correlated significantly with psychosocial functioning. Furthermore, childhood IQ scores not only correlated significantly with adult scores, meaning that IQ remained reasonably stable over time, but also predicted adult outcome in terms of psychosocial functioning. Again, there was some evidence that those with phrase speech by age 4 showed a better outcome as adults (Farley et al. 2009). On the whole, the most robust predictor of a good outcome in adult age was a high score in the adaptive functioning assessment. Moreover, the study confirmed that the gap between cognitive and adaptive ability, which had already been described in follow-up studies in children, continues to widen as subjects enter adulthood (Farley et al. 2009). This has been recently confirmed by Matthews et al. (2015) in a cross-sectional study where they compared a group of 28 ASD adolescents aged between 16 and 19, a group of young ASD adults aged 20–24, and a group of adults with ASD aged 25–58 (Matthews et al. 2015). They found that IQ scores were consistently superior to adaptive behavior standardized scores in all age groups, regardless of cognitive ability (although subjects with higher IQ scores tended to have higher adaptive behavior scores). Moreover, they found that adults had lower standardized scores of adaptive functioning in the domains of socialization and communication skills than adolescents, suggesting that with maturing age, skills in those two domains increasingly deviate from the norm (Matthews et al. 2015). In contrast, daily life skills were a domain of relative strength for all age groups, probably because these are skills that are more apt to be learned, imitated, and rehearsed over time.

Howlin et al. (2013) recently published their findings on a group of 60 adults with ASD and a nonverbal IQ >70, whom they followed up from childhood to a mean age of 44 years (Howlin et al. 2013). They found that IQ remained essentially stable throughout the follow-up period, while language improved substantially in the majority of those subjects who had no speech at the time of the first assessment. In terms of psychosocial functioning, 72 % had failed to obtain any formal educational qualification; 26 % lived independently, although many of them in settings with partial formal support; 55 % were either unemployed or in sheltered or volunteer jobs; and none were married or had ever had an intimate long-term relationship (Howlin et al. 2013). Again, higher IQ predicted a better outcome in adult age. However, the best predictor of adult functioning in this study was the severity of ASD symptoms in childhood, especially social reciprocity deficits, which were predictive of a worse psychosocial outcome in adult age (Howlin et al. 2013). In another recent longitudinal study of 58 individuals with average nonverbal IQ (mean estimated IQ of 88.7) followed up for an average time interval of 37 years, Moss et al. (2015) found that only 5 % were employed in highly skilled professions, while 69 % were either unemployed or in sheltered employment (Moss et al. 2015). Only 12 % lived independently, with 54 % living in residential homes, while 83 % had no close reciprocal relationships whatsoever (Moss et al. 2015).

Most studies on adult outcome of ASD, both longitudinal and cross sectional, included subjects spanning a wide age interval. A single study, by Taylor and Seltzer (2011), focused exclusively on a group of subjects who had recently left high school (Taylor and Seltzer 2011). This allowed for a more detailed and valid insight into the process of transition from adolescence into adulthood, and the factors that might influence it. The study found that 47.1 % of the high-functioning (i.e., without intellectual disability) subgroup in the sample were attending university, and a further 11.8 % were competitively employed. However, 23.5 % had no regular activity whatsoever. This particular subgroup showed ASD symptom severity scores and maladaptive behavior scores that were intermediate between those of their gainfully employed high-functioning peers and those of the lower-functioning group. Moreover, 86 % of them had a comorbid psychiatric diagnosis (Taylor and Seltzer 2011). There thus seems to be a substantial minority of individuals who are formally high functioning but who are actually not functioning at the expected level and are also not benefitting from the formal support services typically offered to the lower-functioning group.

A group of studies have opted to focus on perceived quality of life as a more valid measure of adult outcome of ASD than psychosocial measures such as employment status or autonomy. The first of these was a cross-sectional study by Renty (2006), who set out to study adult outcome in terms of quality of life in a sample of 58 subjects with a diagnosis of high-functioning autism (Renty 2006). They found that, in terms of the latter outcome measures, their sample generally replicated the profile reported by previous studies: only 27.6 % of all individuals had a mainstream paid job, 55.2 % were still living with their parents, and 67.2 % were single (i.e., had no intimate heterosexual relationship, had never been married, or had never cohabited with a partner). This was in spite of a mean full-scale IQ of 103. The regular participation in any form of daytime activity had a positive influence on subjective quality of life – an important point – given that a substantial proportion of ASD adults have no daytime activities whatsoever (Renty 2006). This study's main finding, though, was that quality of life depended much more closely on perceived informal support (mostly from mothers, friends, siblings, fathers, and other relatives, in this decreasing order of importance) and the discrepancy between perceived and needed informal support than on objective ASD-related disability or support actually received (either informal or professional) (Renty 2006). A similar finding was reported, more recently, by Kamio et al. (2013), who also cross-sectionally compared a sample of 154 community-dwelling adults with a high-functioning ASD with the general adult reference population in terms of their self-reported psychosocial quality of life. They found that not only ASD subjects rated their psychosocial quality of life lower than the reference group but also that informal support from the mothers, and an early diagnosis, were both associated with better quality of life (Kamio et al. 2013). In another cross-sectional comparison of young adults with Asperger syndrome with a group of neurotypical individuals, Jennes-Coussens et al. (2006) found that the young men in the Asperger syndrome group rated their quality of life significantly lower than the neurotypical control individuals, both in the domains of employment and social functioning (Jennes-Coussens et al. 2006). Although social networks appeared not to differ in dimension across both groups, professional acquaintances were more prominent in the networks of the Asperger syndrome individuals. Young men with Asperger syndrome spent most of their leisure time engaging in solitary activities, and close to 50 % had never had a girlfriend, allegedly because they felt they lacked the necessary social skills (Jennes-Coussens et al. 2006).

More recently, Barneveld et al. (2014) published their findings from a longitudinal case-controlled study where they assessed objective and subjective quality of life in 169 subjects with a high-functioning ASD followed up for a mean period of 14 years (Barneveld et al. 2014). Again, they found that the overwhelming majority (88 %) of subjects were single (i.e., they were unmarried and did not have an intimate long-term relationship). Only about half (49 %) were on paid employment, and the majority were living either with their parents or relatives (44.8 %), or were institutionalized (21.2 %). Almost two thirds (63 %) had completed at least upper secondary education. The important findings from this study, though, were that both objective outcome and subjective quality of life in the domains of employment, independent living, and marital status were significantly worse in the ASD sample than in three groups of age-matched, childhood-diagnosed subjects with ADHD, disruptive behavior disorders, and affective disorders, respectively. Moreover, the authors found that in this sample of ASD subjects with normal IQ, education level was predictive of a better outcome in terms of gainful employment and independent living (Barneveld et al. 2014). This is a relevant finding, as IQ measures were shown to be unreliable predictors of outcome in these domains in high-functioning subjects. In another recent study, Khanna et al. (2014) cross-sectionally compared health-related quality of life in a large sample of 291 adults with an ASD (comprising mainly, but not exclusively, high-functioning individuals, including 59.5 % with Asperger syndrome) with that of the general US adult population (Khanna et al. 2014). Almost half of these subjects (46.7 %) were still living with their families, 28.5 % were employed full time, and 63.2 % had never married. The study found that physical and mental health-related quality of life was significantly lower in the

ASD group compared to the general adult population. More importantly, a regression analysis found that two modifiable factors – maladaptive coping style and perceived informal support – were predictive of health-related quality of life, with other less modifiable predictive factors being ASD symptom severity, living in an institution, or having a comorbid physical or mental illness (Khanna et al. 2014).

Generally speaking then, the results of more recent studies focusing specifically on adult outcome of high-functioning ASD subjects are in line with the observations not only from earlier studies and shorter-term follow-up studies in children but also with the results of studies on low-functioning ASD. The gross conclusion to be drawn is that outcome in adult life of ASD subjects is modest at best, in terms of psychosocial functioning, adaptive behavior, or quality of life (Tobin et al. 2014). On the other hand, there is a clear tendency within individuals for improvement over time in terms of psychosocial functioning (Howlin et al. 2004; Seltzer et al. 2004; Marriage et al. 2009). IQ at the time of first diagnosis and the development of communicative speech before the age of 6 years are clearly the most replicated predictors of adaptive functioning, psychosocial functioning, and quality of life scores when these children reach school age (Lord and Venter 1992; Howlin and Moss 2012; Magiati et al. 2014). This being said, it is also clear that we still cannot predict adequately the adult outcome of ASD at the individual level. In terms of employment, for instance, in spite of the evidence showing childhood IQ to be the best predictor of gainful employment in adult age, subjects with high IQ scores do not necessarily obtain employment consistent with their education level or cognitive ability (Holwerda et al. 2012). Moreover, the increase, in the last decade, of educational facilities and other indicated interventions for children and adolescents with ASD did not necessarily translate into a better functional outcome in adult age in more modern studies, which would be expected to reflect the higher access of more recent generations of ASD patients to indicated specialized interventions (Howlin et al. 2004; Howlin and Moss 2012; Magiati et al. 2014). The fact remains, nonetheless, that having a normal childhood and adult IQ and good language development are clearly a necessary, though perhaps not sufficient, condition for a positive adult outcome in terms of psychosocial functioning and adaptive behavior. Formal programs such as social skills training, vocational programs, and supported accommodation almost surely have a role to play in modulating the effects of individual prognostic factors (Venter et al. 1992; Nordin and Gillberg 1998; Engstrom et al. 2003; Renty 2006; Marriage et al. 2009). Other factors such as family dynamics, family social-economic status, and informal support from relatives and friends also appear to have a positive influence on adult psychosocial functioning (Venter et al. 1992; Nordin and Gillberg 1998; Engstrom et al. 2003; Renty 2006; Tobin et al. 2014). Severity of ASD in childhood seems to have a poor predictive value with respect to adult functioning and quality of life, although the same may not apply to severity of ASD core symptoms in adolescence and adulthood, as we will see later in this text (Eaves and Ho 2008; Taylor and Seltzer 2011; Khanna et al. 2014). As to factors that negatively affect adult outcome of high-functioning ASD subjects, comorbid epilepsy and psychiatric comorbidity seem to be the most unanimously cited factors (Howlin 2000; Howlin et al. 2004; Billstedt et al. 2005; Eaves and Ho 2008; Farley et al. 2009; Moss et al. 2015).

5.5.2 Longitudinal Evolution of Autistic Core Symptoms from Childhood to Adult Age

A decisive issue in the field of adult outcome of ASD is, of course, whether or not the autistic core phenotype and associated cognitive and psychiatric manifestations change with time as the child moves into adolescence and young adulthood. Again, studies have adopted various methodological approaches to this question, from longitudinal long-term prospective studies to cross-sectional studies comparing behavioral dimensions across samples of children, adolescents, and adults with ASD. In spite of the huge methodological variability, it emerges from most studies that the core symptoms of ASD improve at least partially with growing age, although not necessarily in all subjects (Seltzer et al. 2004; Shattuck et al. 2007). Moreover, this improvement seems to progress nonlinearly, with periods of symptom aggravation (mainly hyperactivity, insistence on sameness, or aggressiveness) interspersed within the general trend to amelioration. Importantly, for the overwhelming majority of subjects, the abatement in symptom severity is seldom significant enough to allow them to function within the age-appropriate level or to warrant a revision of the initial diagnosis (Seltzer et al. 2004).

There is ample evidence that verbal linguistic skills improve significantly in most patients with age, although echolalia and pronoun reversal may persist into adulthood in a significant proportion of cases (probably less so in high-functioning cases) (Billstedt et al. 2007; Shattuck et al. 2007). Other problems that may persist into adulthood, even in high-functioning cases, are literalness, abnormal prosody, poor mimic, and nonverbal communication in general (Nordin and Gillberg 1998; Seltzer et al. 2003; Billstedt et al. 2007; Shattuck et al. 2007). Notwithstanding this, even subjects who had no language at 5 or 6 years of age may eventually have developed reasonably social use of language when they reach adult age (up to 40 % of cases), although the majority will never acquire age-appropriate linguistic skills, regardless of their cognitive ability (Howlin 2003; Howlin et al. 2004).

Social skills and reciprocal social behavior also show a trend to amelioration as subjects grow older, albeit to a much more modest degree than communication and language (Howlin et al. 2004, 2013; Seltzer et al. 2004; Billstedt et al. 2007; Shattuck et al. 2007). As they enter adolescence, ASD subjects tend to become less withdrawn socially, and by adult age a significant proportion will have been able to establish a few friendships or even, in some cases, intimate long-term relationships (Nordin and Gillberg 1998; Howlin et al. 2004; Cederlund et al. 2008; Farley et al. 2009). There is evidence that the typical social subtypes described by Lorna Wing (aloof, passive, and active but odd) undergo some phenotypical change during growth, with aloof subjects often coming out of their isolation to become either passively sociable or active but odd (Wing 1981; Nordin and Gillberg 1998; Seltzer et al. 2004). Nevertheless, this apparent improvement in the tendency to withdraw socially does not necessarily translate into a better performance in terms of socialization, probably because of the retinue of faux pas incidents, social awkwardness, and the generally inadequate approach behaviors that accompanies this transformation (Nordin and Gillberg 1998). Indeed, evidence shows that, as adults, most subjects with an ASD continue to display inappropriate emotional responses, poor eye contact, and one-sided social approaches (Billstedt et al. 2007; Shattuck et al. 2007). In summary, in spite of superficial changes in social behavior, mainly achieved through imitation learning, social deficits in ASD tend to persist as a significant problem into adult age (Magiati et al. 2014). It remains a matter of debate if, as individuals grow, there is a persistent lack of interest for socialization, or whether individuals become increasingly interested in relating with others but simply lack the necessary social know-how, exposing them to be rebuffed and reinforcing social avoidant behaviors (Seltzer et al. 2004).

Finally, with regard to restricted, repetitive behaviors and interests, the available data are somewhat inconsistent, with a few studies showing that improvement with age in this symptom domain is much less marked than in the communication and sociabilization domains and that there may even be some degree of symptom aggravation in terms of complexity of rituals and stereotyped behaviors. Clinically significant symptoms in this domain persist into adulthood in as much as 80–90 % of ASD subjects, according to follow-up studies (Seltzer et al. 2003; Howlin et al. 2004). Limitations in the pattern of self-chosen activities are reportedly one of the most persistent problems in this area, with self-chosen activity often limited to a single repetitive interest (Billstedt et al. 2007). Notwithstanding this, some qualitative improvement may occur in a percentage of patients as they reach adult age, namely, in the frequency and complexity of unusual preoccupations (Seltzer et al. 2003; Billstedt et al. 2007). Moreover, there is some evidence that symptoms in this domain tend to abate with age within adulthood, rather than between childhood and young adulthood (Shattuck et al. 2007).

On the whole, then, there seems to be some, albeit modest, abatement of autistic symptoms with age, with the improvement being highest in communication symptoms, somewhat less in restricted and repetitive behaviors, and least in social skills (Magiati et al. 2014). Improvement seems to be decisively and positively influenced by cognitive and verbal ability, as well as by the occurrence of psychiatric comorbidity and epilepsy, which are associated to less symptomatic improvement or even to symptom aggravation (Howlin et al. 2004; Seltzer et al. 2004; Shattuck et al. 2007; Magiati et al. 2014; Gillberg et al. 2015). In high-functioning individuals and especially in those with a childhood diagnosis of Asperger syndrome, improvement may be sufficient to move the subject out of the ASD diagnostic category. In a recent follow-up study of 50 subjects diagnosed with Asperger syndrome in childhood (at a mean age of 11), Helles et al. (2014) found that only 39 still fulfilled DSM-IV diagnostic criteria as adults (mean age of 30) (Helles et al. 2014). Moreover, all subjects showed a variable but significant degree of improvement in some of the core symptoms of Asperger syndrome, namely, special interests, stereotyped or repetitive speech, nonverbal communication, and clumsiness, while social difficulties and excessive adherence to routines by and large remained unchanged over the follow-up period. Interestingly, in this particularly high-functioning sample, IQ was not predictive of symptomatic improvement or level of functioning, suggesting that IQ may only impact decisively on the adult outcome of ASD for those who start off with a low normal or below normal IQ (Helles et al. 2014).

A few studies have looked for factors that might influence the rate and direction of ASD symptom modification with growth into adult age. In an important study by Taylor and Seltzer (2010), the authors followed up a group of 242 youth with ASD for an average of 10 years until after they left high school, with the aim of capturing the transition from school years to post-high school adult age (Taylor and Seltzer 2010). They found that ASD core symptoms improved steadily over the years, regardless of the presence of intellectual delay and gender. Importantly, the rate of improvement in the ASD core symptomatic dimensions of deficits in socialization and repetitive and restricted behaviors and interests attenuated significantly once the subjects left high school, particularly in high-functioning individuals. Maladaptive behaviors likewise improved during school years, only to stagnate once subjects left school (Taylor and Seltzer 2010). The important conclusion to draw from this study is that ASD deficits will improve as long as the subject remains integrated in a stimulating and organized regular activity, which probably explains why, in individuals with a high-functioning ASD, education, rather than IQ, seems to have a significant influence on adult outcome (Taylor and Seltzer 2010; Barneveld et al. 2014).

In another longitudinal, prospective study of 406 subjects (including cases with and without intellectual disability) aged between 10 and 49, followed up for an average period of 8.5 years, Woodman et al. (2015) found that ASD core symptoms generally became less severe over the course of the follow-up (Woodman et al. 2015). Improvement was particularly marked for repetitive behaviors/stereotyped interests and verbal communication, although social reciprocity deficits and nonverbal communication also showed a significant improvement. Unusual preoccupations, complex mannerisms, and poor use of conventional and instrumental gestures tended to persist over time in this study. The study's most momentous finding, though, was that higher levels of maternal praise and higher-quality relationships between patients and their mothers were both associated to less impairment in social reciprocity and nonverbal communication, as well as a more marked improvement in externalizing and antisocial maladaptive behaviors (Woodman et al. 2015). Conversely, the same group demonstrated that higher levels of expressed emotion, and more specifically higher levels of expressed maternal criticism (two concepts originally forged in the context of psychosis and psychotic relapse), are associated with higher levels of internalizing and antisocial behavioral problems, as well as more prominent symptoms in the domain of repetitive behaviors and restricted interests (Smith et al. 2014). Similarly to families of schizophrenia patients, the levels of expressed emotions are not a static feature of the families' communication stile. They may become aggravated over time, especially in times of transition such as early adulthood, and are also amenable to modification by multifamily group psycho-educational interventions (Smith et al. 2014).

Although less studied, noncore symptoms that are frequently found in ASD, such as clumsiness, unsuitable choice of clothing, unusual responses to sensory, auditory or visual symptoms, or indifference to pain, also tend to persist into adult age in the overwhelming majority of high-functioning cases according to the limited available evidence (Billstedt et al. 2007; Leekam et al. 2007). Sensory abnormalities were present in up to 89 % of high-functioning ASD adults in the study by Leekam et al. (2007), with the majority of subjects showing symptoms in two or more domains. Sensory abnormalities relating to audition, touch, smell or taste, and pain were the most frequent, with visual sensory abnormalities and kinesthetic symptoms (i.e., enjoys being spun round, walks or runs around in circles) being markedly rarer in this age group than in younger high-functioning ASD subjects (Leekam et al. 2007). Self-injurious behaviors leading to moderate or severe self-harm may be present in up to 19 % of ASD adults with normal IQ, with close to one half of these subjects also exhibiting maladaptive behaviors that damage others (Taylor and Seltzer 2010; Moss et al. 2015).

Another aspect that has attracted significant interest in terms of growth-related changes in ASD subjects is cognitive performance. In general, IQ scores tend to remain remarkably stable during growth in high-functioning ASD, with a number of studies reporting a significant correlation between childhood IQ scores and scores obtained in adolescence and adult age (Howlin 2000; Howlin et al. 2004, 2013; Cederlund et al. 2008; Eaves and Ho 2008; Farley et al. 2009; Magiati et al. 2014). Again, subtle changes, with little impact on the general pattern of IQ stability over time, have been reported by some of these studies, namely, a slight improvement in verbal IQ and a slight decrease in performance IQ in those who have higher performance than verbal IQ scores in childhood and the opposite pattern in those who have a nonverbal learning disability profile as children (mostly subjects with a diagnosis of Asperger syndrome) (Howlin et al. 2004).

On the whole, the available evidence consistently shows that, similarly to what has been described in low-functioning autism, autistic core symptoms in high-functioning ASD become attenuated with increasing age. Nevertheless, impairments in social relationships and ritualistic and repetitive behaviors and interests survive into adult age and in most individuals remain a potential limitation, with a significant impact on quality of life and the level of functioning attained in adult age. Moreover, while ASD symptom severity shows a clear tendency to amelioration with age, the opposite occurs with adaptive functioning, with individuals progressively deviating from the adaptive functioning levels of their neurotypical age peers as they grow older. The evolution of each symptom dimension varies widely between subjects, and the rate of change during growth is far from linear, with a general tendency for stagnation once subjects reach young adulthood. Transition into adult age seems to be a particularly vulnerable time, when a decisive split becomes evident between those who will fare well as adults and those who will do little better than low-functioning individuals. It remains disconcertingly difficult to predict, at the individual level, who will fall onto which side of this split, and what are the determining factors. Although intellectual ability is unquestionably a necessary factor for a subject with an ASD to achieve a good outcome as an adult, it is clear that in high-functioning individuals, other factors, such as formal education, informal support from relatives and friends, and the level of expressed emotion in the family environment, play a much more decisive role. Furthermore, many of these are factors that are amenable to intervention and modification, unlike other relevant prognostic determinants such as childhood IQ or childhood ASD symptom severity. Studies assessing the efficacy of interventions in these domains are lacking, though, and this is clearly a worthwhile area for future clinical experimental research.

5.6 Summary

Autism spectrum disorders, though usually diagnosed in childhood, are lifelong conditions with a prevalence in the adult population at least as high as that of schizophrenia. Yet, most mental health professionals working in adult mental health care lack adequate training in detecting and treating this group of disorders. This is particularly worrisome as it is clear that a substantial proportion of more able individuals with an ASD remain undiagnosed until adult age, although not necessarily less impaired than high-functioning individuals diagnosed as children. As adults, regardless of the age of diagnosis and despite some symptom amelioration with age, only a minority of individuals with an ASD and normal or above normal cognitive ability are able to hold full-time remunerated jobs, to live independently, or to raise a family of their own. The majority of high-functioning ASD adults function way below what could be expected in light of their IQ scores and academic achievement during their school years. This is a particularly vulnerable subgroup, with high rates of psychiatric comorbidity and a significant risk of social exclusion.

The diagnosis of ASD in adults requires adequate clinician training and experience, and it is evidently unrealistic to expect to find these skills across all levels of mental health care. The best pathway to diagnosis probably implies widespread screening capacity across several levels of mental health services and clear referral pathways to specialized services for confirmatory diagnostic workup and assessment of adaptive functioning, comorbidities, cognitive profile, and other aspects. Diagnostic assessment ideally includes cross-sectional and retrospective formal structured assessment of development and ASD symptoms based on information provided directly by the patient and, if possible, by relatives who can report on the subject's infancy and childhood.

Predicting individual adult outcome in high-functioning ASD remains an elusive task. Notwithstanding this, there is credible evidence that having an occupation, higher education, adequate family support, and emotional dynamics, as well as better socialization skills, are predictive of a better outcome in all domains of functioning, as well as in terms of quality of life. As ASD gain visibility as a significant mental health problem in adults, new forms of intervention are likely to appear. These should probably prioritize the improvement of adaptive functioning rather than attempt to modify ASD core features. It is important that these interventions take into account the existence and the special needs of a particular subgroup of cognitively able individuals who, though formally labeled as high functioning, are actually functioning at a level that is essentially not much better than that of less cognitively able individuals. New developments are also needed in terms of formal assessment of psychiatric comorbidity in this population, as psychiatric comorbidity is not only the rule in cognitively able adults with an ASD but is also a major factor negatively affecting outcome. Unfortunately, highly impaired adults with a high-functioning ASD seldom receive adequate formal support from mental health and rehabilitation services, as most available programs are predominantly designed to address the needs of either low-functioning individuals with a neurodevelopmental disorder or patients with severe chronic mental disorders such as schizophrenia, leaving these subjects to wander in a sort of no-man's land of adult mental health care.

References

American Psychiatric Association (institution) (2013) Schizophrenia Spectrum and Other Psychotic Disorders. In: American Psychiatric Association (institution) (ed) Diagnostic and statistic manual of mental disorders (DSM-5). 5th edn. APA, Washington DC

Attwood T (2007) The complete guide to Asperger's syndrome. Jessica Kingsley Publishers, London/Philadelphia

Barahona-Corrêa JB, Filipe CN (2016) A concise history of Asperger syndrome: the short reign of a troublesome diagnosis. Front Psychol 6(January):1–7. Available at: http://journal.frontiersin.org/Article/10.3389/fpsyg.2015.02024/abstract

Barneveld PS et al (2014) Quality of life: a case-controlled long-term follow-up study, comparing young high-functioning adults with autism spectrum disorders with adults with other psychiatric disorders diagnosed in childhood. Compr Psychiatry 55(2):302–310. Available at: http://dx.doi.org/10.1016/j.comppsych.2013.08.001

Baron-Cohen S et al (2005) The Adult Asperger Assessment (AAA): a diagnostic method. J Autism Dev Disord 35(6):807–819

Bastiaansen JA et al (2011) Diagnosing autism spectrum disorders in adults: the use of Autism Diagnostic Observation Schedule (ADOS) module 4. J Autism Dev Disord 41(9):1256–1266. Available at: http://link.springer.com/10.1007/s10803-010-1157-x

Bernardo Barahona-Corrêa J et al (2015) From thought to action: how the interplay between neuroscience and phenomenology changed our understanding of obsessive-compulsive disorder. Frontiers Psychol 6(NOV):1–12

Billstedt E, Gillberg C, Gillberg C (2005). Autism after adolescence: population-based 13- to 22-year follow-up study of 120 individuals with autism diagnosed in childhood. J Autism Dev Disord 35(3):351–360. Available at: http://link.springer.com/10.1007/s10803-005-3302-5

Billstedt E, Carina Gillberg I, Gillberg C (2007) Autism in adults: symptom patterns and early childhood predictors. Use of the DISCO in a community sample followed from childhood. J Child Psychol Psychiat Allied D 48(11):1102–1110

Bruder MB et al (2012) Brief report: the medical care of adults with autism spectrum disorders: identifying the needs. J Autism Dev Disord 42(11):2498–2504. Available at: http://www.ncbi.nlm.nih.gov/pubmed/22427260

Brugha TS et al (2011) Epidemiology of autism spectrum disorders in adults in the community in England. Arch Gen Psychiatry 68(5):459–465

Buck TR et al (2014) Psychiatric comorbidity and medication use in adults with autism spectrum disorder. J Autism Dev Disord 44:3063–3071

Carina Gillberg I et al (2007) Cognitive and executive functions in anorexia nervosa ten years after onset of eating disorder. J Clin Exp Neuropsychol 29(2):170–178. Available at: http://www.tandfonline.com/doi/abs/10.1080/13803390600584632#.VhzDLnpViko

Cassidy S et al (2014) Suicidal ideation and suicide plans or attempts in adults with asperger's syndrome attending a specialist diagnostic clinic: a clinical cohort study. Lancet Psych 1(2):142–147. Available at: http://dx.doi.org/10.1016/S2215-0366(14)70248-2

Cath DC et al (2008) Symptom overlap between Autism spectrum disorder, generalized social anxiety disorder and obsessive-compulsive disorder in adults: a preliminary case-controlled study. Psychopathol 41(2):101–110

Cederlund M, Gillberg C (2004) One hundred males with Asperger syndrome: a clinical study of background and associated factors. Dev Med Child Neurol 46:652–660. Available at: http://www.ncbi.nlm.nih.gov/pubmed/15473168

Cederlund M et al (2008) Asperger syndrome and autism: a comparative longitudinal follow-up study more than 5 years after original diagnosis. J Autism Dev Disord 38(1):72–85

Chiang HM et al (2014) A meta-analysis of differences in IQ profiles between individuals with Asperger's disorder and high-functioning autism. J Autism Dev Disord 44(7):1577–1596

Davis E, Saeed SA, Antonacci DJ (2008) Anxiety disorders in persons with developmental disabilities: empirically informed diagnosis and treatment: orders in dd population with practical take-home messages for the clinician. Psychiatry Q 79(3):249–263

Eaves LC, Ho HH (2008) Young adult outcome of autism spectrum disorders. J Autism Dev Disord 38(4):739–747

Engstrom I, Engstrom L, Emilsson B (2003) Psychosocial functioning in a group of Swedish adults with Asperger syndrome or high-functioning autism. Autism 7(1):99–110. Available at: http://www.ingentaselect.com/rpsv/cgi-bin/cgi?ini=xref&body=linker&reqdoi=10.1177/1362361303007001013\n, http://aut.sagepub.com/content/7/1/99.full.pdf+html

Esbensen AJ et al (2009) A longitudinal investigation of psychotropic and non-psychotropic medication use among adolescents and adults with autism spectrum disorders. J Autism Dev Disord 39(9):1339–1349

Farley MA et al (2009) Twenty-year outcome for individuals with autism and average or near-average cognitive abilities. Autism Res 2(2):109–118

Fitzgerald M (2012) Schizophrenia and autism/Asperger's syndrome: overlap and difference. Clin Neuropathol 9(4):171–176

Geurts HM, Jansen MD (2011) A retrospective chart study: the pathway to a diagnosis for adults referred for ASD assessment. Autism 16(3):299–305. Available at: http://aut.sagepub.com/content/16/3/299.abstract

Ghaziuddin M, Zafar S (2008) Psychiatric comorbidity of adults with autism spectrum disorders. Clin Neuropathol 5(1):9–12

Ghaziuddin M, Ghaziuddin N, Greden J (2002) Depression in persons with autism: implications for research and clinical care. J Autism Dev Disord 32(4):299–306

Gillberg C (2002) A guide to Asperger syndrome, 1st edn. Cambridge University Press, Cambridge

Gillberg C et al (2001) The Asperger syndrome (and high-functioning autism) Diagnostic Interview (ASDI): a preliminary study of a new structured clinical interview. Autism 5(1):57–66. Available at: http://aut.sagepub.com/cgi/doi/10.1177/1362361301005001006

Gillberg IC et al (2015) Boys with Asperger syndrome grow up: psychiatric and neurodevelopmental disorders 20 years after initial diagnosis. J Autism Dev Disord. Available at: http://link.springer.com/10.1007/s10803-015-2544-0

Griffith G et al (2012) "I just don't fit anywhere": support experiences and future support needs of individuals with Asperger syndrome in middle adulthood. Autism 16(5):532–546

Harrison PL, Oakland T (2003) Adaptive behavior assessment system, 2nd edn. The Psychological Corporation, San Antonio

Helles A et al (2014) Asperger syndrome in males over two decades: stability and predictors of diagnosis. J Child Psychol Psy. p.n/a-n/a. Available at: http://doi.wiley.com/10.1111/jcpp.12334

Hofvander B et al (2009) Psychiatric and psychosocial problems in adults with normal-intelligence autism spectrum disorders. BMC Psychiat 9:35

Holwerda A et al (2012) Predictors for work participation in individuals with an autism spectrum disorder: a systematic review. J Occup Rehabil 22(3):333–352

Howlin P (2000) Outcome in adult life for more able individuals with Autism or Asperger Syndrome. Autism 4(1):63–83
Howlin P (2003) Outcome in high-functioning adults with autism with and without early language delays: implications for the differentiation between autism and asperger syndrome. J Autism Dev Disord 33(1):3–13
Howlin P, Moss P (2012) Adults with autism spectrum disorders. Can J Psychiatr 57(5):275–283. Available at: http://search.ebscohost.com/login.aspx?direct=true&db=pbh&AN=76476991&site=ehost-live
Howlin P et al (2004) Adult outcome for children with autism. J Child Psychol Psychiat Allied Disciplines 45:212–229
Howlin P, Alcock J, Burkin C (2005) An 8 year follow-up of a specialist supported employment service for high-ability adults with autism or Asperger syndrome. Autism Int J Res Pract 9(5):533–549
Howlin P et al (2013) Social outcomes in mid- to later adulthood among individuals diagnosed with autism and average nonverbal IQ as children. J Am Acad Child Adolescent Psy 53(6):572–581.e1
Hus V, Lord C (2014) The autism diagnostic observation schedule, module 4: revised algorithm and standardized severity scores. J Autism Dev Disord 44(8):1996–2012
Hutton J et al (2008) New-onset psychiatric disorders in individuals with autism. Autism Int J Res Practice 12(4):373–390
Jennes-Coussens M, Magill-Evans J, Koning C (2006) The quality of life of young men with Asperger syndrome: a brief report. Autism Int J Res Practice 10(4):403–414
Jones L et al (2014) Experiences of receiving a diagnosis of autism spectrum disorder: a survey of adults in the United Kingdom. J Autism Dev Disord 44(12):3033–3044. Available at: http://www.ncbi.nlm.nih.gov/pubmed/15003161
Joshi G et al (2010) The heavy burden of psychiatric comorbidity in youth with autism spectrum disorders: a large comparative study of a psychiatrically referred population. J Autism Dev Disord 40(11):1361–1370
Joshi G et al (2013) Psychiatric comorbidity and functioning in a clinically referred population of adults with autism spectrum disorders: a comparative study. J Autism Dev Disord 43(6):1314–1325
Kamio Y, Inada N, Koyama T (2013) A nationwide survey on quality of life and associated factors of adults with high-functioning autism spectrum disorders. Autism 17(1):15–26. Available at: http://aut.sagepub.com/cgi/doi/10.1177/1362361312436848
Kato K et al (2013) Clinical features of suicide attempts in adults with autism spectrum disorders. Gen Hosp Psychiatry 35(1):50–53. Available at: http://linkinghub.elsevier.com/retrieve/pii/S0163834312002782
Kenworthy L et al (2010) Adaptive behavior ratings correlate with symptomatology and IQ among individuals with high-functioning autism spectrum disorders. J Autism Dev Disord 40(4):416–423. Available at: http://link.springer.com/10.1007/s10803-009-0911-4
Khanna R et al (2014) Health-related quality of life and its determinants among adults with autism. Res Autism Spectrum Disord 8(3):157–167. Available at: http://dx.doi.org/10.1016/j.rasd.2013.11.003
Kite DM, Gullifer J, Tyson GA (2013) Views on the diagnostic labels of autism and Asperger's disorder and the proposed changes in the DSM. J Autism Dev Disord 43(7):1692–1700
Klin A et al (2007) Social and communication abilities and disabilities in higher functioning individuals with autism spectrum disorders: the Vineland and the ADOS. J Autism Dev Disord 37(4):748–759
Kreiser NL, White SW (2015) ASD traits and co-occurring psychopathology: the moderating role of gender. J Autism Dev Disord. Available at: http://link.springer.com/10.1007/s10803-015-2580-9
Lai M-C, Baron-Cohen S (2015) Identifying the lost generation of adults with autism spectrum conditions. Lancet Psy 2(11):1013–1027. Available at: http://linkinghub.elsevier.com/retrieve/pii/S2215036615002771

Lai MC et al (2011) A behavioral comparison of male and female adults with high functioning autism spectrum conditions. PLoS ONE 6(6)
Leekam SR et al (2007) Describing the sensory abnormalities of children and adults with autism. J Autism Dev Disord 37(5):894–910
Lehnhardt F-G et al (2011) Autism spectrum disorders in adulthood: clinical and neuropsychological findings of Aspergers syndrome diagnosed late in life. Fortschr Neurol Psychiatr 79(5):290–297
Lehnhardt FG et al (2012) Das psychosoziale Funktionsniveau spätdiagnostizierter Patienten mit Autismus-Spektrum-Störungen – eine retrospektive Untersuchung im Erwachsenenalter. Fortschritte der Neurologie Psychiatrie 80(2):88–97
Lehnhardt F-G et al (2013) The investigation and differential diagnosis of asperger syndrome in adults. Deutsches Ärzteblatt International 110(45):755–763. Available at: http://www.ncbi.nlm.nih.gov/pubmed/24290364
Lord C, Venter A (1992) Outcome and follow-up studies of high-functioning autistic individuals. In: Schopler E, Mesibov GB (eds) High-functioning individuals with Autism. Springer Science + Business Media, New York, pp 187–199
Lord C, Rutter M, Le Couteur A (1994) Autism diagnostic interview-revised: a revised version of a diagnostic interview for caregivers of individuals with possible pervasive developmental disorders. J Autism Dev Disord 24(5):659–685. Available at: http://infantlab.fiu.edu/articles/Lord,Rutter,LeCouteur_1994 JADD.pdf\n, http://link.springer.com/10.1007/BF02172145
Lord C et al (2000) The autism diagnostic observation schedule–generic: a standard measure of social and communication deficits associated with the spectrum of autism. J Autism Dev Disord 30(3):205–223
Lugnegård T, Hallerbäck MU, Gillberg C (2011) Psychiatric comorbidity in young adults with a clinical diagnosis of Asperger syndrome. Res Dev Disabil 32(5):1910–1917. Available at: http://linkinghub.elsevier.com/retrieve/pii/S0891422211001442
Magiati I, Tay XW, Howlin P (2014) Cognitive, language, social and behavioural outcomes in adults with autism spectrum disorders: a systematic review of longitudinal follow-up studies in adulthood. Clin Psychol Rev 34(1):78–86. Available at: http://dx.doi.org/10.1016/j.cpr.2013.11.002
Marriage S, Wolverton A, Marriage K (2009) Autism spectrum disorder grown up: a chart review of adult functioning. J Can Acad Child Adolescent Psychiat 18(4):322–328
Matson JL, Boisjoli JA (2008) Strategies for assessing Asperger's syndrome: a critical review of data based methods. Res Autism Spectrum Disord 2(2):237–248
Matson JL, Goldin RL (2014) What is the future of assessment for autism spectrum disorders: short and long term. Res Autism Spectrum Disord 8(3):209–213. Available at: http://dx.doi.org/10.1016/j.rasd.2013.01.007
Matson JL, Wilkins J (2008) Nosology and diagnosis of Asperger's syndrome. Res Autism Spectrum Disord 2(2):288–300
Matthews NL et al (2015) Adaptive functioning in autism spectrum disorder during the transition to adulthood. J Autism Dev Disord 2349–2360. Available at: http://link.springer.com/10.1007/s10803-015-2400-2
Miguel EC et al (2001) The tic-related obsessive-compulsive disorder phenotype and treatment implications. Adv Neurol 85:43–55
Moss P et al (2015) Self and informant reports of mental health difficulties among adults with autism findings from a long-term follow-up study. Autism Int J Res Pract 1362361315585916. Available at: http://aut.sagepub.com/content/early/2015/05/22/1362361315585916.abstract
Mouridsen SE et al (2008) Psychiatric disorders in individuals diagnosed with infantile autism as children: a case control study. J Psy Pract 14(1):5–12. Available at: http://www.ncbi.nlm.nih.gov/pubmed/18212598
National Institute for Health and Care Excellence (2012) Autism: recognition, referral, diagnosis and management of adults on the autism spectrum. The British Psychological Society and The Royal College of Psychiatrists, London

Nicolaidis C et al (2011) "Respect the way I need to communicate with you": healthcare experiences of adults on the autistic spectrum. J Gen Internal Med Conf S184–S185. Available at: http://shibboleth.ovid.com/secure/?T=JS&CSC=Y&NEWS=N&PAGE=fulltext&D=emed10&AN=70653570\n, http://sfx.kcl.ac.uk/kings?genre=article&atitle="Respect+the+way+I+need+to+communicate+with+you":+Healthcare+experiences+of+adults+on+the+autistic+spectrum&title=Jour

Nordin V, Gillberg C (1998) The long-term course of autistic disorders: update on follow-up studies. Acta Psychiatr Scand 97(2):99–108

Nylander L, Gillberg C (2001) Screening for autism spectrum disorders in adult psychiatric outpatients: a preliminary report. Acta Psychiatr Scand 103(6):428–434. Available at: http://doi.wiley.com/10.1034/j.1600-0447.2001.00175.x

Palmer CJ et al (2014) "Subtypes" in the presentation of autistic traits in the general adult population. J Autism Dev Disord 1291–1301. Available at: http://link.springer.com/10.1007/s10803-014-2289-1

Pilling, S. et al., 2012. Recognition, referral, diagnosis, and management of adults with autism: summary of NICE guidance. BMJ 344(jun27 1):e4082–e4082.

Pugliese CE et al (2015) Replication and comparison of the newly proposed ADOS-2, module 4 algorithm in ASD without ID: a multi-site study. J Autism Dev Disord (September). Available at: http://link.springer.com/10.1007/s10803-015-2586-3

Punshon C, Skirrow P, Murphy G (2009) The not guilty verdict: psychological reactions to a diagnosis of Asperger syndrome in adulthood. Autism Int J Res Practice 13(3):265–283. Available at: http://aut.sagepub.com/content/13/3/265.long\n, http://www.researchgate.net/publication/24280450_The_'not_guilty_verdict'_Psychological_reactions_to_a_diagnosis_of_Asperger_syndrome_in_adulthood

Råstam M (2008) Eating disturbances in autism spectrum disorders with focus on adolescent and adult years. Clin Neuropathol 5(1):31–42

Renty JO (2006) Quality of life in high-functioning adults with autism spectrum disorder: the predictive value of disability and support characteristics. Autism 10(5):511–524. Available at: http://aut.sagepub.com/cgi/doi/10.1177/1362361306066604

Rodgers J et al (2012) The relationship between anxiety and repetitive behaviours in autism spectrum disorder. J Autism Dev Disord 42(11):2404–2409

Rumsey JM, Rapoport JL, Sceery WR (1985) Autistic children as adults: psychiatric, social, and behavioral outcomes. J Am Academy Child Psy 24(4):465–473. Available at: http://www.sciencedirect.com/science/article/pii/S0002713809605665

Russell AJ et al (2005) Obsessions and compulsions in Asperger syndrome and high-functioning autism. Br J Psy 186(JUNE):525–528

Rutter M et al (2007) Early adolescent outcomes of institutionally deprived and non-deprived adoptees. III Quasi-autism. J Child Psychol Psychiat Allied D 48(12):1200–1207

Rydén E, Bejerot S (2008) Autism spectrum disorders in an adult psychiatric population. A naturalistic cross-sectional controlled study Eleonore Rydén and Susanne Bejerot. Clin Neuropathol 5(1):13–21

Ryden G, Ryden E, Hetta J (2008) Borderline personality disorder and autism spectrum disorder in females – a cross-sectional study. Clin Neuropathol 5(1):22–30. Available at: http://www.clinicalneuropsychiatry.org/pdf/04_ryden_hetta.pdf

Sappok T et al (2013) Diagnosing autism in a clinical sample of adults with intellectual disabilities: how useful are the ADOS and the ADI-R? Res Dev Disabil 34(5):1642–1655. Available at: http://linkinghub.elsevier.com/retrieve/pii/S0891422213000413

Seltzer MM et al (2003) The symptoms of autism spectrum disorders in adolescence and adulthood. J Autism Dev Disord 33(6):565–581. Available at: c:\pdf\b\xc27333.pdf

Seltzer MM et al (2004) Trajectory of development in adolescents and adults with autism. Mental Retard Dev Disabil Res Rev 10(4):234–247. Available at: http://www.ncbi.nlm.nih.gov/puebmed/15666341

Shattuck PT et al (2007) Change in autism symptoms and maladaptive behaviors in adolescents and adults with an autism spectrum disorder. J Autism Dev Disord 37(9):1735–1747

Sizoo B et al (2010) Treatment seeking adults with autism or ADHD and co-morbid substance use disorder: prevalence, risk factors and functional disability. Drug Alcoh Depen 107(1):44–50. Available at: http://www.ncbi.nlm.nih.gov/pubmed/19786328

Smith LE, Greenberg JS, Mailick MR (2014) The family context of autism spectrum disorders. Influence on the behavioral phenotype and quality of life. Child Adolesc Psychiatr Clin N Am 23(1):143–155

Sparrow S, Cicchetti D, Balla DA (2005) Vineland adaptive behavior scales second edition: survey forms manual. Pearson, Minneapolis

Spek AA, Scholte EM, Van Berckelaer-Onnes IA (2008) Brief report: the use of WAIS-III in adults with HFA and Asperger syndrome. J Autism Dev Disord 38(4):782–787

Spillers JLH, Sensui LM, Linton KF (2014) Concerns about identity and services among people with Autism and Asperger's regarding DSM-5 changes. J Soc Work Disabil Rehabil (August):37–41. Available at: http://www.ncbi.nlm.nih.gov/pubmed/24816184

Stahlberg O et al (2004) Bipolar disorder, schizophrenia, and other psychotic disorders in adults with childhood onset AD/HD and/or autism spectrum disorders. J Neural Transm 111(7):891–902

Stewart ME et al (2006) Presentation of depression in autism and Asperger syndrome: a review. Autism 10(1):103–116. Available at: http://aut.sagepub.com/cgi/doi/10.1177/1362361306062013

Szatmari P et al (1989) A follow-up study of high-functioning autistic children. J Autism Dev Disord 19(2):213–225

Takara K, Kondo T (2014a) Autism spectrum disorder among first-visit depressed adult patients: diagnostic clues from backgrounds and past history. Gen Hosp Psychiatry 36(6):737–742. Available at: http://linkinghub.elsevier.com/retrieve/pii/S0163834314002084

Takara K, Kondo T (2014b) Comorbid atypical autistic traits as a potential risk factor for suicide attempts among adult depressed patients: a case–control study. Ann Gen Psy 13(1):33. Available at: http://www.annals-general-psychiatry.com/content/13/1/33

Tantam D (2000) Psychological disorder in adolescents and adults with Asperger syndrome. Autism 4(1):47–62. Available at: http://aut.sagepub.com/cgi/doi/10.1177/1362361300004001004

Taylor JL, Seltzer MM (2010) Changes in the autism behavioral phenotype during the transition to adulthood. J Autism Dev Disord 40(12):1431–1446

Taylor JL, Seltzer MM (2011) Employment and post-secondary educational activities for young adults with autism spectrum disorder during the transition to adulthood. J Autism Dev Disord 41(5):566–574

Tobin MC, Drager KDR, Richardson LF (2014) A systematic review of social participation for adults with autism spectrum disorders: support, social functioning, and quality of life. Res Autism Spectrum Disord 8(3):214–229. Available at: http://dx.doi.org/10.1016/j.rasd.2013.12.002

Tsuchiya KJ et al (2013) Reliability and validity of autism diagnostic interview-revised, Japanese version. J Autism Dev Disord 43(2013):643–662

Tyson KE, Cruess DG (2012) Differentiating high-functioning autism and social phobia. J Autism Dev Disord 42(7):1477–1490

Underwood L, McCarthy J, Tsakanikos E (2011) Assessment of comorbid psychopathology. In: Matson JL, Sturmey P (eds) International handbook of autism and pervasive developmental disorders. Springer Science + Business Media, New York/Dordrecht/Heidelberg/London, pp 287–293

Underwood L et al (2015) Assessment and diagnosis of psychiatric disorder in adults with autism spectrum disorder. Adv Ment Health Intellect Disabil 9(5):222–229. Available at: http://www.emeraldinsight.com/doi/10.1108/AMHID-05-2015-0025

Van Wijngaarden-Cremers PJM et al (2014) Gender and age differences in the core triad of impairments in autism spectrum disorders: a systematic review and meta-analysis. J Autism Dev Disord 44(3):627–635

Venter A, Lord C, Schopler E (1992) A follow-up study of high-functioning autistic children. J Child Psychol Psychiatry 33(3):489–597

Wallace GL et al (2015) Real-world executive functions in adults with Autism spectrum disorder: profiles of impairment and associations with adaptive functioning and co-morbid anxiety and depression. J Autism Dev Disord. Available at: http://link.springer.com/10.1007/s10803-015-2655-7

Wing L (1981) Asperger syndrome: a clinical account. Psychol Med 11(1):115–129

Wing L et al (2002) The diagnostic interview for social and communication disorders: background, inter-rater reliability and clinical use. J Child Psy Psychiat 43(3):307–325. Available at: http://www.ncbi.nlm.nih.gov/pubmed/11944874

Woodman AC et al (2015) Change in autism symptoms and maladaptive behaviors in adolescence and adulthood: the role of positive family processes. J Autism Dev Disord 45(1):111–126

Zerbo O et al (2015) A study of physician knowledge and experience with Autism in adults in a large integrated healthcare system. J Autism Dev Disord. Available at: http://link.springer.com/10.1007/s10803-015-2579-2

Zucker NL et al (2007) Anorexia nervosa and autism spectrum disorders: guided investigation of social cognitive endophenotypes. Psychol Bull 133(6):976–1006

Ageing with Autistic-Spectrum Disorder (ASD)

6

Elizabeta B. Mukaetova-Ladinska and Barbara Maier

6.1 Barbara's Story

'I have Asperger and I tell my clients'. This sentence puzzled me while I was checking the Internet site of the German author and famous trainer for communication Vera Felicitas Birkenbihl. 'I have Asperger' sounded to me like 'I have a flu', or some sort of disease. So I searched the World Wide Web for 'Asperger'.

What I found puzzled me even more, because the definition of the Asperger syndrome sounded like the description of my own personality. The more I read about it on the Internet, the bigger my suspicion grew that this could be the explanation for all the difficulties I had throughout my life. And it explained why at the age of 48, I still loved to watch the rotating drum of the washing machine.

It took a lot of phone calls and some persistence to find a clinic that could provide a diagnosis. The process itself was demanding. Besides the standardised tests I had to undergo, the biography was required. I had to remember all the embarrassing and unpleasant situations that my odd and inappropriate quotations and actions had caused. They had made teachers and many persons wonder about me.

The confirmation of my suspicion, the diagnosis of Asperger syndrome (or high-function autism), was a shock and a relief at the same time. I was stunned: how was it possible that none of the medically and psychologically educated persons in my professional environment had recognised me as an autistic person?

E.B. Mukaetova-Ladinska, MD, PhD, MRCPsych (✉)
Institute of Neuroscience, Newcastle University, Campus for Ageing and Vitality, Newcastle upon, Tyne NE4 5PL, UK

Newcastle Integrated Liaison Team, Richardson Unit, Royal Victoria Infirmary, Newcastle upon, Tyne NE1 4LP, UK
e-mail: Elizabeta.Mukaetova-Ladinska@ncl.ac.uk

B. Maier
Kapellenstraße 4, 4591, Molln, Austria

B. Barahona Corrêa, R.-J. van der Gaag (eds.), *Autism Spectrum Disorders in Adults*, DOI 10.1007/978-3-319-42713-3_6

The relief still persists. The wondering about why I had passed the final exams of my professional training as a registered nurse with distinction and on the other hand failed over and over again, especially in social situations, had found a conceivable explanation.

Reading and learning about autism as much as possible was my way of dealing with all the emotions that I felt at that time. In various autobiographies, I found depictions that sounded very strange to me, while others were so familiar and described exactly my experiences. Is that one of the reasons why the condition remains undetected so often?

Autistic persons are so different from each other. The phenomenon autism is often described in literature and movies, but it is not labelled adequately. The specific features of an autistic person are not described in a few words. So there are many autistic persons who are not identified and are leading a life with bigger or smaller difficulties. The consequences, the so-called comorbidities, often are depression and even suicide. The constant efforts to cope, to fit in and to learn, using the intellect, all those things that others manage to do intuitively right, are very strenuous. To differentiate and process all the stimuli of a world that is normal to others is a very tiring challenge. Failures occur despite of all the efforts. They are frustrating and discouraging.

Now I know that some problems are caused by the different types of intelligence that are rather balanced in neurologically typical persons. In contrast, autistic persons have peaks and valleys in this profile. And it has to do with the pace and mode of processing stimuli. When performing certain tasks, autistic persons activate areas in the brain that are different from those activated by 'average persons' performing the same tasks. The motoric problems and the hyper- and hyposensitivity to smells and taste and to tactile, auditory and visual perception suggest that the nervous system is impaired. Does the accumulation of hints to health problems that can be found in various (auto)biographies indicate an impaired immune system as well?

I am 50 now and luckily I could *improve* on some of my weaknesses:

I have gained a certain repertoire of themes for small talk.

I have learned to understand many jokes, proverbial sayings and metaphors. I have also learned to ask frequently, whenever I do not understand something. In my profession and the accompanying psychological coaching, in many classes with psychological content and particularly through the psychotherapy, which I have attended on my own account, I learned to understand humans and their actions a little. But still there are social situations that I need to be explained to me. I still depend on well-meaning persons. I have become very insecure about my communication, and my shyness with people remains.

What has not improved at all is my sensitivity to certain stimuli, for example, certain odours or loud noises. My impression is that over the years, my nervous system is becoming more sensitive, and thus my level of tolerance is getting less.

My daily routines, which define everyday life and provide security, become more and more important. Deviations from this daily rhythm are becoming increasingly challenging.

So the outlook for *the future*, for age with autism, is one I must contemplate with concern.

Will it be known in the future that autism is a social handicap, and will it be generally recognised?

Will it be common knowledge that the autistic perception of the world can be very different from the perception of the so-called neurologically typical?

Will the public know that the thinking processes run differently in us? As a result, our communication skills are different. That means, dealing with us sometimes needs an increased amount of time. Time is money, and money gets less and less where it is needed.

How will it be, when one day the persons that we trust and that support us and assist us in everyday life will not be there anymore? Every new, strange person means stress for me. If we are not very good in taking care of us and our economic situation at a young age, how will that be when we are old? Will there be new and appropriate individuals who do not cheat us?

If I will become dependent on care, will it be respected that I do not want to be massaged, stroked and have applied lotions? Even touches and sometimes hugs can be unbearable? And will I be able to communicate my needs?

Will there be understanding that human voices at times are intolerable for me, as well as certain sounds, and will there be assistance, when one day I will no longer be able to apply earplugs?

And will it be well known that when confronted with too much stimulation, a sensory overload is possible, which can express itself differently depending on the person? Will there be help for prevention, and if it does happen, how will that situation be dealt with? With understanding and competence or with sedatives?

Will it be possible that one day there are jobs for us, allowing us to endure a working life until reaching the legal age for retirement? Will it be possible that the surroundings are adjusted to our needs and that one day our talents and competencies will be recognised and used for the benefit of all? Because, without a doubt, every human being has special capabilities.

6.2 Ageing with ASD

'Adults with autism need to be heard and listened to' stated one of the greatest researchers and practitioners in the field of autism – Sir Michael Rutter. Yet, the voice of autistic-spectrum disorder (ASD) adults is hardly heard. In a recent workshop, one of the ASD adults we interviewed spoke of his fear facing ageing. For him, 'the first transition was difficult, but the second looks even more worrying'

(Mukaetova-Ladinska and Stuart-Hamilton 2016). This statement summarises the great unknowns and insecurity ageing with ASD brings.

Barbara's testimonial clearly identifies several domains for successful ageing of ASD individuals: service provision (including obtaining diagnosis for those adult ASD subjects who have not graduated from the child ASD services), importance of professional services (calling for more research to understand ASD brain neurobiology and functioning), frustrations and discouragements she faced in her adulthood, as well as the self-help and wider understanding of the ASD process. According to her narrative, growing up with ASD consists of achievements [e.g. gaining new social skills with professional help; improving social communication; ability to understand jokes, abstract sayings and metaphors; self-motivation and self-education, searching the Web in an attempt to understand behaviour; being assertive to enquire about things one is not familiar with; improving understanding of 'humans and their actions' and problems coping to fit in (i.e. coping with stimuli and processing normal to the outside world); and facing failures, frustration and discouragements during the long process of relearning to adapt to the world of normotypicals]. This perspective comes from a highly functioning ASD individual, and in face of the lack of research on ageing in intellectually challenged ASD subjects, it is difficult to state whether these can be generalised for the whole ASD spectrum.

6.2.1 ASD Adults: Unmet Needs

Barbara's adulthood achievements appear to be closely linked to an increasing dependence on well-meaning people (family, friends and colleagues) who guide and provide explanation and support. This argues that the societal backup continues to play a major role in supporting ASD adults. However, there are discrepancies between current availability of support provisions for ASD children and their families and those for ASD adults and older people. Does this mean that the support set-up during childhood is sufficient to meet the ASD adults' needs? Are ASD adults being left to fend for themselves or, at best, to depend on support from their families? Has enough been done to educate society to follow this change? If so, have ASD adults' social needs been met, i.e. responsibilities and expectations of being a grown-up, including living independently, employment, being in a relationship, starting a family or losing one's parents and the support one has had throughout the lifetime from a significant carer? Becoming a grown-up also faces persons with an ASD with further emotional struggle of coping with loss, with financial responsibility and with the challenge of interacting and dealing with normotypicals and understanding socially acceptable norms. In addition, there is the emotional turmoil and apprehension faced by families with ASD children: what will the future bring for them, who will look after them when parents are gone? Who will provide the financial security for them in the long term? Will the services be equipped to know their habits and traits (Case Vignette 6.1)? Last but not least, the anguish of not knowing whether service provision in old age will be apt to recognise and manage elderly people with ASD.

Case Vignette 6.1: Depression in Older Parent with an Adult ASD Son

David, 74-year-old man, was referred to Old Age Psychiatry due to ongoing unexplained physical problems. He lost 10 kg in weight over 10 months and was not sleeping, fearing that his chest pain might result in a heart infarct. He was fully investigated for chest pain, shortness of breath and widespread pain and underwent extensive physical examinations with cardiology and pneumology specialists. His ECG, chest X-ray, MRI spine scans and laboratory investigations were all normal. He was treated by his family practitioner with an antidepressant, but continued to be unmotivated and needed lots of encouragement to do routine daily tasks.

The change in antidepressants appeared initially to work well, but the symptoms returned, and David started frequenting the psychiatry services, predominantly complaining of chest and muscle pain. Although initially he was very guarded about his private life, and denied any issues of relevance in his marriage, gradually he started talking about his sons. David and his wife did not have children for a long time and adopted Michael at 3 months old when they were in their 40s. They devoted themselves to their young baby. Michael was not developing well and was diagnosed with ASD at the age of 4 years. The social services offered to take the toddler, but the couple refused and instead adopted another toddler, Peter. As the boys grew up, Peter proved to be a natural leader and excelled in team sports. In contrast, Michael's profound learning disability coupled with aggression, unexpected tantrums and sleepless nights resulted in him going into 24 h care when he was 14 years old. David took this very hard – he was visiting Michael every day. He frequently questioned whether his son recognised him, whether he knew his father was visiting him, but felt it was important for Michael to have a strong connection with his family.

With time, David's wife stopped visiting. David became even more devoted to their older son. He noticed the dynamic in the care home was changing: every year the number of visitors declined (parents dying, moving away, getting separated or becoming unwell), and the service users moved to other facilities due to economic and/or family reasons or getting unwell and dying. David became concerned about Michael's future. He could not share this with his wife, who was now fully occupied with becoming a grandmother and helping their younger son. David had numerous questions: What would happen with Michael when his parents would not be around? Who would visit him? Would Michael miss his parents? Who would pay the bills for his upkeep? Who would notice if Michael was unwell? These were only a few of the questions David had been worrying about. David himself formulated his depressive symptoms being due to 'loving Michael too much'(Fig. 6.1).

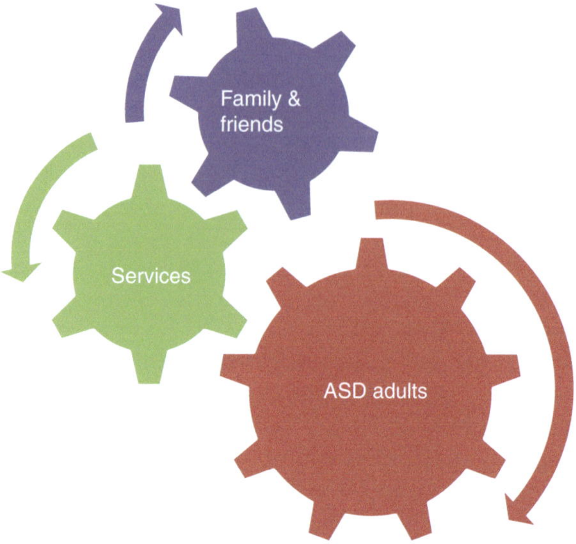

Fig. 6.1 Successful ASD ageing gearbox

6.2.2 ASD Diagnosis in Adulthood

There are numerous social and health differences between ASD adult subjects diagnosed in childhood and those who remain undiagnosed in their adulthood. The second group appears to face more challenges, in terms of seeking the diagnosis relying on the Web, in terms of understanding and knowledge of their families and with regard to having had to cope with their symptoms unaided throughout their lifetime. It is, thus, not surprising that many of the undiagnosed ASD subjects get their first diagnosis by chance, i.e. when referred to psychiatric services as a result of psychiatric comorbidities such as depression, unusual behaviour, memory problems (James et al. 2006; Naidu et al. 2006) or even general health problems (i.e. when investigated or treated for underlying physical issues; Mukaetova-Ladinska and Coppock 2016). Even then, the diagnosis is troublesome.

When should we consider diagnosing adults with ASD? How helpful is it to obtain an ASD diagnosis in adulthood? The diagnosis per se does not only provide a self- and social explanation and understanding of the long-term traits of the ASD person but also facilitates communication, management and insight into their world. In particular, for those of us working in medical settings, the diagnosis of ASD is helpful to manage our mentally and physically ill patients and enables us to implement a person-centred care approach and to optimise their overall medical treatment. Similar benefits should be seen in other aspects of social and economic interactions of ASD individuals and would provide the obvious explanation for some of their behaviour. This in turn should also lead to education of the population for accepting adult ASD individuals.

Table 6.1 Identification and initial assessment of possible autism in adults (after NICE 2012)

Consider assessment for possible autism when a person has:
A. *One or more of the following*:
Persistent difficulties in social interaction
Persistent difficulties in social communication
Stereotypic (rigid and repetitive) behaviour
Resistance to change
Restricted interests
B. *One or more of the following*:
Problems in obtaining or sustaining employment or education
Difficulties in initiating or sustaining social relationships
Previous or current contact with mental health or learning disability services
A history of a neurodevelopmental condition (including learning disabilities and attention deficit hyperactivity disorder) or mental disorder

NICE (2012) provides guidance for identifying and diagnosing ASD adults. Guidelines propose a two-step assessment: identification and initial assessment of possible ASD in adults (Table 6.1) followed by assessments for suspected ASD in adults, based in the traditional ASD diagnosis model of developmental screening and comprehensive diagnostic evaluation (Table 6.2).

When diagnosing adults with ASD, primary care needs to play an important role in screening, detecting and referring these individuals to appropriate specialist services (Lehnhardt et al. 2013; Valkanova et al. 2013; Nicolaidis et al. 2014). The screening questions are mainly around early development and behavioural problems in different settings, i.e. home, school, work placement and/or social interactions. Since gastrointestinal and sensory problems are common in ASD, these should also be enquired after (Valkanova et al. 2013). In addition, the abbreviated Autism-Spectrum Quotient, consisting of ten items, is currently recommended for use as a screening tool for people with suspected ASD (Valkanova et al. 2013; Lehnhardt et al. 2013). This screening tool should help identify those adults who should be referred for further clinical assessments by specialised multidisciplinary services (Valkanova et al. 2013). The above recommendations have yet to be implemented widely in primary care and may help improve the diagnosis of ASD adults in general, including at the level of secondary and tertiary care.

6.2.3 Ageing Out of ASD

The anecdotal examples of some ASD individuals improving with age have been recently confirmed in a number of longitudinal studies conducted in children. One of the earliest studies (Seltzer et al. 2004) indicated that as many as between 10 and 20 % of ASD diagnosed individuals outgrow their original diagnosis. This may be a result of improvement, especially in their restrictive, repetitive behaviours that include stereotypical movements, restricted interests, ritualistic and compulsive

Table 6.2 Assessments of suspected autism in adults (after NICE 2012)

A. *Screening stage:*
1. For adults with possible autism who do not have a moderate or severe learning disability, consider using the Autism-Spectrum Quotient – 10 items (AQ-10)
2. For adults with possible autism who have a moderate or severe learning disability, consider a brief assessment to ascertain the presence of following behaviours (using a collateral information whenever possible from a family member, partner or carer; if two or more of these behaviour are present, offer a comprehensive assessment for autism):
Difficulties in reciprocal social interaction including:
Limited interaction with others (e.g. being aloof, indifferent or unusual)
Interaction to fulfil needs only
Interaction that is naive or one-sided
Lack of responsiveness to others
Little or no change in behaviour in response to different social situations
Limited social demonstration of empathy
Rigid routines and resistance to change
Marked repetitive activities (e.g. rocking and hand or finger flapping), especially when under stress or expressing emotion
3. If two or more of the above categories of behaviour are present, offer a comprehensive assessment for autism
B. *Comprehensive (diagnostic, needs and risks) assessment*
Assessment undertaken by trained, team-based professionals who draw on a range of professions and skills and if possible involvement of a family member, partner, carer or other informant or uses documentary evidence or current and past behaviours and early development
Discussion for the purpose of the assessment and how the outcome of the assessment will be fed back to them (feedback should be individualised and to involve family member or members, partner, carer or advocate, where appropriate, to support the person and help explain the feedback)
During the assessment, enquire about and assess core autism signs and symptoms (difficulties in social interaction and communication and the presence of stereotypic behaviour, resistance to change or restricted interests) that have been present in childhood and continued into adulthood, early developmental history, where possible behavioural problems, functioning at home, at school or at work, past and current physical and mental disorders other than neurodevelopmental conditions, hyper- and/or hypo-sensory sensitivities and attention to detail. Carry out direct observation of core autism signs and symptoms especially in social situations
For more complex diagnosis and assessment of adults, use a formal assessment tool, i.e. the Adult Asperger Assessment (AAA) (includes the Autism-Spectrum Quotient [AQ] and the Empathy Quotient [EQ]), the Autism Diagnostic Interview-Revised (ADI-R), the Autism Diagnostic Observation Schedule-Generic (ADOS-G), the Asperger Syndrome (and high-functioning autism) Diagnostic Interview (ASDI), the Ritvo Autism Asperger Diagnostic Scale-Revised (RAADS-R) (for people who do not have a learning disability) and ADOS-G and ADI-R for people with a learning disability; additional tools to use for a more complex assessment include Diagnostic Interview for Social and Communication Disorders (DISCO) and the ADOS-G or the ADI-R

Table 6.2 (continued)

Take into account and assess for possible differential diagnoses and coexisting disorders or conditions, i.e. other neurodevelopmental conditions (use formal assessment tools for learning disabilities), mental disorders (e.g. schizophrenia, depression or other mood disorder anxiety disorders, including social anxiety disorder and obsessive-compulsive disorder), neurological disorders (epilepsy), physical disorders, communication difficulties (e.g. speech and language problems and selective mutism) and hyper- and/or hypo-sensory sensitivities
Biological tests, genetic tests or neuroimaging for diagnostic purposes are not recommended as a part of the comprehensive assessment. However, they can be used on an individual basis, and using information from the comprehensive assessment and physical examination, and clinical judgement, if there are specific dysmorphic features, congenital anomalies and/or evidence of a learning disability; electroencephalography if there is suspicion of epilepsy; hearing or sight tests, if there is suspicion of hearing or visual impairment; and other medical tests depending on individual signs and symptoms (e.g. sudden onset of challenging behaviour, change in usual patterns of behaviour, sudden change in weight or suspicion that the person might be in pain and is unable to communicate this)

behaviour(s) and self-injuries, which all appear to be less intense and severe and more infrequent as ASD individuals age (Esbensen et al. 2009). This has been noted even by Kanner, in 1973, when he described that some of the ASD individuals had '…positive adult outcomes (since)….they were self-motivated to change'. One of the explanations for this has been attributed to the ageing of the sensory systems, with the decrease in hypersensitivity and increase in hyposensitivity to levels that are usual for the normotypical population (Kern et al. 2006).

Most recent studies similarly described ASD symptoms becoming milder in intensity/severity with age, and even becoming subclinical, only to emerge in a crisis or an adverse environment (Balfe et al. 2011; Fein et al. 2013). Fein et al. (2013) reported that a number of highly functioning ASD children achieve so-called optimal outcomes (e.g. become devoid of ASD symptomatology) as they grow up. According to their definition, 'optimal outcome' requires losing all symptoms of ASD in addition to the diagnosis and functioning within the non-autistic range of social interaction and communication. The optimal outcome subjects did not differ on socialisation, communication, face recognition or most language subscales from their normotypical counterparts. However, this ASD group displayed milder symptoms than the rest of highly functioning ASD subjects early in their development in the social domain, in spite of equally severe difficulties with communication and repetitive behaviours. Clinical progress included improvement in their restricted and repetitive behaviours (Troyb et al. 2014a), having similar academic abilities to those of typically developing age peers (Troyb et al. 2014b), and improved pitch discrimination (Eigsti and Fein 2013). Nevertheless, these optimal outcome ASD subjects continued to exhibit profound difficulties in their executive function, including impulsivity, set-shifting, problem-solving, working memory and planning (Troyb et al. 2014c), thus differing substantially from their neurotypical counterparts.

In an additional review of more than 5000 studies, Magiati et al. (2014) found 25 reports, each comprising between 10 and 725 subjects with ASD diagnosed in childhood and evaluated at least once as adolescents or adults. They similarly found that although IQ and communication skills remain stable over age, there was enormous variability among the participants, concluding that no generalisation is possible regarding the prediction of adult outcomes in ASD. In an other study, van Heijst and Geurts (2015) performed a quantitative meta-analysis of ten studies on adult ASD to address the issue quality of life, defined here as a person's sense of satisfaction and fulfilment in day-to-day life in relation to his or her own goals, values, standards and expectations. Furthermore, a mix of factors influencing the latter was also addressed, e.g. physical health and psychological functioning and independence and social relationship(s). This review was based on data from 482 ASD people and 17,775 control subjects and an additional survey of 24 individuals (51–84 years of age) and 24 control subjects. The findings confirm that life satisfaction was significantly lower for people with ASD than their control counterparts. The authors concluded that even if older people with ASD have gained additional mechanisms/skills to deal with challenges in life, this does not affect (e.g. improve) their quality of life. In their latest work, Geurts and Lever (2014), based on 233 ASD and 125 control individual (19–79 years, IQ>80), found no evidence supporting the idea that ASD symptoms decrease with increasing age. Moreover, even though people with ASD experience more cognitive difficulties as compared to controls, this was not differentially related to age. Similarly, face recognition deficits in adults and elderly with ASD were independent of age (Koolschijn and Geurts 2014). The latter findings were based on 27 ASD individuals aged between 31 and 76 years. While age does seem to have a different effect on experienced quality of life in people with ASD and controls, according to people with ASD themselves, their quality of life remains relatively low.

Further evidence for the neurodiversity potential of the ageing ASD brain comes from animal studies, correlative behavioural and imaging studies as well as a series of transcranial magnetic stimulation (TMS) studies in subjects with autism. Thus, the ageing ASD rodent model shows increased synapses and hyperconnected neuronal circuits (Jasien et al. 2014), and these can be an effective advantage in the ageing process. A recent neuropsychological study similarly provided evidence that ASD modulates cognitive ageing, via sparing of the working memory (Lever et al. 2015). In addition, the lifetime behavioural and eclectic interventions as well as longstanding treatments with antidepressants and antipsychotic medication may also have a modulating effect on several brain regions involved in cognition, emotion and motivation [i.e. amygdala (anxiety, antidepressants use), caudate activity (obsessive-compulsive behaviour), prefrontal cortex and subgenual cingulate (antidepressants, conventional antipsychotics) (reviewed in Crocker et al. 2013) and striatum and nucleus accumbens (conventional antipsychotics, whereas atypical antipsychotic drugs have a subtler and more widespread impact; reviewed in Konradi and Heckers 2001)]. All these findings suggest that at least some ASD individuals have hidden brain potential that in certain instances can be unmasked. This bears resemblance to studies on people with visual and auditory deprivation, where the lost senses are recruited by spared sensory modalities (Merabet and Pascual-Leone 2010), thus confirming that even the adult brain possesses abilities that are normally concealed.

Although TMS, a non-invasive brain stimulation tool, has been predominantly explored as a novel treatment intervention in young ASD subjects, these findings can also be used to confirm that the underlying cortical mechanisms of excitability, connectivity and plasticity that underlie the higher cortical functions in ASD can be modulated in, at least, some ASD subjects, irrespective of their age. Thus, improvement in behaviour (Fecteau et al. 2011; D'Urso et al. 2015), language processing (Fecteau et al. 2011; Casanova et al. 2012, 2014), executive function (Sokhadze et al. 2014), social relatedness (Enticott et al. 2014), reduction in both repetitive-ritualistic behaviours (Sokhadze et al. 2010) and irritability (Baruth et al. 2010; Casanova et al. 2012, 2014) has been demonstrated in some ASD individuals, and this success largely depended on the brain areas that were stimulated (i.e. dorsolateral prefrontal cortex, dorsomedial prefrontal cortex, medial prefrontal cortex, supplementary motor area, right pars triangularis and pars opercularis, temporoparietal junction and superior temporal sulcus, all involved in mentalising ability), with emerging data suggesting that cerebellar stimulation may play a role in improving cognitive functioning in ASD (reviewed in Hoppenbrouwers et al. 2008). In the words of John Elder Robinson, TMS provides an experience of 'emotional awakening, world is brighter, more colourful, and more alive than before…no longer an outsider….gone from feeling like a social outcast to feeling like talking to anyone, most any time. It's a magical thing'.

Conclusion

The unknown faced by ASD subjects throughout their adult life is rarely documented by the ASD subjects, their families, society or the research community. Surprisingly, since the first meeting on Ageing with ASD in Newcastle 2009, the scientific literature resulted in reviews (Piven et al. 2011; Mukaetova-Ladinska et al. 2012; Happe and Charlton 2012; Perkins and Berkman 2012), but very little in terms of clinical research papers (Wallace et al. 2016; Lever and Geurts 2016). The latest research on the ASD hidden brain potential and its ability to be unmasked opens a number of possibilities to be explored not only for ASD adults and their families but the wider (research) community: Can they be generalised for the whole ASD spectrum? How young can ASD individuals react to rTMS? Are the rTMS therapeutic outcomes sustained throughout their adulthood? Can rTMS modify the ASD ageing process? Can the unmasking of hidden brain potential be used positively to prevent or even treat cognitive and behavioural problems associated with the ageing brain and dementia? In answering these questions, the active involvement of ASD adults from the whole spectrum, their life experiences and societal interactions as well as the engagement of the research community are of utmost importance to understand and facilitate successful ageing in ASD individuals.

Acknowledgements We would like to thank Mrs. Margaret Oliver for secretarial support.

References

Balfe M, Tantam D, Campbell M (2011) Possible evidence for a fall in the prevalence of high-functioning pervasive developmental disorder with age? Autism Res Treat 2011:325495

Baruth JM, Casanova MF, El-Baz A, Horrell T, Mathai G, Sears L, Sokhadze E (2010) Low-frequency Repetitive Transcranial Magnetic Stimulation (rTMS) modulates evoked-gamma frequency oscillations in Autism Spectrum Disorder (ASD). J Neurother 14(3):179–194

Casanova MF, Baruth JM, El-Baz A, Tasman A, Sears L, Sokhadze E (2012) Repetitive transcranial magnetic stimulation (rTMS) modulates event-related potential (ERP) indices of attention in autism. Transl Neurosci 3(2):170–180

Casanova MF, Hensley MK, Sokhadze EM, El-Baz AS, Wang Y, Li X, Sears L (2014) Effects of weekly low-frequency rTMS on autonomic measures in children with autism spectrum disorder. Front Hum Neurosci 8:851

Crocker LD, Heller W, Warren SL, O'Hare AJ, Infantolino ZP, Miller GA (2013) Relationships among cognition, emotion, and motivation: implications for intervention and neuroplasticity in psychopathology. Front Hum Neurosci 7:261

D'Urso G, Bruzzese D, Ferrucci R, Priori A, Pascotto A, Galderisi S, Altamura AC, Bravaccio C (2015) Transcranial direct current stimulation for hyperactivity and noncompliance in autistic disorder. World J Biol Psychiatry 16(5):361–366

Eigsti IM, Fein DA (2013) More is less: pitch discrimination and language delays in children with optimal outcomes from autism. Autism Res 6(6):605–613

Enticott PG, Fitzgibbon BM, Kennedy HA, Arnold SL, Elliot D, Peachey A, Zangen A, Fitzgerald PB (2014) Double-blind, randomized trial of deep repetitive transcranial magnetic stimulation (rTMS) for autism spectrum disorder. Brain Stimul 7(2):206–211

Esbensen AJ, Seltzer MM, Lam KS, Bodfish JW (2009) Age-related differences in restricted repetitive behaviors in autism spectrum disorders. J Autism Develop Dis 39(1):57–66

Fecteau S, Agosta S, Oberman L, Pascual-Leone A (2011) Brain stimulation over Broca's area differentially modulates naming skills in neurotypical adults and individuals with Asperger's syndrome. Eur J Neurosci 34(1):1581–1564

Fein D, Barton M, Eigsti IM, Kelley E, Naigles L, Schultz RT, Stevens M, Helt M, Orinstein A, Rosenthal M, Troyb E, Tyson K (2013) Optimal outcome in individuals with a history of autism. J Child Psychol Psychiatry 54(2):195–205

Geurts HM, Lever AG (2014) Self-reports of ASD symptomatology, cognitive failures, & quality of life in adults (19–79 years) with ASD: a cross sectional study 102.005 abstract 2014. International Meeting for Autism Research in Atlanta

Happé F, Charlton RA (2012) Aging in autism spectrum disorders: a mini-review. Gerontology 58(1):70–78

Hoppenbrouwers SS, Schutter DJ, Fitzgerald PB, Chen R, Daskalakis ZJ (2008) The role of the cerebellum in the pathophysiology and treatment of neuropsychiatric disorders: a review. Brain Res Rev 59:185–200

James IA, Mukaetova-Ladinska E, Reichelt FK, Briel R, Scully A (2006) Diagnosing Aspergers syndrome in the elderly: a series of case presentations. Int J Geriatr Psychiatry 21(10):951–960

Jasien JM, Daimon CM, Wang R, Shapiro BK, Martin B, Maudsley S (2014) The effects of aging on the BTBR mouse model of autism spectrum disorder. Front Aging Neurosci 6:225

Kanner L (1973) Childhood psychosis: initial studies and new insights. WH Winston, Washington, p. 209

Kern JK, Trivedi MH, Garver CR, Grannemann BD, Andrews AA, Savla JS, Johnson DG, Mehta JA, Schroeder JL (2006) The pattern of sensory processing abnormalities in autism. Autism 10(5):480–494

Konradi C, Heckers S (2001) Antipsychotic drugs and neuroplasticity: insights into the treatment and neurobiology of schizophrenia. Biol Psychiatry 50(10):729–742

Koolschijn PCM, Geurts HM (2014) The neural correlates of perceptual closure in adults and elderly with autism. 138.049 49 abstract 2014. International Meeting for Autism Research in Atlanta

Lehnhardt F-G, Garwonski A, Pfeiffer K, Kockler H, Schilbach L, Vogeley K (2013) The investigation and differential diagnosis of Asperger syndrome in adults. Dtsch Arztebl Int 110:755–763

Lever AG, Geurts HM (2016) Psychiatric co-occurring symptoms and disorders in young, middle-aged, and older adults with autism spectrum disorder. J Autism Dev Disord 46(6):1916–1930

Lever AG, Werkle-Bergner M, Brandmaier AM, Ridderinkhof KR, Geurts HM (2015) Atypical working memory decline across the adult lifespan in autism spectrum disorder? J Abnorm Psychol 24(4):1014–1026

Magiati I, Tay XW, Howlin P (2014) Cognitive, language, social and behavioural outcomes in adults with autism spectrum disorders: a systematic review of longitudinal follow-up studies in adulthood. Clin Psychol Rev 34(1):73–86

Merabet LB, Pascual-Leone A (2010) Neural reorganization following sensory loss: the opportunity of change. Nat Rev Neurosci 11(1):44–52

Mukaetova-Ladinska EB, Coppock M (2016) Ageing in people with autism Spectrum Disorder (ASD): liaison old age psychiatry perspective. In: Wright SD (ed) Autism spectrum disorder in mid and laterl. Jessica Lingley Publishers, London/Philadelphia, pp 120–140

Mukaetova-Ladinska EB, Perry E, Baron M, Povey C; Autism Ageing Writing Group (2012) Ageing in people with autistic spectrum disorder. Int J Geriatr Psychiatry 27(2):109–118

Mukaetova-Ladinska EB, Stuart-Hamilton I (2016) Adults with Autism Spectrum Disorder (ASD): service user perspective on ageing transition(s). Am J Autism 2(1):1–11

Naidu A, James I, Mukaetova-Ladinska E, Briel R (2006) Diagnosis of Asperger syndrome in a 66-year-old male presenting with depression. Int Psychogeriatr 18(1):171–173

National Institute for Clinical excellence (NICE) (2012) Autism in adults: diagnosis and management. nice.org.uk/guidance/cg142

Nicolaidis C, Kripke CC, Raymaker D (2014) Primary care for adults on the autism spectrum. Med Clin North Am 98(5):1169–1191

Perkins EA, Berkman KA (2012) Into the unknown: aging with autism spectrum disorders. Am J Intellect Dev Disabil 117(6):478–496

Piven J, Rabins P, Autism-in-Older Adults Working Group (2011) Autism spectrum disorders in older adults: toward defining a research agenda. J Am Geriatr Soc 59(11):2151–2155

Seltzer MM, Shattuck P, Abbeduto L, Greenberg JS (2004) Trajectory of development in adolescents and adults with autism. Ment Retard Dev Disabil Res Rev 10(4):234–247

Sokhadze E, Baruth J, Tasman A, Mansoor M, Ramaswamy R, Sears L, Mathai G, El-Baz A, Casanova MF (2010) Low-frequency repetitive transcranial magnetic stimulation (rTMS) affects event-related potential measures of novelty processing in autism. Appl Psychophysiol Biofeedback 35(2):147–161

Sokhadze EM, El-Baz AS, Tasman A, Sears LL, Wang Y, Lamina EV, Casanova MF (2014) Neuromodulation integrating rTMS and neurofeedback for the treatment of autism spectrum disorder: an exploratory study. Appl Psychophysiol Biofeedback 39(3–4):237–257

Troyb E, Orinstein A, Tyson K, Eigsti IM, Naigles L, Fein D (2014a) Restricted and repetitive behaviors in individuals with a history of ASDs who have achieved optimal outcomes. J Autism Dev Disord 44(12):3168–3184

Troyb E, Orinstein A, Tyson K, Helt M, Eigsti IM, Stevens M, Fein D (2014b) Academic abilities in children and adolescents with a history of autism spectrum disorders who have achieved optimal outcomes. Autism 18(3):233–243

Troyb E, Rosenthal M, Eigsti IM, Kelley E, Tyson K, Orinstein A, Barton M, Fein D (2014c) Executive functioning in individuals with a history of ASDs who have achieved optimal outcomes. Child Neuropsychol 20(4):378–397

Valkanova V, Rhodes F, Allan CL (2013) Diagnosis and management of autism in adults. Practitioner 257(1761):13–16, 2–3

van Heijst BF, Geurts HM (2015) Quality of life in autism across the lifespan: a meta-analysis. Autism 19(2):158–167

Wallace GL, Budgett J, Charlton RA (2016) Aging and autism spectrum disorder: evidence from the broad autism phenotype. Autism Res. doi:10.1002/aur.1620

7 Autism in Girls and Women

Patricia van Wijngaarden-Cremers

7.1 Introduction

Men are biologically more brittle, while women are socially vulnerable. This proposition has long been supported by the differences in prevalence of psychopathology between genders at different ages. In childhood (development) psychopathology is seen far more often in boys, while from adolescence onwards, psychopathology appears to be more prevalent in women (Rutter 2008). Yet, this vision has become unsustainable in recent years. Developmental disorders such as attention-deficit hyperactivity disorder (ADHD) and autism spectrum disorders (ASD) are still more often identified in boys than in girls. Disruptive behaviour in boys is indeed striking and therefore raises more concerns and leads more often to act and consequently to more referrals. However in adulthood the prevalence of developmental disorders in both sexes grows very close to each other. This could be because more boys than girls are "cured" of their developmental disorder and have fewer problems in adulthood. On the other hand, it is far more likely that developmental disorders in girls are less well recognized. This has very serious consequences. By not acknowledging a developmental disorders behind a façade of traumatization or addiction or another wrong diagnosis (e.g. borderline personality disorder instead of ADHD or ASD), many women are withheld from adequate treatment and unnecessary suffering for a very long time (van Wijngaarden and van der Gaag 2010).

In this chapter we will discuss the causal mechanisms and especially the role of gender in the development of the phenotypical presentation of ASD. We will also give a great deal of attention to the impact of missing the diagnosis and its consequences. Finally, we will offer suggestions for improving earlier recognition of ASD among girls.

But let us start with a clinical vignette to get the picture.

P. van Wijngaarden-Cremers
Radboud University Nijmegen Medical Centre, Dimence Centre of Developmental Disorders, Deventer, The Netherlands
e-mail: p.vanwijngaarden@dimence.nl

B. Barahona Corrêa, R.-J. van der Gaag (eds.), *Autism Spectrum Disorders in Adults*, DOI 10.1007/978-3-319-42713-3_7

Clinical Vignette

Mary was 22 years old when she was first referred to our clinic. She had already had several unsuccessful treatments in several addiction clinics before she was referred to our clinic for the treatment of substance use disorder, post-traumatic stress disorder (PTSD) and borderline personality disorder. She was addicted to heroin, cocaine and also used cannabis, XTC, speed and alcohol on a regular basis. She first started using drugs when she was 14 years old. Mary had been physically abused by her father. At the elementary school, she had aggressive outbursts, which disappeared at the age of 10, by the time a 16-year-old boy from the neighbourhood began sexually abusing her. Later, in high school, she also was sexually abused by one of her teachers.

After detox, Mary was a very anxious, shy, chaotic, restless and clumsy young woman who had difficulties expressing herself in the group. She didn't interact a lot with the group, yet she was not a real loner. The group members instantly liked her.

One poignant habit of Mary was to take showers many times a day. Both her shyness and her frequent showering were interpreted as a consequence of her history of sexual abuse. During her treatment in our clinic, we did not observe any symptoms to confirm the diagnosis of borderline personality disorder. Due to her chaotic and clumsy behaviour, added to a hetero-anamnestic confirmed history of lifelong concentration problems and hyperactivity, we first performed a standardized clinical assessment on ADHD, which confirmed the presence of ADHD. The ADHD and the PTSD were treated according to the state of the art. Unfortunately, after a short period of improvement, her situation worsened: Mary became afraid of leaving the clinic and spent a great deal of time alone in her own apartment, which her parents had arranged for her, thus avoiding the necessary steps to build up a social life or in fact any activities outside the clinic. She became more and more anxious, with increasing insomnia and nightmares. Coincidentally she developed more compulsive behaviours, such as showering even more often and for a longer time than before, and did it according to a specific and strict ritual. She also started sticking to specific rituals for getting dressed or leaving the apartment. The staff observed these changes and felt increasingly concerned about how to turn this situation for the better.

It was in the face of these concerns that we started to explore with Mary her anxiety, her shyness, her reservations about meaningful friendships and family bonds and why she had not succeeded in looking for, let alone finding, a job. It emerged that she simply didn't know how to live her life. She had difficulties interpreting social situations and was afraid of new situations. Her lack of imagination made it impossible for her to anticipate correctly. It became clear why she was so vulnerable for sexual abuse: She had misinterpreted the intentions of that boy and her teacher. She did not dare to say "no" to the offenders because she thought that she had to comply to meet their expectations and was also afraid to lose their friendship.

At this point it first occurred to us that she could be autistic. Her early history revealed that all these problems had existed all her life, and, after a standardized assessment according to the Dutch guidelines, an ASD diagnosis was confirmed.

This vignette highlights that shyness and a variety of psychiatric symptoms may mask the ASD in women. Intelligent females with ASD, (high-functioning (HF) girls, appear to look carefully at what other girls their age do). They are eager to be accepted, and to reach that goal, they tend to copy the other girls' behaviours and thus try their very best to fulfil the expectations they think others have of them, and this makes them vulnerable, among other things, to sexual abuse. If they cannot manage to meet the supposed expectations because it causes too much anxiety, they disengage from social contact or start using drugs to help them overcome their fear.

7.2 Development and ASD

7.2.1 Development: An Ongoing Interactive Process Between Gene and Environment

Development is an interactional process. As from the prenatal period, and visible from birth, the interaction with the biopsychosocial environment plays an essential role in the development of the individual (Fig. 7.1).

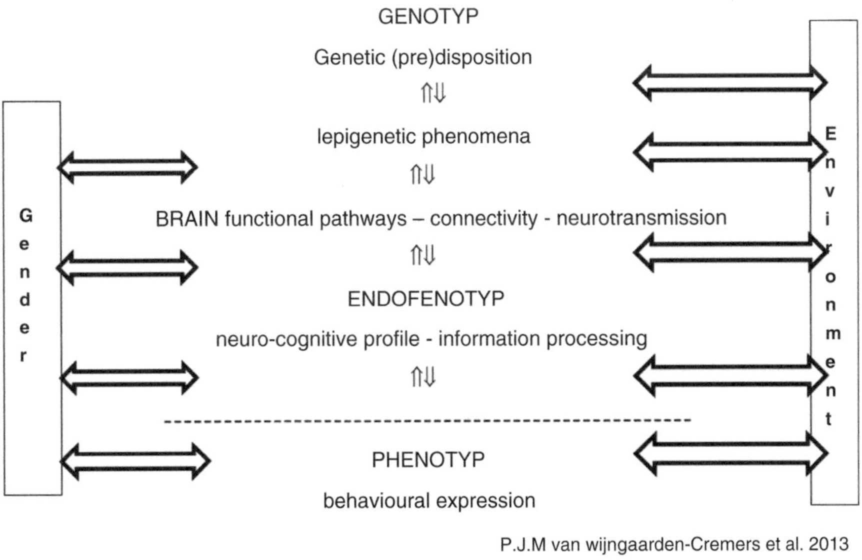

Fig. 7.1 Development: an interactive process

This figure demonstrates that the interactions and experiences between the child and the environment have a direct effect on the configuration of the brain. In return the individual has a strong impact on its environment (the more responsive the baby, the more it is addressed and encouraged). This is clearly visible in babies with autism who respond less and show less social engagement. After 6 months the environment becomes discouraged by lack of responsive reward and will tend to encourage the baby less (Brisson et al. 2012).

Thus development is an ongoing interaction between "*nature and nurture*". Genetic make-up and epigenetic changes influence the structural and dynamic development of the brain. The connectivity within the brain and the repartition of neurotransmitters are a result of this dynamic process. The individual's neurocognitive capacities are likewise the consequence of the interaction between the developing brain and everyday experiences. The outcome of the processes, which is also influenced by gender (Nugent and McCarthy 2011), expresses itself in (psychopathological) cognitions, emotions and behaviours. In other words, genetic and epigenetic deviances lead to "different" brains, which result in "different" behaviours and vice versa.

7.2.2 Gender Differences and Development

In addition to organic distinctive characteristics, other differences in development between men and women exist. At brain level this has implications for the development of networks in the central nervous system, involving the structure of the reward system and stress response patterns. In boys and men, this leads to more "externalizing" violent behaviour and "blaming others", whereas in women it leads to more "internalizing" behaviour and a tendency to blame themselves (Brody and Hall 2008).

These reaction types are strongly determined by evolution. In prehistoric societies genetically "attractive" women were those who focused on social interaction and were able to maintain social cohesion in the communities. "Appealing" men were successful hunters: detail oriented, with focused determination and "functional" in their relationship patterns. Interestingly, these behavioural characteristics are also apparent in the neuropsychological profile: Women have more linguistic skills, are more socially oriented and have weaker visuospatial properties (orientation capability), while men are more detail oriented and have more rigid ways of planning and organizing (executive functions). As human characteristics are distributed according to the well-known Gauss curves, there is of course a large overlap in the distribution.

Gene-environment interactions are highly gender sensitive. There seem to be neurobiological differences between females and males in the development of stress regulation. The much shorter but far more intense reaction of the hypothalamus-pituitary-adrenergic system in (premenopausal) women has an impact on immune reactions but also especially affects the vulnerability for psychopathology. Several studies suggest that stress has a greater negative impact on the psychological health in women (Goel et al. 2014). For instance, stress-related mood disorders (depression, general anxiety) are twice as prevalent in women as in men (Kessler et al.

1993, 2005). Moreover, women are more likely to develop psychopathology (for instance, post-traumatic stress disorder) or autoimmune diseases when facing the same stressful events than men (Breslau 2009; Iteke et al. 2011).

This tendency appears to have been strengthened by the different way in which parents react to their daughters, as compared to their sons. Social environment also plays an important role as it appears that women are far more sensitive to rejection (Stroud et al. 2002), to the absence of social support (Kendler et al. 2005) or to lack of social structure (Haller et al. 1999), whereas defeat has a greater impact on stress regulation in men.

In other words gender plays a role in the vulnerability for developing certain physical and/or mental diseases as well as the way individuals learn how to cope with them and therefore influences physical, mental as well as social health.

In this chapter we want to point out that many developmental disorders are extremes of the normal distribution. Especially in autism spectrum disorders, we are facing the extreme of male behaviour (functionally oriented digital and strict logical thinking, impulsive and externalizing,). As a result, the symptom description of these syndromes is really grafted on the male characteristics. This has had very negative consequences for diagnosing girls and women with an ASD.

7.3 Autism Spectrum Disorders (ASD) in Women

The term autism spectrum disorder (ASD) is used to describe a heterogeneous group of developmental disorders characterized by impairments in social interaction, verbal and non-verbal communication and repetitive and stereotyped behaviours (DSM 5 2013). The prevalence is approximately 1 % in the general population (Fombonne 2009). The overall sex ratio is 4–5 males versus 1 woman (Baird et al. 2011). In individuals with co-occurring intellectual disability, the sex ratio drops to 2:1 or tends to be equal, whereas women are underrepresented in high-functioning individuals with ASD.

ASD show a bimodal distribution in females, with on one hand a group of severely impaired girls in whom the disorder is diagnosed very early in life and on the other hand a group of girls with milder symptoms in whom the disorder is diagnosed much later in life or not at all. Indeed, there is limited but consistent evidence in favour of a specific female phenotype in autism based on severe cases of autism with co-occurring marked intellectual disability that are diagnosed early in life (Ozonoff et al. 2010; Rivet and Matson 2011). Several other studies have shown that girls with milder symptoms and a normal IQ tend to be diagnosed at a later age than boys (Kopp and Gillberg 1992; Goin-Kochel et al. 2006; Siklos and Kerns 2007; Begeer et al. 2013; Russell et al. 2011; Giarelli et al. 2010) or are misdiagnosed (Kopp and Gillberg 1992; Nilsson et al. 1999; Begeer et al. 2013).

Defined (DSM and ICD) criteria are mainly based on male behaviour (qualitative approach) and so are the thresholds for qualifying for the diagnosis (Holtmann et al. 2007; Lai et al. 2011; McLennan et al. 1993; Tsai and Beisler 1983). This is in spite of the fact that the syndrome may appear differently in males as compared to females, which might explain the delays in ASD diagnosis in females, as well as missed or wrong diagnoses in milder female cases (Rivet and Matson 2011). In research, this may have led to an obvious male bias: Boys and men are overrepresented, but results are commonly generalized to both sexes (Lai et al. 2011).

When looking at the literature that focuses on gender differences in ASD, findings seem not always easy to relate to each other, and conclusions can be ambiguous (Lai et al. 2011). However, once the diagnosis of ASD has been established, studies show that there are no differences in the type or severity of the core symptoms and the same type of comorbid conditions accompanying ASD in girls as in boys (Lugnegård et al. 2011; van Wijngaarden-Cremers et al. 2014). This indicates that the ascertainment bias is a real problem in the identification of females with ASD as a group of girls with milder symptoms in whom the disorder is not, or only later, diagnosed.

Masking factors

- Females (including females with an ASD) are more inclined to wanting to meet the standard. They want to be like all the other girls. Therefore they observe and copy other girls and behave like other girls, which allows them to go unnoticed (Attwood 2007; Ozonoff et al. 2010; Sipes et al. 2011; Bolte et al. 2011).
- Females with ASD are more easily and adequately adopted by neurotypical girls, because in this way, they become less isolated and hence draw less attention! Problems mostly occur and increase during adolescence when social interaction becomes more complex and intimacy becomes more important (Kopp and Gilberg 2011; Dworzynski et al. 2012; Lunegård et al. 2011).
- The preoccupations in ASD females are less bizarre. The topics are less disturbing: They focus on animals (horses, cats) or are interested in (classic) literature like many other women. This is less odd than being interested in washing machines or spinning wheels or dinosaurs which is more common in boys (Attwood 2007; Carter et al. 2007).
- Characteristics like shyness and modesty are common in women; aloofness in ASD girls is more likely to be considered "normal" as compared to boys.

This misinterpretation of symptoms leads to misreferrals and ultimately to misdiagnosis (Holtmann et al. 2007). Autistic girls may be diagnosed as having an anxiety disorder, avoidant personality disorder, etc. This implies that ASD is potentially under-diagnosed in girls and women (Mandy et al. 2011). Moreover, girls with "internalizing" problems are referred to professionals less often than boys with similar problems, probably because these behaviours are considered to be "normal" in females (Rucklidge 2010) and cause little disruption.

- Females with ASD may display severe challenging behaviour such as bouts of aggression and rage and self-harm. These disruptive behaviours serve a different goal than in males. In males they are due to gain objects, whereas in females they aim at gaining (the caregivers') attention. This can easily be misinterpreted as a manifestation of borderline personality disorder.

7.4 Implications for Research and Clinical Practice

7.4.1 Implications for Research

Research should take a different approach at targeting genes and endophenotypes (at a different level), namely, by taking development and gender into account as crucial features when studying (developmental {psycho}) pathology. It will also be important to trace antecedents of women diagnosed with autism to look for patterns that may help to understand why their diagnosis was missed for such a long time and which symptoms should raise awareness in clinicians. More research is needed to develop (screenings) instruments that are better adapted to help defining and identifying a female phenotype of ASD.

7.4.2 Implications for Clinical Practice

In terms of ASD in girls and women, clinicians should be well aware of the fact that the phenotypical presentation in females can be very different and is often masked by conditions like anxiety disorders, PTSD and SUD or an inaccurate interpretation of symptoms like social anxiety, obsessive-compulsive disorder or borderline behaviour that may be resulting from copying, attempts to gain (caregivers') attention, or from wrong reinforcement.

Clinicians should be advised that it is not only important to focus on good diagnostics and treatment of ASD but also to be aware of gender influences on health and on how gender plays a role in the patient's ability to cope and adapt. This implies that clinicians have to understand the different factors that influence the development of (psycho)pathology and how gender plays an important role in these interactions. Healthcare workers should realize that women are biologically more vulnerable to stress because of differences at the level of HPA axis activity and subsequently are more likely to develop psychopathology (affective disorders) when facing the same stressful events as man. They should also bear in mind that the social environment plays a different role in men and women. This is illustrated by the fact that women are far more sensitive to rejection, the absence of social support or social structure, whereas defeat has a greater impact on stress dysregulation in men.

In terms of treatment approaches, psycho-education should be adapted in order to help girls and women understand what their condition is and how they can learn to cope with it, by being explicit about the specificities of their diagnosis. Individual approaches should be favoured, and special attention should be given to traumatic experiences that so many women with ASD have endured, having been deceived and misused in their quest for social contact and esteem. In a later stage, contact with akin women may prove helpful. It is interesting to note that direct contact may be stressful, whereas virtual contact via internet chats may prove greatly helpful (van der Aa et al. 2014).

Conclusion

Gender plays an important role in development of psychopathology as well as in the development of coping styles and clearly affects behavioural patterns. Therefore clinicians should develop awareness of these gender influences when assessing girls and women for a possible ASD.

Diagnosing ASD in high-functioning girls and women can be difficult as symptoms like (social) information-processing defects are often masked. Moreover, the clinical picture may be misinterpreted. This consequently may lead to misreferrals to unsuited services and ultimately to misdiagnosis. Thus, knowledge of the specific characteristics of ASD in high-functioning women should receive attention during training and the education of involved professionals.

References

American Psychiatric Association (2013) Diagnostic and statistical manual of mental disorders (DSM 5). American Psychiatric Association Press, Washington

Attwood TB (2007) The complete guide to Asperger's syndrome. jessica Kingsley Publishers, London

Baird G, Douglas HR, Murphy MS (2011) Recognising and diagnosing autism in children and young people: summary of NICE guidance. BMJ 343:d6360

Begeer S, Mandell D, Wijnker-Holmes B, Venderbosch S, Rem D, Stekelenburg F, Koot HM (2013) Sex differences in the timing of identification among children and adults with autism spectrum disorders. J Autism Dev Disord 43(5):1151–1156

Bölte S, Duketis E, Poustka F, Holtmann M (2011) Sex differences in cognitive domains and their clinical correlates in higher-functioning autism spectrum disorders. Autism 15(4):497–511

Breslau N (2009) The epidemiology of trauma, PTSD, and other posttrauma disorders. Trauma Violence Abuse 10:198–210

Brody LR, Hall JA (2008) Gender and emotion in context. In: Lewis M, Haviland-Jones JM, Barrett LF (eds) Handbook of emotions, 3rd edn. Guilford, New York, pp 395–408

Brisson J, Warreyn P, Serres J, Foussier S, Adrien-Louis J (2012) Motor anticipation failure in infants with autism: a retrospective analysis of feeding situations. Autism 16(4):420–429

Carter AS, Black DO, Tewani S, Connolly CE, Kadlec MB, Tager-Flusberg H (2007) Sex differences in toddlers with autism spectrum disorders. J Autism Dev Disord 37(1):86–97

Dworzynski K, Ronald A, Bolton P, Happe F (2012) How different are girls and boys above and below the diagnostic threshold for autism spectrum disorders? J Am Acad Child Adolesc Psychiatry 51(8):788–797

Fombonne E (2009) Epidemiology of pervasive developmental disorders. Pediatr Res 65(6):591–598

Giarelli E, Wiggins LD, Rice CE, Levy SE, Kirby RS, Pinto-Martin J, Mandell D (2010) Sex differences in the evaluation and diagnosis of autism spectrum disorders among children. Disabil Health J 3(2):107–116

Goin-Kochel RP, Mackintosh VH, Myers BJ (2006) How many doctors does it take to make an autism spectrum diagnosis? Autism 10(5):439–451

Goel N, Workman JL, Lee TT, Innala L, Viau V (2014) Sex differences in the HPA axis. Compr Physiol 4(3):1121–1155

Haller J, Fuchs E, Halasz J, Makara GB (1999) Defeat is a major stressor in males while social instability is stressful mainly in females: towards the development of a social stress model in female rats. Brain Res Bull 50:33–39

Holtmann M, Bolte S, Poustka F (2007) Autism spectrum disorders: sex differences in autistic behaviour domains and coexisting psychopathology. Dev Med Child Neurol 49(5):361–366

Iteke O, Bakare MO, Agomoh AO, Uwakwe R, Onwukwe JU (2011) Road traffic accidents and posttraumatic stress disorder in an orthopedic setting in South-Eastern Nigeria: a controlled study. Scand J Trauma Resusc Emerg Med 19:39

Kendler KS, Myers J, Prescott CA (2005) Sex differences in the relationship between social support and risk for major depression: a longitudinal study of opposite-sex twin pairs. Am J Psychiatry 162:250–256

Kessler RC, Berglund P, Demler O, Jin R, Merikangas KR, Walters EE (2005) Lifetime prevalence and age-of-onset distributions of DSM-IV disorders in the National Comorbidity Survey Replication. Arch Gen Psychiatry 62:593–602

Kessler RC, McGonagle KA, Swartz M, Blazer DG, Nelson CB (1993) Sex and depression in the National Comorbidity Survey I: lifetime prevalence, chronicity and recurrence. J Affect Disord 29:85–96

Kopp S, Gillberg C (1992) Girls with social deficits and learning problems: autism, atypical Asperger syndrome or a variant of these conditions. Eur Child Adolesc Psychiatry 1(2):89–99

Kopp S, Gillberg C (2011) The Autism Spectrum Screening Questionnaire (ASSQ)-Revised Extended Version (ASSQ-REV): an instrument for better capturing the autism phenotype in girls? A preliminary study involving 191 clinical cases and community controls. Res Dev Disabil 32(6):2875–2888

Lai MC, Lombardo MV, Pasco G, Ruigrok AN, Wheelwright SJ, Sadek SA et al (2011) A behavioral comparison of male and female adults with high functioning autism spectrum conditions. PLoS One 6(6):e20835

Lugnegård T, Hallerbäck MU, Gillberg C (2011) Psychiatric comorbidity in young adults with a clinical diagnosis of Asperger syndrome. Res Dev Disabil 32(5):1910–1917

Mandy W, Chilvers R, Chowdhury U, Salter G, Seigal A, Skuse D (2011) Sex differences in autism spectrum disorder: evidence from a large sample of children and adolescents. J Autism Dev Disord 42(7):1304–1313

McLennan JD, Lord C, Schopler E (1993) Sex differences in higher functioning people with autism. J Autism Dev Disord 23(2):217–227

Nilsson EW, Gillberg C, Carina Gillberg I, Råstam M (1999) Ten-year follow-up of adolescent-onset anorexia nervosa: Personality disorders. J Am Acad Child Adolesc Psychiatry 38(11): 1389–1395

Nugent BM, McCarthy MM (2011) Epigenetic underpinnings of developmental sex differences in the brain. Neuroendocrinology 93:150–158

Ozonoff S, Iosif AM, Baguio F, Cook IC, Hill MM, Hutman T et al (2010) A prospective study of the emergence of early behavioral signs of autism. J Am Acad Child Adolesc Psychiatry 49(3):256–266.e.251–252

Rivet TT, Matson JL (2011) Review of gender differences in core symptomatology in autism spectrum disorders. Res Autism Spectrum Disord 5(3):957–976

Russell G, Steer C, Golding (2011) Social and demographic factors that influence the diagnosis of autistic spectrum disorders. J. Soc Psychiatry Psychiatr Epidemiol 46(12):1283–93

Rutter M (2008) Developing concepts in developmental psychopathology. In: Hudziak JJ (ed) Developmental psychopathology and wellness: genetic and environmental influences. American Psychiatric Publishing, Washington, pp 3–22

Rucklidge JJ (2010) Gender differences in attention-deficit/hyperactivity disorder. Psychiatr Clin North Am 33(2):357–373

Siklos S, Kerns KA (2007) Assessing the diagnostic experiences of a small sample of parents of children with autism spectrum disorders. Res Dev Disabil 28(1):9–22

Sipes M, Matson JL, Worley JA, Kozlowski AM (2011) Gender differences in symptoms of Autism Spectrum Disorders in toddlers. Res Autism Spectrum Disord 5(4):1465–1470

Stroud LR, Salovey P, Epel ES (2002) Sex differences in stress responses: social rejection versus achievement stress. Biol Psychiatry 52(4):318–327

Tsai LY, Beisler JM (1983) The development of sex differences in infantile autism. Br J Psychiatry 142:373–378 van der Aa CPDM, Pollmann MMH, Plaat A, van der Gaag RJ (2014) Computer-mediated communication in adults with high-functioning Autism Spectrum Conditions. CoRR abs/1410.1087

Van Wijngaarden-Cremers PJM, van der Gaag RJ (2010) Verslaving als ontwikkelingsstoornis. Kind Adolescent 31:174–187

van Wijngaarden-Cremers PJM, van Eeten E, Groen WB, van Deurzen PA, Oosterling IJ, van der Gaag RJ (2014) Gender and age differences in the core triad of impairments in autism spectrum disorders: a systematic review and meta-analysis. J Autism Dev Disord 44(3):627–635

Psychiatric and Neurological Problems in Adults with Autism Spectrum Disorders

8

Carlos Nunes Filipe

8.1 Introduction

Individuals with autism spectrum disorders (ASDs) frequently have neurological and psychiatric comorbidities (de Bruin et al. 2007; Evans et al. 2005; Drmic and Szatmari 2014; Leyfer et al. 2006; Mattila et al. 2010). Psychiatric comorbidities are even more frequent in individuals with ASD than they are in the general population and indeed more frequent than they are in most other clinical groups (Bradley et al. 2004; Drmic and Szatmari 2014; Gadow et al. 2004; Gillott et al. 2001; Joshi et al. 2010) Whereas there are no recognized treatments for autism, there are treatments, namely, pharmacological treatments, with proven efficacy for the majority of neurological and psychiatric comorbid disorders that affect individuals with ASD (Joshi et al. 2010; Mazzone et al. 2012). The differential diagnosis and the correct identification of these comorbidities are therefore of utmost importance.

On average, nearly 70 % of individuals with ASD meet diagnostic criteria for at least one psychiatric disorder (Drmic and Szatmari 2014), with a reported prevalence of more than 80 % (de Bruin et al. 2007; Mattila et al. 2010). Among these, 27–50 % meet criteria for two or more comorbid disorders (Drmic and Szatmari 2014). The occurrence of psychiatric disorders in individuals with ASD, including those with a good functioning, contributes to the deterioration of their quality of life and has a negative impact both on daily functioning and the future life of patients and their family and caregivers (de Bruin et al. 2007; Joshi et al. 2010; Leyfer et al. 2006; Mazzone et al. 2012). Moreover, the co-occurrence of psychiatric or neurological disorders may exacerbate certain symptoms of autism such as ritualistic behaviour, obsessions and social isolation (Quek et al. 2012).

C.N. Filipe
NOVA Medical School, NOVA University of Lisbon, Lisbon, Portugal
e-mail: carlos.filipe@nms.unl.pt

B. Barahona Corrêa, R.-J. van der Gaag (eds.), *Autism Spectrum Disorders in Adults*, DOI 10.1007/978-3-319-42713-3_8

Whereas there are no recognized treatments for autism, there are treatments, namely, pharmacological treatments, with proven efficacy for the majority of neurological and psychiatric comorbid disorders that affect individuals with ASD (Joshi et al. 2010; Mazzone et al. 2012). The differential diagnosis and the correct identification of these comorbidities are therefore of utmost importance and a challenge clinicians must be prepared for. Similarly, it may be difficult to diagnose medical problems, presumably more common in this population than they are in the general population, considering that it is often difficult to implement healthy dietary and hygiene rules and provide regular health care to individuals with ASD (Bilder et al. 2013; Croen et al. 2015; Jones et al. 2015).

The clinical manifestations of comorbid psychiatric and neurological disorders in individuals with ASD are frequently different from those typically observed in the general population. Consequently, a correct diagnosis implies both a good knowledge of the syndromic characteristics of autism and the ability to identify what is and what is not a part of it. It is therefore necessary to distinguish the "primary" manifestations of autism from those of a possible comorbid disorder (Leyfer et al. 2006; Mazefsky et al. 2012). The recognition that a certain group of signs and symptoms is not part of the usual ASD framework of a particular individual should alert the clinician to a possible comorbidity and is decisive to the therapeutic approach and to improve prognosis (Drmic and Szatmari 2014; Leyfer et al. 2006; Mazefsky et al. 2012; White et al. 2009).

The inability, or reduced capacity, that individuals with ASD have to identify and verbalize symptoms of distress and the emotional discomfort that may be associated therewith determine the need to collect detailed information from relatives and caregivers (Leyfer et al. 2006; Mazzone et al. 2012). The possible presence of an intellectual disability can make the diagnosis even more difficult.

Autism is a neurodevelopmental disorder, and, accordingly, its expression develops in continuity throughout life. The onset of a medical, neurological or psychiatric disorder appears, in most cases, as a discontinuity in the personal course. The occurrence of a discontinuity is therefore the first feature that one should be aware of when it comes to making the differential diagnosis between the signs and symptoms related to autism and those due to the appearance of a comorbid disorder (Leyfer et al. 2006; Mazefsky et al. 2012). A gradual or a more or less sudden change of behaviour, associated with a deterioration of the usual adaptive functioning of the individual, is the first warning sign to be considered for the likelihood of a comorbidity in an individual with ASD (Drmic and Szatmari 2014; Mazefsky et al. 2012). The use of psychometric diagnostic scales may be useful (Quek et al. 2012; Joshi et al. 2010; Leyfer et al. 2006; MacNeil et al. 2009; Mattila et al. 2010; Mazefsky et al. 2012), but their use is limited in daily clinical practice. The difficulty and time cost for application of such instruments, the lack of validation for different contexts and languages and the limited accessibility are some of the reasons for the restricted clinical use of comorbidity diagnostic scales in individuals with autism. Moreover, there are nearly no scales specifically designed for people with ASD, and, in most cases, the scales used in this population were designed for the general population or adapted from populations with learning difficulties or psychiatric illness (Gillott et al. 2001; Gillott and Standen 2007; Leyfer et al. 2006; Mazzone et al. 2012; Stewart et al. 2006). It is therefore the clinical experience and the psychopathology knowledge that, on the daily practice, underpin the diagnosis of comorbidity. All available sources of information must be gathered for this assessment, even in the case of adults with ASD. This implies questioning multiple informants, including family members and caregivers, as well as accessing every relevant clinical information (clinical reports, psychological assessments, ancillary tests, etc.) (MacNeil et al. 2009).

The most common psychiatric comorbidities are anxiety disorders, mood disorders (particularly depression), attention-deficit hyperactivity disorder (ADHD) and behavioural problems (Drmic and Szatmari 2014; Joshi et al. 2010; Mattila et al. 2010; Lugnegard et al. 2011; Quek et al. 2012). One should note that behavioural problems are, quite often, just the visible expression of mood disorders and anxiety (Quek et al. 2012). In contrast, substance use disorders and psychotic disorders are uncommon in individuals with ASD (de Bruin et al. 2007; Drmic and Szatmari 2014; Mattila et al. 2010; Lugnegard et al. 2011).

Epilepsies are the most common neurological comorbidities (Maski et al. 2011; Tuchman and Rapin 2002; Tuchman et al. 2009, 2010). Last but not the least, sleep disorders are quite common in individuals with ASD (Croen et al. 2015; Maski et al. 2011).

8.2 Behavioural Problems

8.2.1 Clinical Features

The occurrence of behavioural problems, namely, sporadic or maintained episodes of psychomotor agitation, occasionally with aggressive and/or self-injuring behaviour, is not uncommon in individuals with ASD.

Changes in behaviour are often associated with psychiatric comorbidities, particularly depression and anxiety and, frequently, are the most visible expression of these disorders (Quek et al. 2012). Behaviour problems might also be a manifestation of physical discomfort or pain, specifically in individuals with moderate to severe intellectual disability and language disorder.

Before initiating any therapeutic approach, namely, before using medication (exception made for situations requiring urgent intervention), it is essential to make a full and careful assessment that includes, at least, the following points:

1. Frame the event considering the medical history of the individual and try to understand how different the present behaviour is from the usual behaviour of the subject.
2. Carefully characterize the episodes (frequency, regularity, triggering factors, alleviation factors, daily variation, form of appearance, etc.).

3. Try to unveil the "meaning" of the behaviour. In the case of non-verbal individuals, restlessness may in fact be one of the mechanisms used when struggling for communication.
4. Always exclude the possibility of medical or surgical pathology.

For example, to hit on the head, in the case of a non-verbal ASD person, is often understood as being the manifestation of anger or frustration, but it can also be the consequence of a headache, dental or ear pain.

5. Considering the context of the episodes and their presumed meaning, try to work out behavioural strategies that may lead to their suppression (Sofronoff et al. 2007).
6. Medication should only be used when behavioural strategies have failed or turned out to be insufficient to control the behaviour. In those cases medication should complement, not substitute, the behavioural strategies. As a matter of fact, the use of medication may facilitate the behavioural approach.

8.2.2 Treatment

The development of new drugs with fewer side effects, especially in the last two decades, has been widening the possibilities of psychiatric pharmacological options. For this same reason, the choice of the medication to use in every situation may be difficult. The first choice should fall on any drug with evidence-based effectiveness for both ASD and the comorbid situation. From among these, those drugs with which the clinician has more experience should be given preference over newer, less predictable substances. The lack of an adequate response or the occurrence (or higher risk of occurrence) of undesirable side effects justifies the option for a second-choice medication. In most cases, unfortunately, the available information on the use of medication in ASDs is scarce, and it is the experience and the careful evaluation of the risks and benefits that should guide the option of the physician.

Second- and third-generation antipsychotics are the first-line drugs to control severe behavioural problems in people with autism. One should be conscious, however, of the side effects of these medications, namely, their possible effects on metabolism (increased incidence of hypercholesterolaemia and hypertriglyceridemia, obesity and diabetes II). Therefore, drugs more prone to cause these side effects should be avoided. The use of classical antipsychotics increases the risk of serious motor control disorders (Parkinsonism, tardive dyskinesias, etc.), and, for that reason, their use is also discouraged. Aripiprazole and risperidone have proven to be effective and, in many cases, may even be more effective than first-generation antipsychotics whenever it is necessary to control violent behaviours (Accordino et al. 2016). The suggestion is, therefore, to use them as a first choice, especially when the behaviour changes are associated with anger.

The use of benzodiazepines to control behavioural problems should be cautious, not only because they may induce addiction but also because benzodiazepines are usually less effective than antipsychotics and may elicit idiosyncratic responses and increase irritability.

The use of mood stabilizers such as carbamazepine, sodium valproate and topiramate is an alternative (or possibly a complement in chosen situations) to the use of antipsychotics in order to control impulsivity, reduce emotional lability and reduce the number and severity of disruptive episodes. Topiramate, in particular, has proven to be effective in agitation and impulsiveness control in people with autism, and its association with risperidone can improve both the efficacy of risperidone (some studies have shown a greater effectiveness of risperidone in association with topiramate compared with the use of risperidone in monotherapy) and balance the weight gain induced by the use of the antipsychotic (Rezaei et al. 2010).

8.3 Depression

8.3.1 Clinical Features

Along with anxiety, depression is one of the most frequent psychiatric comorbidities in individuals with ASD (Leyfer et al. 2006; Lugnegard et al. 2011; Quek et al. 2012; Stewart et al. 2006). As a matter of fact, more than half of the individuals with ASD suffer from depression at some moment of their lives. The occurrence of depression is higher in adolescents and adults compared to children with ASD (Drmic and Szatmari 2014; Stewart et al. 2006). Depressive episodes can be prolonged and severe and often tend to be recurrent (Lugnegard et al. 2011). The diagnostic problems in this population are nevertheless important. Depression, even severe depression, tends to go unnoticed or barely be identified in these people. A major difficulty is the atypical symptomatic presentation (Perry et al. 2001; Stewart et al. 2006). The difficulty to access and express feelings, the intellectual disability, when present, and the possible language disorders associated with ASD often modify and mask the syndromic expression of affective disorders in this population. The presence of a depressive episode in ASD, instead of being characterized by depressed mood, apathy, motor retardation, lack of initiative or social isolation (which may also be present...), may be manifested by irritability, impulsivity, agitation and aggression (Perry et al. 2001; Quek et al. 2012; Stewart et al. 2006). Behavioural changes, even though maladjusted and aggressive, may be the only way a person with ASD manages to express the grief and sorrow he feels but does not understand. They reflect a desperate way to communicate with a world whose language he/she cannot access. For this same reason, some symptoms of depression that are common in the general population, such as feelings of worthlessness, guilt, decreased ability to concentrate or suicidal ideation, are uncommon in people with ASD (Stewart et al. 2006). The collection of information from family and caregivers assumes here a special importance. Changes in sleep patterns (which can manifest either by increased sleep time or insomnia) and modification of eating habits (particularly marked decrease in appetite and food refusal) are manifestations that can be associated with depression and may be warning signs in individuals with ASD. Refusal to participate in those activities that were previously performed with pleasure, easy fatigue and the apparent lack of energy are some other signs that may alert us to the presence of depression.

Some alarm signs and symptoms, often associated with depression in individuals with ASD, are listed below (Perry et al. 2001; Stewart et al. 2006):

- Reduction of facial expression
- Tearfulness
- Restlessness
- Self-harm
- Easy fatigue and loss of energy. Long periods spent lying down or leaning back
- Seeking for refuge in the bedroom
- Loss of daily routines and decrease in self-care, as well as neglecting personal hygiene
- Incontinence episodes in a patient who previously had a good control of sphincters
- Pejorative comments about oneself, such as "I'm stupid" and "I cannot do anything well ..."
- Loss of communication skills
- Poor performance in everyday tasks, seeming to be distracted, confused or having memory loss
- Frequent references to the death of family members, friends or known people, exaggerated interest for funerals and cemeteries
- Modification of the sleep pattern (which can be either increased periods of sleep or insomnia)
- Modification of eating habits (namely, a noticeable decrease in appetite or food rejection)
- Weight loss
- Refusal to participate in activities that were previously performed with satisfaction

In the case of individuals with ASD, the occurrence of a depressive episode can lead to a decrease in attention towards the subject's restricted interests or a decrease in time spent in activities previously considered obsessive by others. This is likely to be erroneously interpreted as an improvement in behaviour when in reality it reflects a global and widespread lessening of interests and pleasure (anhedonia) (Stewart et al. 2006). During a depressive episode, the decrease of the individual's attention towards his usual restricted areas of interest is not the result of their replacement by other new interests, to which the individual would devote the same enthusiasm. Instead, it reflects a reduction, or even an absence, of interest for anything at all.

In all cases, the previous usual behaviour of the individual sets an important base of reference to control current behaviour. A behavioural change, whenever it takes the appearance of any of the above-mentioned manifestations, should alert therapists and caregivers to the possibility of being the expression of a depressive episode.

The occurrence of negative life events can trigger the occurrence of a depressive episode in individuals suffering ASD, in the same way as in the general population. The susceptibility, the frequency and the severity of the depressive episodes tend to be, however, higher in individuals with ASD when compared with general population. Intellectual disability and low social status are factors that can decrease the threshold for depression. The high difficulty of adjustment to changing situations of everyday life and repeated discrimination, stigma and abuse are factors that determine an increased risk of anxiety and depression in people with ASD. Stress, fatalities, low socio-economic status, lack of social support and age are factors of greater risk. A higher cognitive ability is not necessarily a protective factor but may instead be a risk factor for depression, as it allows comparison with other people, insight into the patients' own limitations and awareness of a difference, sometimes difficult to understand. Cognitive competence eventually enables the comparison between the individual and others, friends and colleagues, with whom he had, up to a certain age, parallel school and life trajectories. Adolescence and early adulthood are periods of increased risk of mood disorders, especially for those individuals with ASD and good cognitive competence (White et al. 2009). Difficulties of integration and social recognition, emotional problems and academic or professional failure, lifestyle changes (change of school, change of colleagues, etc.), significant losses (death or the absence of significant others) and the emergence of medical or surgical illnesses (especially chronic or prolonged diseases, involving changes in lifestyle) are all situations that increase the risk of depressive and anxiety episodes.

8.3.2 Treatment

The response of young adults and adults with ASD to antidepressant medication is, in our experience, as good as that of the general population. Despite the lack of evidence to support the efficacy of SSRIs in the treatment of depression and anxiety in children with ASD (Drmic and Szatmari 2014), that is not the case for the adult population (Perry et al. 2001; Stewart et al. 2006). In adults with ASD and comorbid depression, therapy with antidepressant medication is associated with both an improvement in mood and a reduction of aggressive behaviour, leading to the recovery of autonomy and self-care skills (Stewart et al. 2006).

Selective serotonin reuptake inhibitors (SSRIs) are, in general, the first-line antidepressants to be used.

Medication should start with low dosages and be slowly increased to the recommended maximum or until an adequate therapeutic response is achieved. Attention should be given to the fact that an increased sensitivity to medication is common in this population and that, quite often, there are idiosyncratic or paradoxical effects. As in the general population, SSRI antidepressants can switch the mood from depression to mania or hypomania, so it is always necessary to make a careful follow-up after initiation of antidepressant medication.

Along with drug therapy, social and family support measures are of great importance.

Psychotherapy, on the other hand, when delivered by experienced therapists with a good knowledge of symptomatic and psychopathological characteristics of ASDs, may be helpful. It aims, in the first instance, to understand and frame the depressive situation. A second aim should be to seek to mobilize the resources both of the individual and his environment, in order to help reorganize the forthcoming life of the individual, according to the new conditions that he will have to face. The framework of interpersonal relationships is crucial here, assuming that the quality of these relations is a protective factor against depression.

Finally, it is important to keep in mind that the aim of any therapeutic intervention is obviously not the "normalization" of the behaviour but the return of the individual to his baseline condition, i.e. the pattern of behaviour and the level of functioning displayed by the subject prior to the depressive episode.

8.4 Anxiety

8.4.1 Clinical Features

Alongside depression, anxiety is one of the most common comorbidities in individuals with ASD, regardless of the cognitive capability (Drmic and Szatmari 2014; Joshi et al. 2010; Gillott et al. 2001; MacNeil et al. 2009; White et al. 2009). The inflexibility of behaviour and the ever present concern with order and routine, characteristics of ASD, lead to the fact that changes, however small, happening in the environment or in the daily routine, can induce marked stress and unexpected anxiety (Gillott et al. 2001; Joshi et al. 2010). Moreover, individuals with ASD have difficulty understanding the environment and anticipating the near future. Consequently, whenever it is necessary to deal appropriately with changes and unexpected situations, in particular if they involve dealing with unpleasant events, the individual hesitates. Social anxiety is also common and can be very conspicuous in individuals with ASD (Gillott and Standen 2007; Gillott et al. 2001; Joshi et al. 2010; Lugnegard et al. 2011). The estimated prevalence of obsessive-compulsive disorder (OCD), on the other hand, varies among studies (11–35 %) (Joshi et al. 2010). This variation certainly reflects the fact that many of the symptoms of OCD are common to ASD. However, the qualitative expression of repetitive behaviours in both disorders is different: in OCD the most common obsessive behaviours are typically washing or cleaning, counting, ordering, checking and collecting, and these are usually driven by obsessive thoughts, urges and intrusive and unwanted concerns, like distressing scruples, fear of disasters or infestation. In ASD, the most commonly observed obsessive behaviours are hand flapping, watching spinning objects, ordering and classifying, repeating words, phrases or sounds and concerns with specific issues (Joshi et al. 2010). These are neither driven by unpleasant obsessive thoughts nor aimed at preventing any feared situation. In OCD, thoughts and behaviours are generally referred to as being strange to the individual who feels them, they are unpleasant and efforts are made to resist them, i.e. they are egodystonic; in ASD, repetitive behaviours are not felt by the individual as strange or leading to anxiety; on the contrary they are felt as natural and calming, that is, they are egosyntonic. Only in those cases in whom repetitive and stereotyped behaviours are a source of distress to the patient should a diagnosis of comorbid OCD be considered and, if confirmed, treated accordingly.

Anxiety often worsens during adolescence in ASD, given the increasing complexity of the social environment and the individual's awareness of his or her own difficulties and disability (White et al. 2009). In most cases, these anxiety problems tend to extend into adulthood (Gillott and Standen 2007).

Stereotypies (e.g. echolalia, twirling, rocking, eye blinking and hand flapping) tend to increase in situations of anxiety, as does psychomotor agitation (e.g. running from one side to the other, talking too much and endlessly repeating the same questions) (Gillott and Standen 2007; Guillott et al. 2001). The presence of anxiety symptoms may decrease tolerance as well as the ability to handle stressors of everyday life. This may ultimately manifest as maladaptative coping strategies, like aggressive or self-injurious behaviours (Gillott and Standen 2007). In all cases it may prove worthwhile to distinguish between the individual characteristic ASD manifestations and the possible expression of comorbid anxiety symptoms (MacNeil et al. 2009).

8.4.2 Treatment

Anxiety is, in its origin, an adaptive response to stress. Therefore, before starting a therapeutic intervention, it is important to evaluate if, and to what degree, the anxiety manifestations cause discomfort and/or affect the life of the patient and his family (White et al. 2009).

Looking at anxiety as an anticipatory response, a useful strategy may be to prevent it by creating predictable situations and environments for the daily functioning of the individual. Creating routines and inform, whenever possible, of the upcoming occurrence of changes, anticipating them, is the first and most effective measure to prevent the occurrence of episodes of anxiety in individuals with ASD. The identification of stress factors, by applying functional behaviour analysis, may be crucial to treatment. The use of cognitive and behavioural psychotherapy techniques in these cases produces very good results (Lang et al. 2010; MacNeil et al. 2009; White et al. 2009). The use of desensitization techniques and relaxation techniques are other examples of behavioural procedures that can help to reduce and control anxiety. The application of these techniques must be mediated by experienced therapists holding a good knowledge about the particularities of individuals with ASD.

The use of anxiolytic drugs may also be indicated. This medication, however, should be used cautiously. In particular, fast-acting and short-term effect anxiolytic medications should be used just in behaviourally uncontrolled acute situations. In many cases it is preferable to use long-lasting effect medications (e.g. SSRIs or buspirone), to reduce background anxiety levels down to a level that allows the individual to control anxiety (White et al. 2009).

8.5 Attention-Deficit Hyperactivity Disorder

8.5.1 Clinical Features

Along with behavioural problems, anxiety and depression, ADHD is the most frequent diagnosis in children with ASD, particularly whenever a broad syndromic construct of ASD is used for diagnosis (Leyfer et al. 2006; Mattila et al. 2010). Given that ADHD is a developmental disorder that often extends into adulthood, certainly many adults with ASD also qualify for a diagnosis of ADHD. The diagnosis of ADHD in adults with ASD is nevertheless controversial (Mazzone et al. 2012). Many signs and symptoms that characterize ADHD are common findings in people with ASD, and the differential diagnosis of ADHD in this population can be very difficult. It is also not surprising that, as both ASD and ADHD are neurodevelopmental disorders, there is an overlap area, not only syndromic but also possibly etiological. In line with this, several authors have been describing disorders that combine ADHD symptoms with ASD symptoms. An example is DAMP (deficits in attention, motor control and perception) described by Scandinavian authors as a disturbance of attention and motor coordination together with perceptive deficits, establishing a possible continuum with ASD (Gillberg 2003). In spite of this, it is of great importance to diagnose and treat ADHD in individuals with ASD. This diagnosis is of utmost importance in individuals with autism and good functional and cognitive competences, in which the constant restlessness and inability to maintain focused attention, even for short periods, significantly interfere with their academic, professional or social activities.

8.5.2 Treatment

In those cases where it is possible to presume comorbid ADHD, treatment should be considered, as ADHD is a disorder that can be successfully treated. Proper treatment of ADHD reduces the symptoms of the disorder and may potentiate the ability of the individual to use his different capabilities. Psychostimulant medications are the first-line drugs for the treatment of ADHD in adults (Kooij et al. 2010). The efficacy and safety of these substances, namely, of methylphenidate, have been widely proven. In the case of comorbidity with ASD, the use of methylphenidate must be particularly cautious, starting with very low dosages of fast-acting methylphenidate (e.g. 2.5–5 mg) and gradually increasing the dosage and daily coverage duration of the therapy, while continuously monitoring the clinical response.

8.6 Epilepsy

8.6.1 Clinical Features

Epilepsy is a particularly frequent neurological comorbidity in autism, with a percentage of 20–30 % (varying across studies from 6 % up to about 50 %) of individuals with ASD suffering or having suffered epileptic seizures (compared to a lifetime prevalence of 0.5–1 % in the general population) (Maski et al. 2011; Tuchman and Rapin 2002; Tuchman et al. 2009, 2010; Yasuhara 2010). Epilepsy is also referred to as being an important cause of mortality in autism (Bilder et al. 2013).

Epilepsy can be present regardless of the functional or cognitive level of the individual, but it is much more common in cases of non-verbal autism and in individuals suffering from intellectual disability and motor deficits (Tuchman and Rapin 2002; Tuchman et al. 2009, 2010; Yasuhara 2010). In these cases the prevalence of epilepsy can reach 40 % (Tuchman et al. 2009). It should be noted that the lifetime prevalence of epilepsy in ASD is much higher than in severe intellectual disability without autism, which leads us to conclude that there is a positive correlation between epilepsy and autism but not with intellectual disability. The fact that children with autism have a higher risk of developing epilepsy has raised the possibility of epilepsy and autism might share underlying neuropathological mechanisms that could account for both disorders (Giannotti et al. 2008; Tuchman and Rapin 2002; Tuchman et al. 2009). Finally, in cases of developmental autistic regression, there may be an increased risk of epilepsy, though the interpretation of available research data remains controversial (Giannotti et al. 2008; Tuchman et al. 2009, 2010).

Age of appearance of the first seizures and age of peak frequency has a bimodal distribution, with peaks occurring in early childhood and, later, in adolescence, particularly during puberty (Maski et al. 2011; Tuchman et al. 2009). Independently of the peak periods of occurrence, seizures can arise at any age. Epilepsy is also a major cause of mortality in autism (Maski et al. 2011). All types of epilepsy have been reported in autism, but the most frequent are partial complex seizures. Attention should be given to the fact that it can be difficult to identify the occurrence of complex partial seizures in individuals with ASD, particularly in those having a low cognitive and functional level (Maski et al. 2011). There is a natural tendency to consider the observed behavioural changes (e.g. gaze deviation, repetitive complex movements, lack of response to call) as being autistic manifestations, rather than clinical manifestations of a seizure.

Electroencephalographic changes are also quite common in individuals with ASD without seizures, including spikes and sharp waves, most often appearing in the central and frontal derivations (Kawasaki et al. 1997; Tuchman et al. 2009; Yasuhara 2010). Up to 85 % of patients with ASD may show epileptiform discharges in the EEG (Yasuhara 2010). These findings increase in frequency with the number of EEGs performed on the same individual and are also particularly frequent in sleep recordings. The clinical implication of these EEG alterations is questionable (Maski et al. 2011; Tuchman et al. 2010). Considering, however, that some authors did show a correlation between the suppression of epileptiform discharges on EEG and an improvement in psychosocial function, namely, a reduction of mood instability, impulsivity and aggression in people with ASD, the use of anticonvulsant therapy may merit consideration in these cases, taking into account the clinical context and the individual developmental trajectory (Maski et al. 2011; Tuchman et al. 2010). Still, the clinical utility of performing an EEG in an individual with ASD and without clinical seizures is unclear (Tuchman et al. 2010).

Finally, not all epileptic seizures are detectable on the scalp EEG, namely, those that originate in the deep structures of the brain, in the inner surfaces of the frontal lobe or in the depth of the sulci. For this reason, it is the careful observation of behavioural changes, namely, sudden changes of the usual behaviour of the individual with a suggestive sequence and typical ictal clinical characteristics that may point to the occurrence of epileptic seizures. Fluctuations in language, performance or behaviour, a significant loss of social and communicative skills or a functional or cognitive regression, for which no clear explanation can be found, are some of the symptoms that should alert the clinician to the possible presence of epileptic seizures (Tuchman et al. 2010). In these cases, it may be helpful to perform video monitoring, ambulatory 24 h EEG or video/EEG recordings.

8.6.2 Treatment

The basic principles of choice and implementation of anticonvulsant therapy are not basically different for individuals with ASD and epilepsy in comparison with those having epilepsy without autism. Thus, anticonvulsive medication choice should take into account the type of seizures, the EEG findings, the tolerance to medication, the combination of drugs that are being used and the possible side effects of different medications (Maski et al. 2011). The aim is to eliminate seizures without compromising cognitive and behavioural functions or affecting them as least as possible (Tuchman et al. 2010).

8.7 Sleep Disorders

8.7.1 Clinical Features

Sleep disorders are very frequent in individuals with ASD. The prevalence of sleep disorders in children with ASD is reported to be superior to that observed both in children with typical development and in children with intellectual disabilities without autism (Cortesi et al. 2010; Robinson-Shelton and Malow 2016). Sleep problems tend to persist and may extend into adulthood (Cortesi et al. 2010). Insomnia, one of the most common sleep disturbances observed in this population, may tend to worsen with age (Mattila et al. 2010). The most common insomnia patterns observed in ASD are sleep-onset delay and frequent night awakenings, often accompanied by night walking and short duration of sleep time (Blackmer and Feinstein 2016; Robinson-Shelton and Malow 2016). The night waking periods may have a prolonged duration of several hours, during which the individual acts as if he was acting in daytime (Cortesi et al. 2010). Apart from insomnia, daytime sleepiness and changes in circadian rhythms are also common (Cortesi et al. 2010; Maski et al. 2011). Sleep disorders are more common in people with ASD and moderate to severe intellectual disability, compared to those with milder degrees of cognitive disability (Cortesi et al. 2010; Giannotti et al. 2008).

The causes of sleep disorders in ASD are variable from individual to individual and result from the interaction between different biological, psychological, environmental and psychosocial factors (Cortesi et al. 2010; Robinson-Shelton and Malow 2016). Accordingly, some of the most commonly referred causes of insomnia in individuals with ASD are the inability to settle down to sleep, the obsessive fixation on events of the day and the hypersensitivity to environmental stimuli (Cortesi et al. 2010; Blackmer and Feinstein 2016).

Changes in the circadian cycle of sleep and wakefulness are very common in ASD and can be manifested by delayed sleep phase disorder, by advanced sleep phase disorder or free-running sleep and by daytime sleepiness (Cortesi et al. 2010; Giannotti et al. 2008; Maski et al. 2011; Tuchman et al. 2009). Disturbances in sleep architecture have also been reported (Cortesi et al. 2010).

One possible cause for these disorders might have to do with low levels of endogenous melatonin (Melke et al. 2008; Maski et al. 2011), possibly secondary to a genetic defect identified in some individuals with ASD (Melke et al. 2008). The decrease in melatonin concentrations could determine a disturbance in the circadian sleep/wake cycle and contribute to the phenotypic manifestations of autism as well as to the appearance of behavioural disorders in people with ASD (Maski et al. 2011; Melke et al. 2008).

Sleep disorders are common manifestations of many psychiatric conditions, such as anxiety and mood disorders. Besides, many other medical disorders can manifest as sleep disturbances, namely, some respiratory and endocrine diseases, among others. Thus, in the case of persistent sleep disturbances, it is important to investigate if they are ASD related or instead the expression of another comorbid somatic disorder (Cortesi et al. 2010; Maski et al. 2011; Robinson-Shelton and Malow 2016).

Given the high prevalence of sleep disorders in autism, it is crucial that during the clinical assessment of an individual with ASD, whether child or adult, questions are formulated to evaluate quality of sleep (Maski et al. 2011; Mattila et al. 2010; Robinson-Shelton and Malow 2016; Mazurek and Sohl 2016). These questions should also be addressed to family members and caregivers living with the individual. Identifying and treating sleep disorders can result in an improvement of both the individual's sleep and his daytime behaviour, leading to a global improvement in the quality of life of his family (Cortesi et al. 2010; Mazurek and Sohl 2016).

8.7.2 Treatment

Given the implications these conditions may have, both in daily living and in the physiological development of the individual, it is of utmost importance to treat sleep disorders. After ruling out the presence of comorbid disorders that may determine the observed sleep alterations, it is important to try to synchronize the circadian rhythm. Synchronization with sunlight and physical activity is the first measure to be implemented. The use of behavioural techniques may be sufficient to regulate the circadian cycle of sleep and wakefulness. Implementation of sleep hygiene measures should also be part of the first-line approach (Cortesi et al. 2010; Blackmer and Feinstein 2016; Robinson-Shelton and Malow 2016).

Thus, in all cases of sleep disturbances, the following sleep hygiene measures should be implemented:

- Promote exposure to daylight.
- Implement regular schedules to go to bed and wake up. Avoid going to bed too soon.
- Optimize sleep environment and prevent noise and excessive light during night-time.
- Avoid naps during the day.
- Promote the maintenance of social routines and occupational activities during the day.
- Promote physical exercise. Do not practice exercise too late (physical exercise should end at least 4 h before bedtime).
- Do not have a computer, TV or other sources of light and noise in the bedroom.
- Adjust the schedule of administration of medication that can negatively impact sleep.

Oral administration of melatonin at bedtime can be very useful for the synchronization of the circadian cycle of sleep and wakefulness in people with ASD, assuming that its production is often decreased (Cortesi et al. 2010; Blackmer and Feinstein 2016; Maski et al. 2011; Robinson-Shelton and Malow 2016).

The use of sleeping pills, in particular benzodiazepines (particularly having fast-acting and short-duration effect), should be avoided and, if required, should be used only for a short period of time. These drugs alter the architecture of sleep, cause habituation and may have paradoxical effects, including increased irritability and worsening insomnia. The use of antiepileptic drugs such as gabapentin or antidepressants such as mirtazapine, amitriptyline and trazodone to promote and maintain sleep has been used with good results, and is supported by some degree of evidence (Robinson-Shelton and Malow 2016).

References

Accordino RE, Kidd C, Politte LC, Henry CA, McDougle CJ (2016) Psychopharmacological interventions in autism spectrum disorder (2016). Expert Opin Pharmacother 7:1–16

Bradley EA, Summers JA, Wood HL, Bryson SE (2004) Comparing rates of psychiatric and behavior disorders in adolescents and young adults with severe intellectual disability with and without autism. J Autism Dev Disord 34:151–161

Bilder D, Botts EL, Smith KR, Pimentel R, Farley M, Viskochil J, McMahon WM, Block H, Ritvo E, Ritvo RA, Coon H (2013) Excess mortality and causes of death in autism spectrum disorders: a follow up of the 1980s Utah/UCLA autism epidemiologic study. J Autism Dev Disord 43(5):1196–1204

Blackmer AB, Feinstein JA (2016) Management of sleep disorders in children with neurodevelopmental disorders: a review. Pharmacotherapy 36(1):84–98

Cortesi F, Giannotti F, Ivanenko A, Johnson K (2010) Sleep in children with autistic spectrum disorder. Sleep Med 11(7):659–664
Croen LA, Zerbo O, Qian Y, Massolo ML, Rich S, Sidney S, Kripke C (2015) The health status of adults on the autism spectrum. Autism 19(7):814–823
de Bruin EI, Ferdinand RF, Meester S, de Nijs PFA, Verheij F (2007) High rates of psychiatric comorbidity in PDD-NOS. J Autism Dev Disord 37:877–886
Drmic IE, Szatmari P (2014) Emotional dysregulation and comorbidity in Autism Spectrum Disorder (ASD). CEPiP 1:119–131
Evans DW, Canavera K, Kleinpeter FL, Maccubbin E, Taga K (2005) The fears, phobias, and anxieties of children with autism spectrum disorders and down syndrome: comparisons with developmentally and chronologically aged matched children. Child Psychiatry Hum Dev 36:3–26
Gadow KD, DeVincent CJ, Pomeroy J, Azizian A (2004) Psychiatric symptoms in preschool children with PDD and clinic and comparison samples. J Autism Dev Disord 34(4):379–393
Giannotti F, Cortesi F, Cerquiglini A, Miraglia D, Vagnoni C, Sebastiani T, Bernabei P (2008) An investigation of sleep characteristics, EEG abnormalities and epilepsy in developmentally regressed and non-regressed children with autism. J Autism Dev Disord 38(10):1888–1897
Gillberg C (2003) Deficits in attention, motor control, and perception: a brief review. Arch Dis Child 88(10):904–910
Gillott A, Furniss F, Walter A (2001) Anxiety in high-functioning children with autism. Autism 5(3):277–286
Gillott A, Standen PJ (2007) Levels of anxiety and sources of stress in adults with autism. J Intellect Disabil 11(4):359–370
Jones KB, Cottle K, Bakian A, Farley M, Bilder D, Coon H, McMahon WM (2015) A description of medical conditions in adults with autism spectrum disorder: a follow-up of the 1980s Utah/UCLA Autism Epidemiologic Study. Autism 20(5):551–561
Joshi G, Petty C, Wozniak J, Henin A, Fried R, Galdo M, Kotarski M, Walls S, Biederman J (2010) The heavy burden of psychiatric comorbidity in youth with autism spectrum disorders: a large comparative study of a psychiatrically referred population. J Autism Dev Disord 40(11):1361–1370
Kawasaki Y, Yokota K, Shinomiya M, Shimizu Y, Niwa S (1997) Brief report: electroencephalographic paroxysmal activities in the frontal area emerged in middle childhood and during adolescence in a follow-up study of autism. J Autism Dev Disord 27(5):605–620
Kooij SJ, Bejerot S, Blackwell A, Caci H, Casas-Brugué M, Carpentier PJ, Edvinsson D, Fayyad J, Foeken K, Fitzgerald M, Gaillac V, Ginsberg Y, Henry C, Krause J, Lensing MB, Manor I, Niederhofer H, Nunes-Filipe C, Ohlmeier MD, Oswald P, Pallanti S, Pehlivanidis A, Ramos-Quiroga JA, Rastam M, Ryffel-Rawak D, Stes S, Asherson P (2010) European consensus statement on diagnosis and treatment of adult ADHD: The European Network Adult ADHD. BMC Psychiatry 10:67
Lang R, Regester A, Lauderdale S, Ashbaugh K, Haring A (2010) Treatment of anxiety in autism spectrum disorders using cognitive behavioral therapy: a systematic review. Dev Neurorehabil 13:53–63
Leyfer OT, Folstein SE, Bacalman S, Davis NO, Dinh E, Morgan J (2006) Comorbid psychiatric disorders in children with autism: interview development and rates of disorders. J Autism Dev Disord 36:849–861
Lugnegard T, Hallerback MU, Gillberg C (2011) Psychiatric comorbidity in young adults with a clinical diagnosis of Asperger syndrome. Res Dev Disabil 32:1910–1917
MacNeil BM, Lopes VA, Minnes PM (2009) Anxiety in children and adolescents with autism spectrum disorders. Res Autism Spectrum Disord 3:1–21
Maski KP, Jeste SS, Spence SJ (2011) Common neurological co-morbidities in autism spectrum disorders. Curr Opin Pediatr 23(6):609–615
Mattila ML, Hurtig T, Haapsamo H, Jussila K, Kuusikko-Gauffin S, Kielinen M, Linna SL, Ebeling H, Bloigu R, Joskitt L, Pauls DL, Moilanen I (2010) Comorbid psychiatric disorders associated with Asperger syndrome/high functioning autism: a community and clinic-based study. J Autism Dev Disord 40:1080–1093

Mazefsky CA, Oswald DP, Day TN, Eack SM, Minshew NJ, Lainhart JE (2012) ASD, a psychiatric disorder, or both? Psychiatric diagnoses in adolescents with high-functioning ASD. J Clin Child Adolesc Psychol 41(4):516–523

Mazurek MO, Sohl K (2016) Sleep and behavioral problems in children with autism spectrum disorder. J Autism Dev Disord 46(6):1906–1915. doi:10.1007/s10803-016-2723-7

Mazzone L, Ruta L, Reale L (2012) Psychiatric comorbidities in Asperger syndrome and high functioning autism: diagnostic challenges. Ann Gen Psychiatry 11(1):16

Melke J, Goubran Botros H, Chaste P, Betancur C, Nygren G, Anckarsäter H, Rastam M, Ståhlberg O, Gillberg IC, Delorme R, Chabane N, Mouren-Simeoni MC, Fauchereau F, Durand CM, Chevalier F, Drouot X, Collet C, Launay JM, Leboyer M, Gillberg C, Bourgeron T (2008) Abnormal melatonin synthesis in autism spectrum disorders. Mol Psychiatry 13(1):90–98

Perry DW, Marston GM, Hinder SA, Munden AC, Roy A (2001) The phenomenology of depressive illness in people with a learning disability and autism. Autism 5(3):265–275

Quek L-H, Sofronoff K, Sheffield J, White A, Kelly A (2012) Co-occurring anger in young people with Asperger's syndrome. J Clin Psychol 68(10):1142–1148

Rezaei V, Mohammadi MR, Ghanizadeh A, Sahraian A, Tabrizi M, Rezazadeh SA, Akhondzadeh S (2010) Double-blind, placebo-controlled trial of risperidone plus topiramate in children with autistic disorder. Prog Neuro-Psychopharmacol Biol Psychiatry 34(7):1269–1272

Robinson-Shelton A, Malow BA (2016) Sleep disturbances in neurodevelopmental disorders. Curr Psychiatry Rep 18(1):6

Sofronoff K, Attwood T, Hinton S, Levin I (2007) A randomized controlled trial of a cognitive behavioural intervention for anger management in children diagnosed with Asperger syndrome. J Autism Dev Disord 37(7):1203–1214

Stewart ME, Barnard L, Pearson J, Hasan R, O'Brien G (2006) Presentation of depression in autism and Asperger syndrome: a review. Autism 10(1):103–116

Tuchman R, Rapin I (2002) Epilepsy in autism. Lancet Neurol 1(6):352–358

Tuchman R, Moshé SL, Rapin I (2009) Convulsing toward the pathophysiology of autism. Brain Dev 31(2):95–103

Tuchman R, Alessandri M, Cuccaro M (2010) Autism spectrum disorders and epilepsy: moving towards a comprehensive approach to treatment. Brain Dev 32(9):719–730

White S, Oswald D, Ollendick T, Scahill L (2009) Anxiety in children and adolescents with ASD. Clin Psychol Rev 29:216–229

Yasuhara A (2010) Correlation between EEG abnormalities and symptoms of autism spectrum disorder (ASD). Brain Dev 32(10):791–798

Adult Outcomes and Supported Employment Strategies

9

Sandra Pinho

9.1 Introduction

When reviewing literature on adult outcomes in autism spectrum disorders (ASD), words like "unemployed," "underemployed," "malemployed," "poor," and "very poor" outcomes abound. In fact, the constellation of symptoms that characterizes ASD, with pervasive deficits in reciprocal social communication and interaction and restricted and repetitive patterns of behavior and interests, as described in DSM 5 (American Psychiatric Association 2013), persists into adulthood and is deemed to affect the completion of developmental challenges in transition to adult life, like securing and sustaining competitive employment, getting and maintaining a group of friends, making arrangements for independent living, and diversifying occupational and leisure activities.

This seems to be true across countries and over time, with reviewed literature from 2004 to 2015 reporting realities in the USA, Australia, the UK, and Germany leading to the "same old place": "unemployment," "underemployment," "malemployment," "poor," and "very poor" outcomes. Work, in special, is one of the most valued roles in adult life, and it represents multiple challenges for youth and adults with ASD. As Baldwin and colleagues put it, these challenges may include understanding complex job application materials, thinking "on their feet" in an interview, acclimatizing to new procedures and routines, remembering and following instructions, responding flexibly to unexpected situations, planning and juggling multiple tasks, communicating effectively with coworkers, interacting socially, and managing sensitivities in the workplace (Baldwin et al. 2014).

In this chapter, I will present some established facts on adult outcomes in ASD based on a review of literature published in English language in the past 10 years. It

S. Pinho
CADIn – Centro de Apoio ao Desenvolvimento Infantil, Department for Intervention in Adolescence and Adulthood, Cascais, Portugal
e-mail: sandra.pinho@cadin.net

B. Barahona Corrêa, R.-J. van der Gaag (eds.), *Autism Spectrum Disorders in Adults*, DOI 10.1007/978-3-319-42713-3_9

is not an exhaustive review but rather an attempt to draw the big picture of the struggle of people with ASD, their families, professionals, and agencies to ascertain a right that the United Nations considered a mandatory human right: that is, the right to employment for people with disability. I will finish presenting a model for supported employment in ASD. This model was developed mostly based on clinical practice with ASD, but it also aligns with recent investigation in this field.

9.2 ASD Outcomes: The Big Picture

In the UK, Howlin et al. (2004) conducted a follow-up study of 68 individuals meeting the criteria for autism and with a performance IQ of 50 or above. They found out that although a minority of adults had achieved relatively high levels of independence, most remained very dependent on their families or formal support services. Few lived alone and had close friends or permanent employment. Communication generally was impaired and reading and spelling abilities were poor. Stereotyped behaviors or interests frequently persisted into adulthood. Ten individuals had developed epilepsy. Overall, only 12 % were rated as having "very good" outcome; 10 % were rated as "good" and 19 % as "fair." The majority was rated as having "poor" (46 %) or "very poor" (12 %) outcome. Representing at the time one of the largest follow-up studies of autism in adult life, the results were nevertheless disappointing, as it would appear that the huge increase in educational facilities for children with autism over three decades had not necessarily resulted in significant improvements in outcome for adults (Howlin et al. 2004).

Lawer et al. (2009) compared the experiences of individuals with autism spectrum disorders in the US vocational rehabilitation system with the experience of others who use this system. The goal of the vocational rehabilitation system provided by the US Department of Education is to maximize the employment outcomes by providing services such as assessment and diagnosis, counseling, job search assistance, assistive technology, and on-the-job training. Any individual with a disability who requires help attaining employment is eligible for these services, which are aimed at creating the necessary skills and supports for individuals to be employed. Depending on the extent of their disability, individuals can be placed in noncompetitive or competitive employment. Competitive employment occurs in integrated settings, with or without supports, and is associated with wages at or above the federal minimum. Noncompetitive employment does not have the same wage requirement and can include sheltered employment in nonintegrated settings. While sheltered employment is often a stepping stone to successful competitive employment, it usually includes less social interaction and income. The study results showed that relative to other individuals served by the vocational rehabilitation system, individuals with ASD were more likely to be denied services because it was believed that their disability was too severe for them to benefit from these services. Furthermore, among those who received services, people with ASD received a more expensive set of services than those with other impairments, similar to the costs of services offered to individuals with intellectual disability (ID). Finally, competitive employment rates among people with ASD did not differ from those with specific learning disabilities (SLD) or ID and were much higher than those people with other impairments. Further analyses suggested that successful competitive employment for people with ASD and ID may depend on the presence of on-the-job supports, which include job coaching, follow-up and follow along, and job retention services (Lawer et al. 2009). It is important to acknowledge that individuals who use vocational rehabilitation services return the investment through taxes within 2–4 years, on average (Mawhood and Howlin 1999 cited by Lawer et al. 2009). In a study aiming to assess the cost-effectiveness of supported employment compared with standard care (day services) for adults with autism in the UK, Mavranezouli et al. (2014) concluded that although initial costs of such schemes are higher than standard care, they decrease over time and ultimately supported employment results not only in individual gains in social integration and well-being but also in reductions of the economic burden to health and social services and the wider society. The authors recommend that the programs be individualized but include common core elements of prior and on-the-job training, advocacy, and long-term support to ensure job retention.

Taylor and Seltzer (2010) examined 242 youth with ASD to determine whether exiting school was associated with alterations in rates of change in autism symptoms and maladaptive behaviors. Results indicated overall improvement of autism symptoms and internalized behaviors over the study period but slowing rates of improvement after exit. Youth who did not have an intellectual disability evidenced the greatest slowing in improvement. This study was the first to shed light on how exiting school – an important turning point in the lives of all youth including those with ASD – impacts the autism behavioral phenotype. Although autism symptoms and maladaptive behaviors were generally improving while adolescents and young adults with ASD were in the secondary school system, improvement slowed significantly after high school exit for internalizing behaviors and all but one of the autism symptom sub-domains. The authors considered that this slowing of improvement in the autism behavioral phenotype following high school exit reflected the less stimulating nature of adult occupational and day activities compared to those experienced in school. The most pronounced slowing of improvement after high school exit was observed for young adults with ASD who did not have ID. This stood in contrast to behavioral phenotypic change while these youth were in high school. Those with ASD who did not have ID improved more in both autism symptoms and maladaptive behaviors while they were in high school compared to those with comorbid ID. After high school exit, however, improvement in symptoms and behaviors slowed more for those without ID, with trajectories that appeared similar to youth with comorbid ID. The disruptive influence of high school exit for young adults without ID may be related to difficulties finding appropriate educational and occupational activities after exit. Nearly three fourths (74 %) of young adults with ASD and comorbid ID were receiving adult day services in the years immediately following high school exit compared to only 6 % of those without ID (Taylor and Seltzer 2010).

In another paper by Taylor and Seltzer (2011), the authors describe a group of post-high school educational and occupational activities for 66 young adults with

ASD who had recently exited the secondary school system in the USA. Analysis indicated low rates of employment in the community, with the majority of young adults (56 %) spending time in sheltered workshops or day activity centers. Again, young adults with ASD without an intellectual disability were three times more likely to have no daytime activities compared to adults with ASD who had an intellectual disability. The authors suggest that more autism-focused adult services are needed that will allow youths with ASD who do not have intellectual disabilities to achieve their maximum level of independence and develop sustainable careers. The current US developmental disability services do not appear to be accommodating the unique needs of individuals with ASD without ID. There might be a group of youths with ASD in the mid-level of functioning – not severe enough to receive adult day services but too severe to function independently – who are falling through the cracks during the transition to adulthood (Taylor and Seltzer 2011). On a more optimistic note, the authors remark that nearly 50 % of youths with ASD without ID were pursuing a postsecondary educational degree, suggesting that this is a viable option for many youths with ASD who do not have ID.

Despite this optimistic note, bad news came from Australia some years later. Drawing on data from a national survey, Baldwin et al. (2014) reported employment activities and experiences for 130 adults with Asperger disorder (AD) and high-functioning autism (HFA) in Australia. It is important to start with the note that this study sample constituted just over half (54 %) of the original research population from which it was drawn: namely, adults with AD and HFA participating in the "We Belong" survey project, who had left full-time education. The remainder of this group (n = 119) had no paid job at the time of completing the survey used in the study. While it was the express intention of the study to focus on adults in employment, secondarily the study emphasized that unemployment is a significant issue for high-functioning adults on the autism spectrum in Australia too. The findings highlighted the comparatively high education attainments of the study population. The proportion of participants holding a post-school qualification (86 %) was substantially higher than the 57 % reported for the general adult Australian population. Objectively speaking, the educational credentials of adults with AD and HFA should place them in a favorable position in the labor market. It is well established that, in the general population, higher levels of education are linked to increased earnings across the life span, a lower probability of unemployment, greater access to on-the-job training, and higher job satisfaction. Nevertheless, the study adds weight to existing evidence of underemployment and malemployment for adults with autism and specifically for those without ID. In particular, it strongly highlights the issue of "over education" as a concern for this group. Close to half (45 %) of the adults surveyed in this study were working in jobs for which they were overqualified. This rate of overqualification is more than twice that estimated by (Black 2013 cited by Baldwin et al. 2014) for the Australian workforce as a whole (21 %).

In an analysis of a large national US sample (n = 500), Shattuck et al. (2012) examined rates of postsecondary education and employment participation of individuals with ASD. They found that youth with ASD had a lower rate of employment relative to those in the speech/language impairment (SLI), learning disability

(LD), and mental retardation (MR) categories. The rate of postsecondary education among those with an ASD was lower than for those in the SLI or LD categories but higher than for those in the MR category. Young people with ASD had the highest risk of being completely disengaged from any kind of postsecondary education or employment. This risk remained larger than 50 % for the first 2 years after high school.

Gray et al. (2014) conducted a longitudinal study that followed a community sample of children and adolescents with autism into adulthood. The authors found that social outcomes in relation to community inclusion and living skills were modest in the majority of cases. More than half (61 %) of the individuals in their study were living with their parents. Only 9 % were living independently. While 99 % of the sample was engaged in some form of daytime activities, for the majority these consisted of a day program or sheltered workshop. Only 18 % were in paid employment. Although only one person in the study was not engaged in some form of organized activity, a significant number were only engaged for fewer than 20 h per week. Those with a more severe degree of intellectual disability (ID) were more likely to be living in care, and those with an average IQ were more likely to be living independently. The same pattern was true for daytime activities; individuals with either a mild degree of ID or a borderline-average IQ were more likely to be in paid employment or undertaking postsecondary school study. Although child and adolescent behavior and emotional problems did not contribute to adult outcomes in terms of living arrangements and activities, they did predict a lower number of hours spent weekly on these activities. With respect to living skills, children and adolescents with mild-borderline IQ or average IQ had better outcomes at follow-up. Neither gender nor behavior and emotional problems were associated with adult living skills. Both paid employment and postsecondary education were associated with better living skills.

I would like to finish this "Big Picture" section of this chapter with two studies that explored the perspectives of people with ASD on this scenario.

Hurlbutt and Chalmers (2004) interviewed six adults with Asperger syndrome (AS) about their experiences regarding employment. Repeatedly, problems interfering with employment emerged. All adults who were interviewed had difficulty finding work matching their ability levels and had difficulty maintaining jobs. This was the result of poor communication between employee and employer or coworkers, social skill deficits, and sensory issues. The authors also noted that problems and difficulties encountered in the world of work can have a devastating effect on mood, mental health, and self-esteem for adults with AS. Depression, anxiety, and anger are very common in adults with AS and often the result of employment issues. To help adults with AS in obtaining and maintaining work, the authors present the following recommendations:

1. Adoption of the supported employment model and the master and apprentice model
2. Taking into account the strengths and interests of the employee, as well as the need for flexibility and job complexity when matching person to job

3. Emphasizing the advantages of hiring individuals with AS to the potential employer
4. Providing tutoring/mentoring in the workplace
5. Evaluating the need for reasonable accommodations and implementing them
6. Providing structure, order, routines and clear rules, and assignments in the workplace
7. Helping the employee with AS to prepare for any needed changes in the workplace or job definition
8. Breaking tasks into steps to alleviate feeling of being overwhelmed (Hurlbutt and Chalmers 2004)

Giarelli et al. (2013) inquired 14 adolescents with Asperger syndrome (AS) about their expectations, perceived barriers, and perceived facilitators to transition to community and adulthood. Adolescents were asked to describe what they believed was a successful transitioning or, specifically, what it meant to them. Most of the participants ($n = 10$; 70 %) hoped for employment and the remainder ($n = 4$, 30 %) hoped to attend college. Additionally, 30 % expressed a dream to find a partner, marry, and raise a family.

The adolescents in the study seemed to have a realistic knowledge of their disorder and described four general barriers to their successful transitioning: (1) behavioral problems, (2) associated features (such as limited attention span and focus, anxiety, and unstable mood and meltdowns), (3) other personal factors, and (4) institutional characteristic (worksite or college) factors. In the category of behavioral problems, the following were perceived as barriers: (a) inability to socialize comfortably, (b) "getting stuck," and (c) inability to make casual conversation. The three most often associated perceived barriers were (1) limited attention span and focus, (2) anxiety, and (3) unstable mood and meltdowns. The adolescents interviewed in this study also spoke of other personal factors that did not fall into the category of associated or core characteristics. These included perceived low self-image, difficulties in motor control, and lack of motivation. The three institutional barriers most often reported were (1) inflexibility of the environment, (2) inadequate orientation for the work experience, and (3) coworker negativity (Giarelli et al. 2013).

Conceptual categories of perceived bridges or facilitators were:

1. Accommodations in the community (e.g., individualized routines, orientation program, and promoting coworker's understanding of the special needs and issues faced by people with AS)
2. Cognitive abilities (e.g., use technical skills, attention to details, focus, memory)
3. Personal qualities (e.g., tolerant, polite, cooperative)
4. Mentor's qualities (e.g., models appropriate behavior, assists to manage work-related problems, accepts difference, and is tolerant) (Giarelli et al. 2013)

As studies reviewed show, there is much work to do in supporting transition to adulthood and adult functioning in ASD individuals, especially those without intellectual disability. Albeit typically showing educational credentials that should place them in a favorable position in the labor market, the current developmental disability services do not appear to be accommodating their unique needs, and this seems to configure a group that is falling through the cracks during the transition to adulthood.

9.3 Helping People with Neurodevelopmental Disorders to Succeed in the Workplace: Supported Employment in ASD

Selection and recruitment processes are all about placing the right person in the right job. Vocational rehabilitation services and professionals concerned with the selection and recruitment of candidates with ASD can help in three fronts: (1) supporting candidates with ASD to find job offers that fit their strengths and qualifications, (2) supporting companies in recruiting candidates with ASD that fit their job descriptions and requirements, and (3) analyzing the requirements for the job and comparing them to the profile of candidates with ASD.

The generalized deficits encountered in ASD mean that some types of work are likely to be unsuited for the majority of adults with ASD. For example, they may not cope well in jobs that require immediate and rapid processing of requests or demands, such as a cashier, a cook, a waiter, or a receptionist. They are also more likely to struggle in busy or noisy environments, such as fast food restaurants and factories. On the other hand, there are jobs in which adults with ASD may perform extremely well, notably, those requiring visual thinking, systematic information processing, or precise technical abilities (e.g., architect, librarian, computer programmer). Nevertheless, care must be taken not to stereotype the vocational interests and capabilities of this group, as studies have shown that adults with ASD are in fact employed across a broad range of occupations, including those more counterintuitive to popular conceptions of the "autistic mind" such as sales, creative arts, and the military (Baldwin et al. 2014).

Nevertheless, most commonly used selection techniques do not guarantee equal opportunities for people with disabilities, especially if they affect psychological/neurological functions as it is the case with ASD. As shown in the previous section of this chapter, numerous research studies have found that adults with ASD experience challenges in securing and sustaining competitive employment. As a group, they are more likely to be unemployed (without a job), underemployed (in jobs that underutilize their knowledge, skills, and experience), or malemployed (in jobs for which they are expressly unsuited) than the population in general. Related to this, they demonstrate a comparatively high level of job switching, resulting in fragmented work histories that may limit their potential for ongoing employment and career development (Baldwin et al. 2014).

As we saw, studies have repeatedly shown that there is a lower rate of activity and employment among people with disabilities in comparison to the general active population, as well as an increased rate of unemployment. In a 2007 study conducted in Portugal, researchers found that that people with a disability were clearly discriminated in accessing work, as were people with mental health problems generally. In particular, people with moderate difficulties in comprehension, interpersonal skills, memory, concentration, adaptive skills, grooming, and clothing seemed to face particularly increased barriers in their work inclusion (Employment of People with Disabilities – An approach to equal opportunities. Ministry of Solidarity and Social Security 2012).

Taking these data into account, it is evident that curriculum analysis will hinder candidates with ASD in the first step of every selection process. Moreover, the selection interview is a compulsory stage in every selection process in which the interviewer assesses the candidate's oral level, nonverbal communication, and the way he or she communicates and relates to others. So, this is a selection element that is very likely to hinder candidates with challenges in social interaction and communication, as it is the case for candidates with ASD. Finally, skills and personality tests, also widely used in selection processes, compare individual performance to a previously established norm and will invariably declassify any "atypical" candidates. If reasonable adjustments are not implemented in the selection processes for these candidates, we will not be able to guarantee equality of employment opportunities for them.

Mark Romoser (2000), an individual with high-functioning autism, writes, in a humorous and ironic demonstration of self-advocacy: The job of anyone working in personnel management is to look at a steady stream of applicants, almost always neurotypical (that is, without autism), and to reject those who are deemed not to fit in that particular corporate culture. When an applicant who has autism shows up, the human resources agents task is almost too easy. She or he just pushes the button underneath the desk, yell "Next!" a trapdoor opens up, and we fall out a chute back onto the street. (Romoser 2000)

As legislation contemplates that the selection process is adapted to the communication/expression profile of the candidate, vocational rehabilitation services should address employers' awareness of ASD and suggest reasonable adjustments for the selection process (e.g., interview adjustments and on-the-job experience). On the other hand, these services should offer some support to candidates in preparing for a job interview and, if necessary, provide accompaniment by a service professional when the ASD subjects go to an interview.

Research suggests that up to 90 % of job losses in individuals with disabilities are due to deficits in social communication (Elksin and Elksin 2001 cited by Strickland et al. 2013), emphasizing the critical importance of skills in this domain. The initial job interview is the first hurdle to getting into the workplace. Thus, social competence in this setting is a specific skill critical to a positive occupational outcome. For that reason, many job interviews include questions that are designed to evaluate the interviewee's social problem solving and teamwork skills. In some cases, social skills and behavioral tendencies are rated more frequently in the interview than any other construct. Socially based skills, including response content, composure, and even appearance, influence how the interviewer perceives and evaluates a candidate.

Strickland et al. (2013) evaluated the effectiveness of an Internet-accessed training program that included Theory of Mind-based guidance, video models, visual supports, and virtual reality practice sessions in teaching appropriate job interview skills to individuals with high-functioning autism spectrum disorders. The results suggested that the tested intervention package is a useful method for working with youth with ASD who are at risk for poor performance in job interviews. It was notable that the program was more effective in teaching "content" rather than "delivery" skills; that is, participants were able to produce more appropriate verbal responses to interview questions following intervention, but the features that accompany those responses (e.g., posture, eye contact, or facial expression) did not improve to the same degree. The authors suggest that efforts to target "delivery" skills as well as "content" skills may require additional time or more feedback to achieve the same degree of improvement (Strickland et al. 2013). The study also revealed several important limitations in participants' responses to questions in a job interview. Many of the participants' responses to such questions as "Tell me a little bit about yourself" and "What are some of your strengths?" suggested a failure to recognize that the information provided ("content" skills) is viewed more favorably when it has some relevance to the work setting. Certain responses that revealed highly personal information (e.g., medication usage, relationship problems, therapy experiences) and responses to questions designed to assess participants' ability to work with a group (teamwork) or their ability to cope with stressful situations suggested that ASD participants did not consider the perspective of the interviewer and therefore failed to use knowledge of the interviewer's expectations to craft a favorable response. In other words, their responses were indicative of their inability to use Theory of Mind skills to their own benefit (Strickland et al. 2013). To address these social cognition and social communication skill issues, the study authors recommend that practitioners repeatedly engage individuals in opportunities to rehearse appropriate responses under conditions that approximate what the individual will encounter in a real situation (Strickland et al. 2013).

Morgan et al. (2014) evaluated the efficacy of the interview skills curriculum (ISC), a manualized 12-week group-delivery intervention for young adults with ASD. This intervention aims to increase social-pragmatic skills essential to a successful job interview. Twenty-eight adults (18–36 year) were randomly assigned to one of two groups: ISC or waitlist control. Results revealed that the experimental group showed larger gains in social-pragmatic skills observed during a mock interview than the control group. However, the authors did not test the effectiveness of their intervention in terms of successful real-world employment.

Smith et al. (2014) assessed the feasibility and efficacy of virtual reality job interview training in adults with autism spectrum disorders. The feasibility results suggested that participants were (1) largely compliant with attendance at training sessions (>90 %), (2) engaged with the simulated interviews during these sessions (>500 min of training out of a maximum of 600 min.), and (3) reported that the virtual reality job interview training (VR-JIT) was easy to use, enjoyable, and helpful, instilled participants with confidence, and prepared them for the future interviews. The efficacy results suggested that when compared to the treatment as usual group, the VR-JIT (virtual reality job interview training) group had: (1) significant improved job interview skills that were characterized by moderate-to-large effect sizes, (2) enhanced job interview self-confidence, and (3) a progressive increase in simulated interview scores across trials and increasing levels of difficulty. This study provides initial evidence that VR-JIT may be a feasible and efficacious program to enhance practical job interview skills for adults with ASD and that job interview role-play performance can be improved with virtual reality training (Smith et al. 2014).

9.4 Developing a Supported Employment Model in ASD

When a candidate is selected and integrated into a workplace, legislation considers the possibility and the responsibility of making reasonable adjustments in the workplace, in order to promote equal opportunities. At this stage, vocational rehabilitation services can help by (1) supporting the employer, (2) supporting the employee, and (3) supporting the communication between employer and employee.

In supporting the employer, three concerns should be addressed: (1) ASD awareness training; (2) selection of a tutor/mentor in the workplace, who is asked to plan activities, support, train, evaluate, give feedback, and nurture the employee with ASD; and (3) making reasonable adjustments (e.g., stable job placement, substituting phone communication for mail communication). Care should be taken, as minimizing change is not necessarily helpful. Individuals with autism need predictability in their environment and not necessarily repetition. For some individuals with autism, engaging in the exact same routine on the job everyday appears to have negative effect on their motivation and work performance (Lawrence et al. 2010).

In supporting the employee with ASD, our model recommends three areas of intervention: (1) training in soft skills (communication, interpersonal, time and money management, emotional regulation skills, and adaptive behavior essential to the labor market), (2) managing performance anxiety in the workplace, and (3) managing time and task prioritization.

Finally, in supporting the communication between the employer and the employee, we recommend regular visits to the workplace.

There is limited but encouraging evidence demonstrating the efficacy of supported employment models in ASD. Garcia-Villamisar and Hughes (2007) examined the effects of a supported employment program on measures of executive functions for 44 adults with autism, assessed at the beginning and at the end of the program period. Although at the start of the vocational program there was no group difference for any cognitive measures, repeated measure analysis of variance demonstrated that by the end of the program, the supported employment group showed higher scores for executive functions when compared to the unemployment group. Results in this study suggest that vocational rehabilitation programs have beneficial impact upon cognitive performance in people with autism. Active engagement in the work setting can help people with autism to improve their cognitive skills. In other words, "work is therapy" (Black 1988, cited by Villamisar and Hughes 2007).

Lattimore et al. (2006) suggested that jobsite training, assumed to be the best practice for teaching vocational skills to workers with disabilities, is likely to be more effective if supplemented with simulation training, at least with subjects who have autism and severe to profound intellectual disability. Their results suggested that adults with autism tended to acquire work skills in a community job more quickly when jobsite training was supplemented with simulation training. In a further analysis (Lattimore, Parsons, and Reid 2008) of the effectiveness of simulation training on work performance in subjects with ASD, the authors found that simulation training enhanced job performance in newly assigned tasks when it is provided prior to on-the-job training. Moreover, simulation training seems to be beneficial even when the work tasks require equipment that cannot be transported to a simulation site for training. A single day of intensive training in a simulation setting was also found to be beneficial in another study conducted by this team (Lattimore, Parsons and Reid 2008). Their results support the utility of simulation training with adults who have severe autism.

Allen et al. (2012) evaluated audio cueing to facilitate community employment of individuals with autism and intellectual disability performing in WalkArounds. Three adolescents with both ASD and ID participated in their study. Participants were, in a first stage, trained and observed at the factory and warehouse where the WalkArounds were manufactured. One portion of the warehouse was arranged into an analogue of a typical aisle at a major discount retailer (e.g., wide aisles, shelves with items for sale on both sides of the aisle, costumers walking by). To help simulate a discount retail store setting, 3–5 volunteers of varying ages were recruited to periodically walk up and down the aisles and past the participant in a WalkAround on a variable interval 15 s schedule. Volunteers were also scheduled to engage in common shopper behaviors, rotating randomly between (1) ignoring the WalkAround, (2) asking a question, (3) responding to any initiations by the WalkAround, (4) walking past the WalkAround while talking on a cell phone, (5) looking at the items on the shelves, and (6) asking for a hug. Job skills targeted for acquisition were grouped into three categories and coded separately: (1) head actions, including nodding or shaking the head, moving the ears, and wagging the tongue; (2) arm/hand actions, including waving, shaking hands, giving high fives, and clapping the arms against the side; and (3) leg/torso actions, including posing for pictures, shaking the tail, shaking the body, and jumping up and down. To perform the job successfully, participants were expected to use multiple target skills for a minimum of 30 % of the time, a criterion that was deemed by the employer to be necessary for the WalkAround to appear "life-like" and engaging to customers. The job required the maintenance of skills over time and also the generalization of those skills to a novel, untrained costume in an untrained setting (actual large discount department store). During baseline, each of the participants showed relatively stable, low rates of multiple target behavior use. With the introduction of the audio cueing, the rates of multiple skills use increased immediately and substantially for each participant. Furthermore, each of the participants was able to perform above criterion in both an untrained costume and an untrained environment. When audio cues were removed in a return to baseline withdrawal, rates of multiple skills use decreased to baseline levels or lower. The results of this investigation demonstrate that individuals with ASD and ID can perform a job usually performed by neurotypical individuals, in a hectic, socially demanding work environment if provided with appropriate supports.

Employment has been demonstrated to improve quality of life in individuals with ASD, and it is thought to promote personal dignity by allowing access to the same opportunities enjoyed by the rest of society. Employment also has a significant cost impact on the economy, resulting in less reliance on government funds and greater contribution in taxes. Finally, there is good evidence to support the potential benefits to employers and companies when they hire individuals with ASD, as these are often more reliable and dependable than more typical part-time employees.

In Europe, Vogeley et al. (2013) comment that the German health and social care systems are not adequately prepared for the proper support of this population. This leads them to suggest that supported employment programs should be developed for adults with HFA that specifically address their needs and requirements. Such programs should comprise (1) the adequate assessment of HFA, including neuropsychological profile and individual matching of the persons' preferences with requirements in the workplace; (2) on-the-job coaching activities that include systematic communication and social interaction training; and (3) instruction of coworkers, including colleagues and supervisors, about weaknesses and strengths of HFA.

With respect to job coaching, based on their experience with adults with HFA, Vogeley et al. (2013) recommend that a successful intervention should probably comprise a period of 12 months, of which at least 3 months should focus on education and training in a group off-the-job setting with a group size of up to six patients and a schedule of one session per week. This should be followed and complemented by a period of 9 months of training on the job, with individual contacts at least once weekly (Vogeley et al. 2013).

Regarding instruction of coworkers, the authors remark that individuals with ASD are more likely to lose their job because of problematic social interactions rather than the inability to perform work tasks. The capacity to process socially relevant information is an essential component of professional environments, which force jobholders to cooperate with colleagues and clients and to coordinate their own activities with those of others. Autism affects the capacity to interact and communicate with others in a fundamental way, as intuitive, fast, and pre-reflexive components of communication are lacking. Education of coworkers to promote knowledge and acceptance of weaknesses and strengths of HFA is therefore a necessary prerequisite for integrating people with HFA in work environment (Vogeley et al. 2013).

Wehman et al. (2014) examined employment outcomes for youth with ASD between the ages of 18–21 years in a randomized clinical trial integrated within Project SEARCH plus ASD supports. Project SEARCH is a 9-month internship model where youth with developmental disabilities who are in their last year of high school are embedded in a large community business such as a hospital, government complex, or banking center. In this study, experimental subjects rotated though numerous internships in two different suburban hospitals. They had the opportunity to practice multiple job skills, such as stocking, filing, cleaning, and transporting materials and documents in various hospital units (nursing, family center, material management, central sterile, surgical services, physical rehabilitation, laboratory services, pharmacy, employee wellness, etc.). In addition, experimental subjects were provided with ASD-specific supports: (1) onsite intensive systematic instruction using principals of applied behavior analysis, (2) onsite support and consultation from a behavior/autism specialist, and (3) intensive staff training in ASD and the Project SEARCH model. The control group consisted of students in their last year of high school who were receiving educational supports and services specified in their individualized educational programs (IEPs). Results were quite positive and encouraging. The treatment group attained employment at the rate of 87,5 % ($n = 21$) upon completion of the Project SEARCH plus ASD program, whereas only 6,25 % ($n = 1$) of subjects in the control group were able to obtain employment. This difference in employment rates was still evident after 3 months. There were also significant differences in the reported need for employment supports, according to the Employment Subscale of the Supports Intensity Scale (Thompson et al. 2004a). After only 3 months of internship, the intensity of support needs in the treatment group decreased significantly. Furthermore, in addition to achieving employment at a statistically higher rate, participants in the treatment group achieved employment in competitive jobs that have not traditionally been considered as accessible for youth with ASD.

In an innovative approach to coaching, Gentry et al. (2015) tested the efficacy of personal digital assistant (PDA) training at the beginning of job placement of adults with ASD. The results showed that training in the use of a PDA as an assistive technology significantly reduces the need for job coaching support by workers with ASD without reducing functional performance on the job. PDA-based applications and strategies included (1) task reminders, (2) task lists, (3) picture prompts, (4) video-based task-sequencing prompts, (5) behavioral self-management adaptations, (6) way-finding tools, and (7) communication with the job coach via Wi-Fi when available in the jobsite. The reduction in job coaching hours shown in the study was large enough to offset the cost of the assistive technology intervention, translating into lower costs for the vocational rehabilitation agency.

Conclusion

It is our hope that practice and investigation in the field of employment in people with ASD can continue to develop so as to change history for these persons all over the world. If the story of many "neurotypical" employees is one of casualness, the story of many employees with disabilities is as follows:

I had to prohibit my son M. from waking up at 6 a.m. on Sundays to do homework! The other day, I found him doing homework at 7 a.m.! (Testimony of M's mother; M is a young adult with Asperger syndrome)

It doesn't matter how many times I say to H that he does not have to finish all the tasks I give him in the same day… it looks as if he absolutely needs to finish his task before going home, otherwise he gets extremely anxious. (Testimony of H's tutor; H is an adult with Asperger syndrome)

The fact is that workers with disabilities, when challenged, are usually more assertive and persistent than workers without disabilities, because they feel the need to prove themselves and work is more than a means to guarantee individual survival, it is also a way of social acceptance, and this aspect is more valued for these adults, who seek to have their full capability recognized through work.

Nevertheless, studies reviewed showed a population that still craves access to adult rights like occupation, home, or employment, especially those with ASD without intellectual disability, who seemed even more alienated from general community. A shade of hope comes up when studies analyzing supported employment strategies and techniques show that much can be achieved with reasonable adjustments that, albeit more expensive in the beginning, will pay at the long run as cost-effectiveness of supported employment compared with day care decreases over time resulting in individual and society gains.

Let's keep this train going so as to cut the prefixes "in" and "un" from the words "incapable" and "unemployed" that still abound in the lives of youth and adults with ASD.

References

Allen K, Burke R, Howard M, Wallace D, Bowen S (2012) Use of audio cuing to expand employment opportunities for adolescents with autism spectrum disorders and intellectual disabilities. J Autism Dev Disord 42:2410–2419

American Psychiatric Association. (2013). Diagnostic and statistical manual of mental disorders (5th ed.). Washington, DC: Author

Baldwin S, Costley D, Warren A (2014) Employment activities and experiences of adults with high-functioning autism and Asperger's disorder. J Autism Dev Disord 44:2440–2449

García-Villamisar D, Hughes C (2007) Supported employment improves cognitive performance in adults with autism. J Intellect Disabil Res 51(2):142–150

Gentry T, Kriner R, Sima A, McDonough J, Wehman P (2015) Reducing the need for personal supports among workers with autism using an iPod touch as an assistive technology: delayed randomized control trial. J Autism Dev Disord 45:669–684

Giarelli E, Ruttenberg J, Segal A (2013) Bridges and barriers to successful transitioning as perceived by adolescents and young adults with Asperger syndrome. J Pediatr Nurs 28:563–574

Gray K, Keating C, Teffe J, Brereton A, Einfeld S, Reardon T, Tonge B (2014) Adult outcomes in autism: community inclusion and living skills. J Autism Dev Disord 44:3006–3015

Howlin P, Goode S, Hutton J, Rutter M (2004) Adult outcome for children with autism. J Child Psychol Psychiatry 45(2):212–229

Hurlbutt K, Chalmers L (2004) Employment and adults with Asperger syndrome. Focus Autism Other Dev Disabil 19(4):215–222

Lattimore L, Parsons M, Reid DH (2006) Enhancing job-site training of supported workers with autism: a reemphasis on simulation. J Appl Behav Anal 36:91–102

Lattimore LP, Parsons MB, Reid DH (2008) Simulation training of community job skills for adults with autism: A further analysis. Behavior Analysis in Practice 1:24–29

Lawer L, Brusilovskiy E, Dalzer M, Mandell D (2009) Use of vocational rehabilitative services among adults with autism. J Autism Dev Disord 39:487–494

Lawrence DH, Alleckson DA, Bjorklund P (2010) Beyond the Roadblocks: Transitioning to Adulthood with Asperger's Disorder. Archives of Psychiatric Nursing 24(4):227–238

Mavranezouli I, Megnin-Viggars O, Cheema N, Howlin P, Baron-Cohen S, Pilling S (2014) The cost-effectiveness of supported employment for adults with autism in the United Kingdom. Autism 18(8):975–984

Morgan L, Leatzow A, Clark M (2014) Interview skills for adults with autism spectrum disorder: a pilot randomized controlled trial. J Autism Dev Disord 44:2290–2300

Romoser M (2000) Malemployment in autism. Focus Autism Other Dev Disabil 15(4):246–247

Shattuck P, Narendorf S, Cooper B, Sterzing P, Wagner M, Taylor S (2012) Postsecondary education and employment among youth with an autism spectrum disorder. www.pediatrics.org/cgi/doi/10.1542/peds.2011-2864

Smith M, Ginger E, Wright K, Wright M, Taylor J, Humm L, Olsen D, Bell M, Fleming M (2014) Virtual reality job interview training in adults with autism spectrum disorder. J Autism Dev Disord 44:2450–2463

Strickland D, Coles C, Southern L (2013) JobTIPS: a transition to employment program for individuals with autism spectrum disorders. J Autism Dev Disord 43:2472–2483

Taylor J, Seltzer M (2010) Changes in the autism behavioral phenotype during the transition to adulthood. J Autism Dev Disord 40:1431–1446

Taylor J, Seltzer M (2011) Employment and post-secondary educational activities for young adults with autism spectrum disorders during the transition to adulthood. J Autism Dev Disord 41:566–574

Thompson JR, Bryant BR, Campbell EM, Craig EM, Hughes CM, Rotholz DA, Schalock R, Silverman W, Tassé M, Wehmeyer M (2004a) Supports Intensity Scale (SIS). Washington, DC: American Association on Mental Retardation

Vogeley K, Kirchner J, Gawronski A, Tebartz van Elst L, Dziobek I (2013) Toward the development of a supported employment program for individuals with high functioning autism in Germany. Eur Arch psychiatry Clin Neurosci 263(2):S197–S203

Wehman P, Schall C, McDonough J, Kregel J, Brooke V, Molinelli A, Ham W, Graham C, Riehle J, Collins H, Thiss W (2014) Competitive employment for youth with autism spectrum disorders: early results from a randomized clinical trial. J Autism Dev Disord 44:487–500

The Institutional and Community Care for Adults with Autistic Spectrum Disorders

10

Jan-Pieter Teunisse

10.1 A Life-Span Perspective

In the Netherlands, like in many countries worldwide, organizing the best possible care and support and guidance for individuals with autism is a matter of concern to which much thinking has been devoted.

The life-span perspective prevails nowadays, whereas in the past autism spectrum disorders (ASD) were mostly perceived as a developmental disorder, mostly limited to childhood and youth. Currently there is solid awareness of the fact that these youngsters will need to have and find their place in society. A seminal report by our Health Council "Autism: being 'different' all lifelong" (Gezondheidsraad 2009) illustrated this perspective. The report summarized the state of the services and provisions for individuals with autism and their relatives at that point and strongly advised several ministries and stakeholders to take the life-span perspective seriously into consideration:

To ensure continuity of care, the commission would favour the appointment of "lifespan-carers" well acquainted with the situation and possibilities within healthcare, education, the working-places and community support, able to provide practical help at different stages as life progresses.

J.-P. Teunisse, PhD (✉)
HAN University of Applied Sciences, Research Group Autism Through the Lifespan, P.O. Box 6960, 6503 GL, Nijmegen, The Netherlands

Dr. Leo Kannerhuis, Centre for Autism, Department of Research Development & Innovation, P.O. Box 62, 6865 ZH, Doorwerth, The Netherlands
e-mail: JanPieter.Teunisse@han.nl

B. Barahona Corrêa, R.-J. van der Gaag (eds.), *Autism Spectrum Disorders in Adults*, DOI 10.1007/978-3-319-42713-3_10

10.2 An Evolving Society: Moving from a Welfare State to a Participation Society

It is important to note that, in this report, ASD was not only approached from a treatment perspective but that special emphasis was put upon dignified participation in society. In our country this accounts not only for individuals with ASD, but to all individuals, as our society is moving from a compassionate supportive society to a society where all are expected to take responsibility for their own functioning and place in society. In parallel with this, the central government is gradually handing over the organization of care delivery to local authorities and communities. The government no longer automatically takes care of citizens in need but encourages them to organize and coordinate their own support. Instead of taking over, the authorities encourage those in need to solve their problems by themselves (self-management) and to call on help within their own social network (family, friends, and neighbors). Only as a last resort are professionals from the health system or social welfare called upon to intervene. In this perspective, professionals should no longer act as the experts who will take over and solve the problem but will merely help to clarify what is the matter and help the citizen in need to solve his own problems. Support and coaching are provided in the setting where the individual is, lives, or works and no longer in the premises of the healthcare and social welfare. Professionals are expected to reach out for users in need and to work in multidisciplinary teams within the local communities. The focus is shifting from emphasis on problems and limitations, to the challenge of striving toward optimal functioning taking into account the individual's possibilities. The urge to evolve from a welfare state to a participation society is a joint effort stemming both from politicians and policy makers as well as from citizens themselves (Newman and Tonkens 2011). This movement was initiated when the costs of social welfare went rising beyond affordability. Therefore, the need for budgetary cuts was the primary motivation for policy makers to induce change, as self-supporting citizens that live independently are far cheaper to society than those depending on social security and institutional care. On the other hand, citizens felt too much patronized and felt too little room for developing their own initiatives and solutions out of the rigid welfare box. The emancipation movements (women's, patients', workers') have played a crucial part in striving for inclusiveness, a more evenly shared decision-making, and real possibilities to build a meaningful existence for each individual in the community.

10.3 Autism in the Participation Society

There is thus a broad support for this societal shift. Both policy makers and citizens welcome this movement toward devolving autonomy and responsibility to citizens, including those in need of support or facing personal limitations and problems.

Yet, should we not also be concerned with the potential risks of marginalization that are inherent to this shift of paradigm, especially when we take adults with ASD into consideration. The "participating society" is based on the assertiveness of active citizens, who know what they want and are very well capable of organizing a network to assist and eventually support and care for themselves. These are people who definitively want to be in charge of their lives and can organize care if necessary. But do people with ASD, hindered by limitations in their cognitive coping competencies (as a result of a limited theory of mind and central coherence and poor executive functions), fit into this picture of the resilient citizen? The whole transition is based on the assumption that individuals in the community are capable of finding their way when they need help or assistance and are able to seek help in their near environment if necessary. This is exactly what most people with ASD are not able to achieve. The essence of ASD is a social-communicative disorder, and the consequence is that one cannot reasonably expect from a person with ASD to take initiative to seek help when needed. The transition of responsibility for care and support from professional organizations to the general public is based on the assumption that the people are well prepared to make the necessary connections and communicate about the kind and amount of care they need. Individuals with ASD are, in general, dependent on structure and are limited in their capacity to assess situations within their context.

According to Lawson (2003) individuals with ASD tend to perceive the world as a scientific lab where everything is regulated according to completely logical and unchangeable laws and rules: B will always follow A. Thus people with ASD need structure and a highly predictable environment with explicit rules and strictly reliable arrangements. Unfortunately, the real social world is very different: it is an open system, with its own dynamics, subject to variation and too many implicit, hidden rules. A may be followed by B or C and eventually tomorrow even D. This makes the world utterly unpredictable for individuals with ASD. They often do not know what to do, let alone decide whom to ask and what to ask. They clearly do not have, nor master, the competencies required to be an active citizen or patient who can stand up for him- or herself.

10.3.1 Self-Determination

Another problematic area for individuals with ASD is the capacity to "self-regulate" (self-determine) one's life, a central notion in the transition toward a "participating society."

The Field and Hoffman model (1995, see Fig. 10.1) of self-determination defines requirements and competencies that, clearly, individuals with ASD will not easily meet. Self-awareness and self-esteem appear to be crucial conditions to be able to achieve some form of autoregulation. One has to be able to imagine what one would like to achieve or reach in the future in a concrete and realistic fashion. As individuals with ASD often lack imagination, this seems to be quite problematic. Moreover, self-determination requires that one has the capacity to generate realistic options from which to choose. Not all of one's dreams are reachable, and one needs to have the competencies to delimitate and consider all the circumstances involved that can be of influence. This holds true in general, but it is clear that this is beyond many

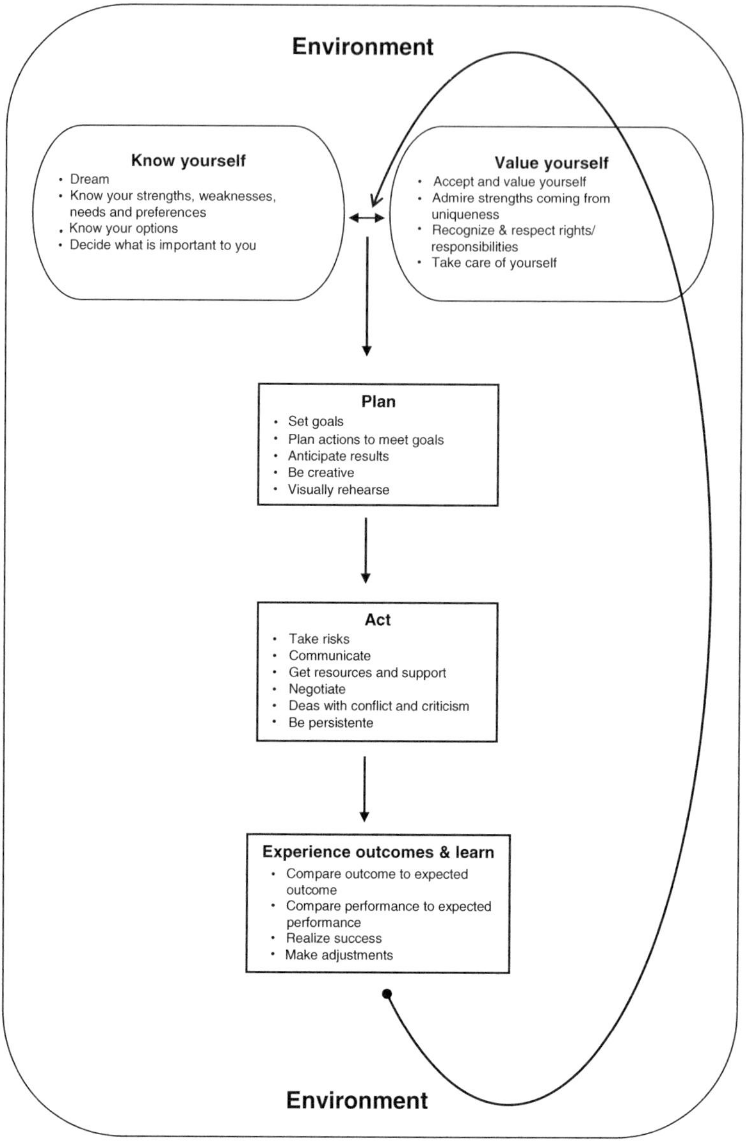

Fig. 10.1 The model of self-determination of Field and Hoffman (1995)

people with ASD due to their weak central coherence and the inference it has on their judgments. Moreover, it is not only a question of knowing oneself but also of accepting oneself in a fair manner. The confrontation with one's personal limitations can be frustrating, leading to a depressed mood and to feelings of helplessness and an even further lack of initiative. The individual must have accepted his condition and know his possibilities and limitations in order to avoid a situation in which one becomes blocked. Once self-awareness has led to self-esteem, one has to master the competencies of being able to reflect on the future and take action in consequence. One has to be capable of setting goals, define small steps in order to reach them, and grow in the process in order to be able to govern one's own life. In other words, self-determination relies on executive functions such as planning, organizing, flexibility, and coping in the sense of problem solving and the capacity to work together with others. These are altogether, by definition, weak aspects in individuals with autism.

10.3.2 The Professional as Guide

Does all this imply that the transition to a participatory society is a step backwards for individuals with ASD? Not necessarily. The principles of participating and being in charge of one's own life are greatly valuable for people with ASD too. People with long-lasting psychiatric conditions such as ASD are far less positive about their lives than the rest of the population (van Hoof and Boevink 2004). Their negative perception specifically refers to a lack of control over their own life and feeling marginalized by society. Many of them report being in need of support in various areas of their lives so as to gain control without becoming too dependent on others. They long for more self-confidence, for having more overview in their lives, and for assistance in building and maintaining social contacts and relationships. They want to accede to purposeful occupations, preferentially paid employment, as well as ways to hold on to them. However, attaining those goals is a great challenge and requires adequate guidance and help. In that sense it is important to realize that "being in charge of one's own life" does not imply by any means that one should do everything by himself. Others can prove greatly helpful providing insight into the ASD individual's own strengths and weaknesses; moreover they can help to discover what goal one really wants to reach and in that process may provide a interlocutor that helps to discover which options are realistic. The professional can become the guide that helps the person with autism and his near and dear ones to define a plan for the future and help them tease out which options are realistic. The professionals' knowledge of and experience with autism help them to build favorable conditions and mobilize the people that can help to make it possible. That does not imply that they take over from the person with ASD but rather that they help them to be in charge by helping to optimize the circumstances.

10.3.3 "Balancing on the Line of Life"

The type of advisory support that we just described above fits in with the concept of life-span guidance. This concept is described in detail in the report *Balancing on the line of life* by Verschuur et al. (2014) that provides concrete guidelines for the carers and a model for the organization of such provisions and financial bases for such guidance across the life-span. This report stems from the working group "From the

Autistic Perspective" (*Vanuit Autism Bekeken*, VAB) commissioned in 2013 by the Ministry of Health in the Netherlands for a period of 3 years to look into what needs to be done to improve the quality of life of individuals with ASD, with a special focus on their integration and participation in society. The working group was a mixed party including users and carers and professionals, all committed to the vision that individuals with autism should be allowed to develop at their own pace, with the perspective of being integrated in their own right in our society. This led to a set of guidelines and a business case (2015), i.e., an estimation of the financial and societal costs and benefits of introducing this new organization of care, including insights in the effort and means that municipalities should afford to ensure the fair inclusion of individuals with autism. The core idea in this report is that guidance and support should proactively focus on the context in which the individual with ASD lives and should foster cooperation between all the stakeholders involved (family, professionals, and organizations). The guidance and support focuses on stimulating development in different areas, to ensure a good balance, striving for further development and a new balance in consequence. Specific attention should be given to the developmental tasks linked to each developmental stage, meeting the needs of the person with ASD. In that sense "life-span guidance" does not aim at achieving a good enough "Disease management" but is far more concerned with tailoring a "life-plan" adapted to the possibilities of the individual with autism rather than worrying about the disorder and its subsequent limitations (Teunisse 2009). Life guidance is closely linked to the notion of "empowerment." Everything in the "life-span" guidance plan aims at reducing dependence on professional support by providing the individuals with tools and skills that enable them to be self-reliant in conjunction with their social network, in a relevant context with specialized support, and making use of modern ICT means of communication. The principles exposed in the VAB report are likewise applicable to the provision of life-span guidance, knowledge, and support means throughout life to the carers and families of individuals with an ASD, with the same aim of flexibly fostering as much independence as possible.

The Ten Essentials of the "Capability Approach" (http://www.iep.utm/edu/ge-capab/#H3)

1. *Life* – able to live to the end of a normal-length human life and to not have one's life reduced to not worth living.
2. *Bodily health* – able to have a good life which includes (but is not limited to) reproductive health, nourishment, and shelter.
3. *Bodily integrity* – able to change locations freely, in addition to having sovereignty over one's body which includes being secure against assault (e.g., sexual assault, child sexual abuse, domestic violence, and the opportunity for sexual satisfaction).
4. *Senses, imagination, and thought* – able to use one's senses to imagine, think, and reason in a "truly human way," informed by an adequate education. Furthermore, the ability to produce self-expressive works and engage in religious rituals without fear of political ramifications. The

ability to have pleasurable experiences and avoid unnecessary pain. Finally, the ability to seek the meaning of life.

5. *Emotions* – able to have attachments to things outside of ourselves; this includes being able to love others, grieve at the loss of loved ones, and be angry when it is justified.
6. *Practical reason* – able to form a conception of the good and critically reflect on it.
7. *Affiliation*
   A. *Able to live* with and show concern for others and empathize with (and show compassion for) others and the capability of justice and friendship. Institutions help develop and protect forms of affiliation.
   B. *Able to have self-respect* and not be humiliated by others, that is, being treated with dignity and equal worth. This entails (at the very least) protections of being discriminated on the basis of race, sex, sexuality, religion, caste, ethnicity, and nationality. In work, this means entering relationships of mutual recognition.
8. *Other species* – able to have concern for and live with other animals, plants, and the environment at large.
9. *Play* – able to laugh, play, and enjoy recreational activities.
10. *Control over one's environment*
    A. Political – able to effectively participate in the political life which includes having the right to free speech and association.
    B. Material – able to own property, not just formally but materially (that is, as a real opportunity). Furthermore, having the ability to seek employment on an equal basis as others and the freedom from unwarranted search and seizure.

10.3.4 Capability Approach

The VAB working group included a large number of high-functioning individuals with an ASD. These relatively capable individuals with ASD stressed the necessity of providing help aimed at achieving the highest possible degree of "normal" integration in society. Their aim is to live as normally as possible, and all forms of help and guidance should support them in this goal. They stress not only the importance of measurable effects of this support but also in particular the relevance, to their own personal lives, of the help given. The type of intervention that fits best to the needs of the user cannot be measured nor seen on itself but should be evaluated in the context of a specific individual's life. Care is part of somebody's life as a meaningful part of it. Yet this makes things complicated in terms of accountability to health insurance agencies or the municipalities that provide the financial means to make these forms of intervention possible. Insurance companies and municipalities will typically ask for hard figures. Outcome of treatment and guidance should be made clear by figures that show the effect size of the interventions as measured by, e.g., routine outcome monitoring (ROM), to ensure that community funds are well spent. This puts many care providers in a difficult situation. Along with fundamental questions on the limited value and validity of outcome measurement as a basis for financing care interventions, let alone supportive processes, it appears in practice very difficult to provide sound input for the ROM measures. Managing costs by these means is therefore quite uncertain, as the outcome is influenced by many factors. In the case of a lasting and chronic condition like ASD, an evidence-based approach relying on measurable outcomes often leads to disappointing conclusions, while the person himself and his carers definitively see the outcome as a positive development. From their perspective, a positive outcome is essentially a question of empowerment and self-esteem, rather than a reduction of the complaints or signs of ASD. Such an outcome means that individuals with ASD will definitively have gained more possibilities to live their lives as they would wish to. According to Nobel Prize laureate Amartya Sen (2001), this is the way we should approach the welfare of people: the enhancement of the possibilities to live one's life in dignity. The individual is free to choose if and which possibilities (in Sen's terms "capabilities") he wants to use and how he values them. Philosopher Martha Nussbaum (2011) defined ten essential capabilities in this so-called capability approach that can be used to appraise the value of support and guidance to an individual. This could open a window of opportunity to assess the core value of "life-span guidance" (enhancing the capacity for self-governance over one's life), though Sen and others question the universality of the list of capabilities because they are too closely linked to the specific circumstances for each individual (Sen 2005).

10.3.5 Redefining Health in a Positive Way

"Life-span guidance" is very much in line with recent changes in the definition of health. Whereas the old WHO definition stresses upon a total state of well-being more than the absence of diseases, the new proposed definition of health takes a positive approach in defining health "*as the ability to adapt and to self manage*" (Huber et al. 2011) in the context of the physical, emotional, and social challenges one faces during one's life (Huber et al. 2016). Here again it is not the disease that is stressed but rather the individual that is placed at the center of the stage. Emphasis is put on promoting health instead of combating disease. Thus, in line with the capability approach, Huber proposes to drop health as a goal to pursue and swap it for one's right to "make the best out of it." The concept of "positive health" encompasses indicators for success along six dimensions: physical, mental, spiritual/existential, quality of life, socio-cultural participation, and daily functioning, each of which is subdivided into different "aspects." Moreover, Huber proposes to define health as a condition that can exist despite disease (which does not necessarily mean that diseases should not be given attention).

10.3.6 Living the Life One Would Wish For

From the perspective of the "capability approach" and the "positive health" stance, the central question is how care and support for people with ASD can contribute to enhancing their capability of living the life they want. Support is needed when it appears that individuals with ASD lack the capabilities to function properly, often as a result of demands in society that they cannot meet. They drop out because they are not able to shape their lives as they would wish and become too much dependent on others. As they are experienced, these shortcomings may induce behavioral problems, depression, and anxiety. If these secondary problems are too prominent or acute, they will ask for focused treatment in the first place. However, even during these treatments, setting goals from the perspective of a meaningful and reachable life is a key issue when striving toward sustainable mental health.

10.4 Treatment- and Guidance-Aimed Assessment

Once the acute problems are under control, focus can be laid on rehabilitation toward a life perceived as "normal" for the individual in question, thus shifting attention from disease to the person. ASD has obviously to be taken into account but only as one of the many characteristics of that individual. How does ASD manifest in that individual? Where are his strengths and which factors determine vulnerability for relapse? Answers to these questions may be found in the regular psychiatric, psychological, or neuropsychological diagnostic assessment procedures and instruments, but they need to be translated in a practical and pragmatic manner into the everyday context of the person with ASD. Thus the "treatment- and guidance-aimed assessment" is a basic prerequisite for the plan that the person with ASD will elaborate, together with his "life-span" coach, to define proactively what should be done and developed in order to achieve the goals expressed.

10.4.1 The Informal and the Professional Network

The person with ASD should actively participate in composing his own roadmap for the future as a comprehensive working plan. But all relevant individuals within the informal as well as the professional network should be involved. Several methods are available to make this possible such as person-centered planning (PCP, Holburn and Vietze 2002), family group conferences (van Pagée 2003), and wraparound (Malysiak 1997). What these approaches have in common is that they include all the people and organizations/institutes asking or offering assistance in setting goals and concrete actions. In a method like PCP, it is the aspirations and needs of the person with ASD that are given primacy, well in line with the core values of the capability approach and the contemporary conceptualization of positive health. This involves not only reviewing the treatment and guidance history (to learn from experience) but also reviewing the other milestones in the individual's life course, his fears, wishes, and dreams, as well as identifying all those people who play an important role in the individual's life. This is a solid base on which goals can be formulated that will contribute to working toward a more meaningful life. The different methods determine how the goals will become reachable and who will contribute in what manner. But it is crucial that the person with ASD himself makes the plan and that it is not, explicitly or implicitly, filled in by other participants in the process. The plan must help to develop and confirm self-management by the person concerned. The overall plan should always include a contingency plan for eventual crises and relapses. Moreover the necessary prerequisites for making the plan possible should be timely addressed. Finally, the question should be addressed regarding which people or parties might still need to be included.

10.4.2 Care and Supportive Networks

Interestingly, this new approach implies that a new, individual network of care and support is created, tailored to the individual's needs. Such a network is not a professional chain cooperation where one refers to one another. Rather, the organization of care and support demands that organizations and individuals should link with each other in a smarter way, where the personal goal of self-governance and self-management should be, and remain, the leading principle. From the authorities' point of view, the question of accountability is of great importance: in other words, how can networks be organized in such a way that makes it absolutely clear who is responsible for what in this process. The commission "Treatment Responsibility in Mental Health Care" (2015) concluded that the recent developments – in which care and support become more personalized while being mostly implemented by multidisciplinary teams – have made clear that "this transition undeniably asks for a fundamental shift of the professional's role from being responsible for treatment content to being responsible for governance and coordination of the treatment process in agreement with the user" (page 38). The commission concludes that the term "governance practitioner" for this professional should be favored. This professional bears responsibility for the governance of coordinated care and support given to a patient, according to the multidisciplinary working plan. The "governance practitioner" plays the central role in the multidisciplinary team in coordination with the individual concerned. This way of organizing care should ensure the quality of the service and give governing power to one individual within the different services involved. Tailoring such cooperation arrangements is currently an intensive effort countrywide, including the elaboration of contracts and arrangements to make it possible for all users.

10.4.3 How Can e-Health Contribute: Patient Portals

Secured digital patient-portals can greatly contribute to enable and ease the functioning of these personalized networks. The personal file of the patient is included.

All professional and informal network members involved are, with explicit permission of the patient, included and can easily communicate between each other in a safe and transparent manner. The individual concerned determines which information will be shared with whom. All have access to the personal work plan, thus preventing useless duplications, interferences, and fragmentation of care and support. Some will remain passive and silent unless they are called upon when the situation requires their competences and/or participation. E-Health and other learning methods can be included, aimed at fostering self-management and independence. The "life-span coach" will help the user to benefit optimally from the digital possibilities and provide advice and guidance as to which possibilities this virtual pathway to low threshold cooperation has to offer.

10.5 A Shift of Paradigm in Care and Research

The dissemination and implementation of new concepts of care and support for individuals with ASD from the perspective of "life-span guidance and coaching" open windows of opportunity to a dignified position in its own right in the emerging "participation" society, where individuals are asked to contribute to self-management in other chronic diseases and forms of invalidity. This asks for major shifts and the necessity to integrate the now still often separate (financial) worlds of healthcare and social well-being. The effect monitoring of these new care and support models also demands for reconsideration of current accountability habits. The supportive role of multidisciplinary networks of both professionals and family/friends/neighbors/voluntary workers for the support and encouragement of vulnerable individuals will need to be cost effective and questionable. Outcome measures for isolated treatment as well as those for the efforts made by those in the network to foster the individual's capacities for independence and self-management will need to be evaluated. A scientific approach developed in the USA in recent decennia, Positive Behavior Support (PBS), may prove helpful. PBS stems from research projects in developmental disorders and has three sources of inspiration: applied behavioral analysis, the normalization/inclusion movement, and giving priority to personalized values (Carr et al. 2002). It encompasses pragmatic research in complex natural settings in the midst of the community. Thus, PBS has proved that along with causality analysis through repeated manipulation of carefully defined independent variables, there is also room for correlational analyses and naturalistic observations and case studies allowing for the application of qualitative research methods in this field. Carr et al. (2002) have elaborated PBS in nine well-defined and correlated characteristics including: (1) lifestyle changes, (2) life-span perspectives, (3) ecological validity, (4) stakeholder participation, (5) social validity, (6) systematic changes, (7) multicomponent interventions, (8) flexibility in methodological approaches, and finally (9) application of multiple theoretical frameworks.

This illustrates that there is a paradigm shift occurring not only in the approach to care and support of adults with ASD but also in the field of research into effective and meaningful treatment and guidance approaches. However, there remains a long way to go in order to achieve and implement the theoretical and philosophical principles on which these approaches are based. The first step should be to bring together individuals with ASD and their relatives with carers and scientists, a step that was achieved in the Netherlands by founding the working party "From the Autistic Perspective"(VAB) as well as two academic workshops for ASD.

References

Carr EG, Dunlap G, Horner RH et al (2002) Positive behavior support: evolution of an applied science. J Posit Behav Interv 4:4–16

Field S, Hoffman A (1995) Development of a model for self-determination. Career Dev Except Individ 17:159–169

Gezondheidsraad (2009) Autismespectrumstoornissen: Een leven lang anders. Gezondheidsraad, publicatienr, Den Haag 2009/09

Holburn E, Vietze PM (2002) Person-centered planning: research, practice and future directions. Brookes, Baltimore

Huber M, Knottnerus JA, Green L et al (2011) How should we define health? BMJ 343:d4163. doi:10.1136/bmj.d4163

Huber M, van Vliet M, Giezenberg M et al (2016) Towards a 'patient-centred' operationalisation of the new dynamic concept of health: a mixed methods study. BMJ Open 6:e010091. doi:10.1136/bmjopen-2015-010091

Lawson J (2003) Depth accessibility difficulties: an alternative conceptualization of Autism Spectrum Conditions. J Theory Soc Behav 33:189–202

Malysiak R (1997) Exploring the theory and paradigm base for wraparound. J Child Fam Stud 6(4):399–408

Newman J, Tonkens E (2011) Participation, responsibility and choice: summoning the active citizen in Western European welfare states. Amsterdam University Press, Amsterdam

Nussbaum MC (2011) Creating capabilities: the human development approach. Belknap Press of Harvard University Press, Cambridge

Sen A (2001) Development as freedom, 2 edn. Oxford University Press, Oxford

Sen A (2005) Human rights and capabilities. J Hum Dev 6(2):151–166

Teunisse JP (2009). Weerbaar bij veranderingen: naar een levensloopbenadering voor mensen met autisme. Intreerede van het lectoraat 'Levensloopbegeleiding bij autisme'. Arnhem, Han University Press

van Hoof F, Boevink W (2004) Meedoen: maatschappelijke ondersteuning van mensen met psychische handicaps. Trimbosinstituut, Utrecht

van Pagée R (2003) Eigen Kracht (Family Group Conference in Nederland): van model naar invoering. SWP, Amsterdam

Verschuur A, Noback A, Thissen A, Post M, Teunisse JP (2014) Balanceren op de levenslijn: Een werkdefinitie van levensloopbegeleiding voor mensen met autisme en hun naasten. Werkgroep Vanuit Autisme Bekeken, Utrecht

Suggested Reading

Commissie Hoofdbehandelaarschap GGZ (2015). Hoofdbehandelaarschap GGZ als noodgreep. Ministerie van Volksgezondheid, Welzijn en Sport, Den Haag

Werkgroep Vanuit Autisme Bekeken (2015) Maatschappelijke businesscase: Levensbrede aanpak bij autisme. Werkgroep Vanuit Autisme Bekeken, Utrecht

Sense and Sensibility: Forensic Issues with Autism Spectrum Disorders

11

David Murphy

11.1 Introduction

Whilst it is widely accepted that the majority of individuals with an autism spectrum disorder (ASD) lead law-abiding and productive lives, individual experiences can vary enormously. In some circumstances, poor outcomes might result in individuals with an ASD finding themselves in contact with the psychiatric and nonpsychiatric services of the criminal justice system (CJS). For individuals with an ASD, although contact with the CJS is more likely to be as a victim or witness of crime, some may have contact as a result of being a perpetrator of some form of offending behaviour. However, it is also possible that the same individual may fall into all of these categories. Whatever the circumstances, once within the CJS, such individuals are typically recognised to present with difficulties and needs that challenge mainstream services.

An examination of the contemporary literature suggests that interest in individuals with an ASD who offend and who become involved with forensic services has increased significantly over recent years. Indeed, there is now a substantial and growing body of research papers, case reports and books devoted to the topic. Attempting to review the entirety of these publications within a single book chapter would be overwhelming, as well as could lead to a rather confused understanding of this diverse and complex group of individuals. Many of the reviews that have been attempted could also be argued to be limited by being very select in their inclusion of studies and make similar observations. Although still biased in interpretation, the aim of this chapter will be to explore the topics that have created the most debate in

D. Murphy
Broadmoor High Secure Psychiatric Hospital, Crowthorne, Berkshire RG45 7EG, UK

Autism Diagnostic Research Centre (ADRC), Unity 12, 9 -19 Rose Road, Southampton SO14 6TE, UK
e-mail: david.murphy@wlmht.nhs.uk

B. Barahona Corrêa, R.-J. van der Gaag (eds.), *Autism Spectrum Disorders in Adults*, DOI 10.1007/978-3-319-42713-3_11

the literature and are most clinically relevant. In addition, some important gaps in our current knowledge will be highlighted, along with suggestions for further research. It is also important to state that although the chapter reflects the English CJS, much of the research cited is international, and the topics discussed are applicable to a wide range of countries and cultures. In addition, the use of the term individuals with an ASD will be used to refer to a broad group of adults such as those with Asperger's syndrome and high-functioning autism. Where there may also be issues linked to intellectual disability, this will be highlighted.

11.2 Media Portrayal of Offenders with ASD

An important place to start any discussion of forensic issues with ASD is how individuals who offend are presented within the media. An examination of the available literature reveals that this has been a neglected topic of research. Certainly most of us do not need to think very hard to recall individuals with an ASD who have been accused of offending and who have attracted a great deal of media attention. For example, within the UK, a high-profile case which generated a great deal of interest was that of Gary McKinnon, who in 2002 was charged with computer-related crimes after hacking into the US military and NASA computer systems, apparently in an attempt to look for evidence of UFOs. Another high-profile case within the UK is that of Nicky Reilly who in 2009 was given a life sentence after being convicted of a failed suicide bomb attempt to blow up a busy restaurant within the context of anti-Western beliefs and wishes to become a martyr. Within the USA, examples of individuals thought to have an ASD and who carried out mass shootings have also been reported, such as Adam Lanza who killed 20 children and 6 adults at Sandy Hook Elementary School in 2012. Other cases such as the worldwide coverage of the Norwegian mass murderer Anders Behring Breivik who was convicted in 2011 of the murder of 77 people are also reported by some to involve ASD.

The influence of the media in shaping our views of ASD and offending should not be understated. However, despite some evidence to suggest that the media is important in influencing public attitudes about disability or mental health conditions (e.g. Lyons 2000) and that the media can be more powerful in shaping beliefs than actual experience (e.g. Philo 1997), there has been very little formal examination of how individuals with an ASD who offend are portrayed in the media. There is a general consensus among clinicians that the media's portrayal of individuals with an ASD who offend can be distorted and leads to public stigma, stereotyping and misunderstanding, as well as the view that such individuals are prone to certain types of offending. Some formal evidence to support this comes from Huw and Jones (2010) in their study of how individuals with autism were portrayed in UK newspapers between 1999 and 2008. Three categories were identified including 'the burden of autism', 'sensationalising' and 'misconceptions and misuse of a label'. The authors also suggest that autism was typically portrayed in a rather standardised and homogenised way that failed to recognise the diversity of the spectrum.

From a CJS point of view, there is recognition that the media's portrayal of individuals with an ASD who offend can have the potential to influence the attitudes, views and decision-making of those working within the legal profession, as well as members of the jury. For example, an interesting study by Berryessa (2014a) describes telephone interviews with 21 California Superior Court judges asking their views of how the media portrays ASD and criminality. The majority of judges asked expressed the view that whilst the general media reports of ASD could be both positive and negative, they felt that the coverage of ASD and criminality was often misleading and created false associations between ASD and violent behaviour.

In summary, whilst individuals with an ASD who commit unusual and particularly violent offences appear to attract rather sensationalist and distorted media attention, it is unclear whether this is always negative. It can be seen from cases such as Gary McKinnon's that whilst some stereotypes are reinforced, considerable public sympathy was also generated and this may have had a significant influence on the dropping of his extradition from the UK to the USA 10 years after being charged. Even the case of Nicky Reilly was reported sympathetically as someone vulnerable and who was taken advantage of. Impressions suggest the portrayal of offenders with an ASD in the media, like most vulnerable groups, is a complex and often contradictory one.

11.3 How Many Individuals with an ASD Offend and What Is the Prevalence of ASD Within Forensic Services?

To date, attempting to obtain an estimate of how many individuals with an ASD engage in law-breaking behaviours and are subsequently involved in the CJS has proved to be a difficult task. Those studies that have been completed also vary significantly in their methodology, from relying on self-report to examining formal conviction records and screening for those detained in various forensic establishments. Most studies have also tended to examine individuals already convicted and detained. Indeed, virtually nothing is known about individuals with an ASD who offend but who do not come into contact with the CJS or who get diverted into the healthcare system. For example, there may be a reluctance by carers to report vulnerable individuals to the CJS, especially so if they have a co-morbid learning disability. Supporting Wing's (1997) comment that the great majority of individuals with an ASD are law abiding and often display a 'literal, pedantic adherence to the letter of the law', Ghaziuddin et al. (1991), examining papers published between 1944 and 1990, found that within 132 published case studies of people with Asperger's syndrome, only three described a history of violence. I suspect, however, that a more contemporary review would result in a higher figure.

In terms of any link between ASD and criminal behaviours, Hans Asperger's original observations also provide some interesting observations, with some children with the disorder being said to display 'mischievous and malicious acts'

(Asperger 1944, translated by Frith 1991). Subsequent analysis, however, of 177 of his former patients using information from the Austrian Penal Register found that they did not differ in the percentage of recorded convictions compared with the general male population (1.30 % compared to 1.25 %, respectively). Specifically, eight individuals were identified who between them had 33 convictions that resulted in 23 custodial sentences (Hipper et al. 2009).

Within the UK, one study that attempted to comment on the rate of offending among a community sample of individuals with an ASD is described by Woodbury Smith et al. (2006). Of the 102 individuals with an ASD initially asked, only half agreed to participate, and a further 20 individuals had to be excluded as they were not considered to meet sufficient ASD diagnostic criteria. A final 25 individuals were asked to complete a self-report offending questionnaire that rated 52 behaviours that could subsequently lead to arrest, prosecution or conviction (including some non-violent offences such as breaking into gas or electricity meters, making obscene telephone calls or taking illicit substances). The UK's home office offender index was also examined to look for any formal convictions among the individuals. In comparison to a matched control group who worked for a local company, 12 individuals with an ASD reported engaging in some form of illegal behaviour compared to 16 of the control group. In addition, an examination of the home office offender index revealed that two individuals with an ASD were listed, compared to none in the control group. Whilst the sample size and some methodological issues (such as not identifying individuals diverted into the forensic mental health system) make it difficult to interpret the findings clearly, nevertheless the results suggest that individuals with an ASD are not more likely to offend compared to the general population. In another UK study, Allen et al. (2008) examined the number of adults with an ASD across 98 different services in South Wales (with a general population of around 1.2 million). From these services, 126 individuals with Asperger's syndrome were identified, 33 of whom had offended or whose behaviour could have resulted in contact with the CJS. Among these, seven were reported as not having been processed/arrested, five had been imprisoned, one had been hospitalised, and three were living in the community. Although the authors recognise some methodological limitations of the study, such as failing to include some prisons and some individuals also having a learning disability, the results were interpreted as suggesting a low incidence of offending within the sample.

Perhaps because of the relative stability of the patient population, high-security psychiatric care within the UK has been the focus of early prevalence estimates. For example, Scragg and Shah's (1994) examination of one high-secure psychiatric hospital found after an initial screen of patient files to identify possible cases followed by interviews with primary nurses and obtaining patients consent that from 17 individuals identified (from a total 392 male patients), 6 met the diagnostic criteria for Asperger's syndrome (representing a prevalence rate of 1.5 %). An additional three possible cases were identified raising the prevalence rate to 2.3 %. The conclusion from this study was that Asperger's syndrome was over-represented compared to the general population prevalence rate. A significant limitation of this study, however, was that the diagnostic process was not based on contemporary best practice. It is also important to highlight that not only the admission criteria to high-security psychiatric care have changed over the 20 years since the study was completed but also that the current total patient population in high-security psychiatric units is approximately two thirds of that examined by Scragg and Shah. Similar points can also be put against another prevalence study of ASD in all three of England's high-security psychiatric hospitals (Broadmoor, Rampton and Ashworth) completed by Hare, Gould, Mills and Wing (1999). Within this study, a total of 31 individuals with an ASD were identified (1.6 % of total patient population). In contrast, Myers (2004), examining a number of forensic and specialist settings in Scotland, found the prevalence of ASD to be quite low (around 0.93 % in prisons, 0.46 % in secure units and 1.39 % in mental health units). However, Myers also noted that many prison staff raised concerns that the number of individuals formally identified probably fell short of the actual number.

International studies of offending in ASD appear broadly consistent with UK estimates. For example, within Sweden, Siponmaa et al. (2001) retrospectively examined the psychiatric assessments of 126 young offenders aged between 15 and 22 years old who were referred for psychiatric assessment after committing a serious offence. Based on examining case files, it was found that 15 % of the sample could be classified with an ASD and a further 12 % with probable ASD. Within Japan, Kugmagami and Matsuura (2009) examined the occurrence of ASD in four family courts. In one court that dealt with 'unusual' offences, 18.2 % cases of ASD were found among the 93 cases examined. Within three other courts, 3.3 % of 335 cases were said to have ASD. Mourisden et al. (2008) in another case record study within Denmark of 313 individuals compared to 933 matched controls found that among those who had received a diagnosis of childhood autism, 0.9 % had received a conviction in adulthood and that those with a diagnosis of atypical autism and Asperger's syndrome had 8.1 % and 18.4 % conviction rates, respectively.

Supporting the conclusions of some review papers (e.g. King and Murphy 2014), there appears to be no robust evidence to suggest that individuals with an ASD engage in more law-breaking behaviours than individuals without an ASD. Whilst some studies suggest an over-representation of individuals with an ASD in some forensic environments, notably high-security psychiatric hospitals, various methodological issues including obtaining a reliable diagnosis and completing research with shifting forensic populations, as well as ethical issues such as obtaining consent, limit the interpretation of these studies and make future accurate studies a challenge. To date, there is no information on the socio-economic status or ethnicity of offenders with an ASD. It is also significant that most of the studies to date have exclusively examined men.

11.4 What Do We Know About Women with an ASD Who Offend?

There is a growing recognition that girls and women with an ASD who offend and are involved with the CJS have been a neglected group. A frequently ignored but interesting series of studies examining the possible prevalence of offending among women with an ASD is by Sula Wolff and colleagues. Writing before Lorna Wing's seminal paper on Asperger's syndrome in 1981, Wolff and Chick (1980) examined the adult offending outcome of a group of 32 girls initially diagnosed with a schizoid personality disorder but who were subsequently thought highly likely to have had Asperger's syndrome. At 27 years old, it was found that, as a group, they reported a similar level of delinquent behaviour and excessive drinking compared to a group of men who were also diagnosed with schizoid personality disorder in childhood. In a further examination of the Scottish criminal records office for recorded offences of these 32 girls, it was found that 34.5 % of the sample had recorded convictions compared with 15.5 % of controls. The mean number of offences committed was also said to be 4.9 and 1.6, respectively. Approximately one third of these women had also received custodial sentences compared to none of the controls. It was concluded that compared to the 5 % recorded convictions for the general population, women with a childhood diagnosis of schizoid personality disorder had exceptionally high rates of criminality (Wolff and Chick 1980; Wolff and McGuire 1995; Wolff 1995).

Another study of the prevalence of ASD in women patients in an English high-security psychiatric hospital was by Crocombe et al. (2006). In this study that might now be considered redundant because there are no longer any women detained in this particular hospital, it was found that of the 51 women patients screened, 6 were considered to have a definite ASD and a further 5 a possible ASD. Examining the offence details of the patients, it was also found that three had offences linked to arson, one to violence and one to threats to kill/hostage-taking. One patient had no formal conviction and had been transferred to high-secure psychiatric care due to management difficulties in her previous care environment. Four of the women with an ASD had been diagnosed with schizophrenia and two with personality disorder. In another study examining the offending rates among a large group of individuals with an ASD in Denmark, Mourisden et al. (2008) found, after examining the Register of Criminality, that whilst gender appeared to be related to criminal activity in a control group of individuals without an ASD, this was not the case in the ASD group. Indeed, women with an ASD displayed similar rates of offending compared to men with an ASD. Males in the control group, however, were found to have significantly higher rates of convictions than females. Clearly much remains to be examined with regard to how many women with an ASD offend and may become involved with forensic services, as well as how we might best address any specific needs. It seems likely that some of the uncertainty with these questions may also be linked to the broader issue of obtaining an accurate ASD diagnosis in girls and women (e.g. Dworzynsky et al. 2012; Gould and Ashton-Smith 2011).

11.5 Types of Offences Committed by Offenders with an ASD

Another aspect of exploring any forensic dimension to ASD is whether individuals with an ASD are anymore prone to commit specific types of offences. Although some case descriptions suggest a 'robust association between ASD and violent behaviour' (e.g. Mawson et al. 1985), much seems to depend on the group of individuals being asked. For example, examining Asperger's original cohort, Hippler et al. (2010) found that among the 33 convictions for eight individuals identified, the most common offences were property related. Only three cases of bodily injury, one case of robbery and one case of violent and threatening behaviour were found. This contrasts with the findings of Tantum (2012), who described a study of 1100 individuals who had attended his ASD clinic and found that 53 % of them reported that they had been interviewed by the police concerning violence against a person (not all of which led to a prosecution) and that 12 % had been interviewed by the police concerning a sexual offence (again, not all of which led to a prosecution). Property offences were found to be less common. Although Tantum's findings suggest relatively high rates of problem behaviours, it is unclear why individuals attended the clinic, and it is possible that the findings reflect the characteristics of a special group of individuals with an ASD who required help due to some form of specific difficulty.

Within high-security psychiatric care, it has been found that whilst patients with an ASD had offences ranging from fire setting, wounding with intent (linked to a perceived 'rejection' by another person), unlawful killing, threats to kill and violence in general, they tended to have lower violence ratings for their index offences compared to patients with schizophrenia and a personality disorder (i.e. less likely to have offences leading to their admission to secure care linked to grievous bodily harm or homicide). In addition, as a group, individuals with an ASD were less likely to have a history of alcohol and illicit substance misuse (Murphy 2003). In a Swedish study comparing male offenders referred for a psychiatric assessment with a diagnosis of ASD or anti-social personality disorder, Wahlund and Kristiansson (2006) also found that those with an ASD were less likely to have been intoxicated at the time of their offence and less likely to have used a weapon compared to those with an anti-social personality disorder.

Across England's three high-secure hospitals, whilst homicide offences among ASD patients have been found to occur at a rate consistent with the base rate for other patients, sexual offences were underrepresented (Hare et al.1999). Where sexual offences are reported in numerous case examples (e.g. Chesterman and Rutter 1993; Murrie et al. 2002; Kugmagami and Matsuura 2009), motivations are typically unusual including with co-morbid paraphilia (e.g. Kohn et al 1998, Cooper et al. 1993; Milton et al. 2002). Some studies have found arson to be over-represented among offenders with an ASD (e.g. Hare et al. 1999; Siponmaa et al. 2001).

A UK community study of self-reported offending in ASD found that whilst drug offences were unlikely, criminal damage was high relative to a control group. There were no significant differences in reported offences relating to theft or violence (Woodbury Smith et al. 2006). Within Allen et al. (2008) study, among the 16 individuals who consented to be interviewed, 13 had histories of violent conduct, 12 histories of threatening behaviour, 8 property destruction, 4 drug offences, 4 theft, 3 sexual offending, 1 fraud, 1 motoring offences and 1 murder.

Several individuals seen by the author have used the Internet to offend, whether by downloading underage indecent material, harassment or pursuing a deviant interest/preoccupation (Murphy 2011). Such offences appear to be increasing, and more research is required into the prevalence and specific vulnerabilities of individuals with an ASD to use computer technology to offend. Some individuals seen by the author have also been convicted of terrorism-related offences and joint enterprise (where an individual may be found guilty for another person's crime if they are present and knowingly assist or encourage the crime and agree to act together with the primary offender for a common purpose). To date, both these offence categories have also been under-researched in this population. Further research is also required in the possible link between ASD and some rare but extreme acts of violence. For example, in a study widely cited in the media, Allely et al. (2014) in a review of the academic literature, legal and journalistic sources examined the presence of ASD and head injuries among individuals linked to serial killings or mass murders. From 239 cases of extreme violence identified, 106 were said to have evidence of an ASD and/or a head injury. Fifty-eight of these were mass murderers, and 48 were serial killers (who had killed three or more individuals).

In summary, current evidence does not support the view that individuals with an ASD are prone to commit certain types of offences. However, for some individuals, there can be a complex interaction between environmental circumstances and individual difficulties that make some offence types more likely. Indeed, a few authors, such as Berney (2004), suggest that offences including obsessive harassment/stalking, inexplicable violence, computer crime and offences arising from misjudged social relationships among individuals should raise questions about the possibility of an ASD diagnosis among perpetrators. Whilst large-scale studies of offenders with an ASD might offer some information on any trends of offence types, results will only reflect breaches in local laws or jurisdictions and not an individual's specific vulnerabilities towards specific problem behaviours. Of greater clinical significance is understanding the reasons why an individual has engaged in a specific behaviour and developing a formulation of the underlying precipitating and vulnerability factors.

11.6 What Difficulties Associated with Having an ASD Might Be Related to Offending?

Whilst there are individuals with an ASD whose offending may be unrelated to their ASD, for many the associated difficulties appear to play a central role. For example, Wing (1981) proposed that low levels of empathy (notably perspective taking difficulties) may make some individuals with an ASD vulnerable to offending. Howlin (1997) suggested that there are four possible factors associated with having an ASD that make individuals particularly vulnerable towards offending. These include increased social naivety, the need for routines or over-rigid adherence to rules, a lack of understanding with social situations (including poor negotiating skills) and pursuing an obsessional interest, exacerbated by a failure to appreciate the implications of behaviour.

Clinical experience and a growing body of case descriptions (e.g. Murrie et al. 2002; Haskins and Silva 2006) and literature reviews (e.g. Gómez de la Cuesta

2010; Lerner et al. 2012) all highlight a number of key features associated with having an ASD that appear to increase an individual's vulnerability towards some offending behaviours. Of those difficulties associated with having an ASD considered particularly influential are the cognitive difficulties such as with theory of mind (including empathy and perspective taking – notably with appreciating rather than necessarily recognising the views of others resulting in an egocentric view of the world), central cohesion (difficulties with appreciating the whole context of a situation rather than often irrelevant details) and in different dimensions of executive functioning (such as with planning and organisation, cognitive rigidity, appreciating the consequences of one's actions as well as generalising learning from one situation to another) Woodbury (2005). Cognitive dysfunction combined with social naivety may be problematic for some individuals vulnerable to exploitation by others (perhaps because of a failure to recognise when one is being used and failing to think through the potential consequences for oneself and others), as might be a failure to deal with sensory hypersensitivity. Difficulties with recognising and appreciating the perspectives of other individuals can also lead to 'malicious' behaviour perhaps in order to generate a reaction in others strong enough to register. Harassment and stalking behaviour may be linked with social naivety, combined with limited empathy and a poor awareness of social norms in developing relationships. Sexual frustration and inappropriate outlets, combined with poor empathy and interpersonal naivety may also be problematic for some cases. For others, cognitive dysfunction within the context of pursuing a preoccupation or deviant interest may lead to problems (e.g. Barry-Walsh and Mullen 2004). However, whilst the relative intensity and nature of a preoccupation are important, it may be the function of a preoccupation that is crucial (e.g. Woodbury Smith et al. 2010), i.e. whether the preoccupation or interest is a prosocial means to meeting other individuals or serves to gratify a deviant personal need. In a comparison of non-forensic and a high-secure psychiatric care sample of individuals with an ASD, it was found that the latter group tended to pursue more solitary and deviant interests than the former whose interests were more social (Mundy and Murphy 2003). Other individuals with offending linked to preoccupations (notably a preoccupation with another person) may also have repressed anger expression difficulties (Murphy 2014). In extreme situations, a lack of internal central cohesion and presence of 'compartmentalising' characteristics may lead to the development of inner preoccupations and maladaptive fantasies (e.g. Silva et al. 2004).

A less explored but important area of potential offending in ASD is an individual's vulnerability towards developing dysfunctional and restricted coping strategies for dealing with feelings of resentment and which in turn may lead to the belief that there was no alternative way of behaving. In terms of interpersonal violence, some individuals with an ASD can experience a profound alienation from other adults and develop maladaptive coping strategies such as fantasies for dealing with emotional regulation difficulties and interpersonal anxiety. Many individuals may also experience intense feelings of being wronged in some way and become hypersensitive to perceived incidents of personal criticism, perhaps leading to rumination, feelings of revenge or a wish to 'prove a point' (e.g. Murphy 2010).

In summary, whilst many of the cognitive, communication, sensory and emotional regulation difficulties associated with ASD can all potentially have an influence on an individual's offending behaviour, it is typically a combination of these, within the context of their immediate environment and other people, that determine actions. Understanding these difficulties informs any intervention and risk reduction programme. However, as Bjørkly (2009) notes, whilst individuals with Asperger's syndrome who commit violent offences appear to be influenced by factors specific to the disorder, supporting evidence is based on limited data. Some caution is therefore required before describing any characteristics that may distinguish the violence of individuals with Asperger's syndrome from other diagnostic groups.

11.7 Role of Psychiatric Co-morbidity

Several studies and reviews highlight psychiatric co-morbidity as a risk factor for violence among individuals with an ASD. For example, Newman and Ghaziuddin (2008) in a review of 37 cases of violent offending and Asperger's syndrome found psychiatric co-morbidity to be present among most. However, it is significant to highlight the range of psychiatric co-morbidity found, including depression, obsessional neurosis, schizoaffective disorder and paraphilia. Other studies suggest that co-morbid psychosis and illicit substance misuse may be particularly problematic for increasing the vulnerability of an individual with an ASD towards interpersonal violence (e.g. Palermo 2004; Långstrom et al. 2009). In Allen et al.'s (2008) community study of offenders with Asperger's syndrome, schizophrenia, depression, anxiety, attention deficit disorder and personality disorder were all said to have been present for a significant number.

Whilst psychiatric co-morbidity appears to be present among many individuals with an ASD who offend, it is sometimes unclear whether this predates any offending and, if so, how it directly influences offending behaviour. If psychiatric co-morbidity is present, it is unlikely to operate without the additional influence of the cognitive, communication, sensory and emotional regulation difficulties. It is possible that for some individuals, the presence of a psychiatric disorder such as psychosis may further compromise cognitive capacity. For example, for individuals with a psychosis without an ASD, poor performance in a social perceptual theory of mind task (the revised eye test) assessed during the admission to high-secure psychiatric care was associated with higher risk and needs ratings 3 years later (Murphy 2007a).

Included as a risk factor within many formal risk for offending assessment tools is psychopathy. Generally accepted to describe a collection of personality features and behaviour characterised by callousness, lack of remorse and irresponsibility, research consistently finds a strong association between the presence of psychopathic characteristics among individuals and an increased likelihood of future violence (e.g. Hare 1999). Although some authors have highlighted the similarities between some features of ASD and some features of psychopathy (e.g. Fitzgerald 2003), the available research does not suggest that individuals with an ASD are more likely to be rated with psychopathy as measured using the Hare Psychopathy

Checklist-Revised (PCL-R) (Hare 2003) (the accepted gold standard method of assessing psychopathy). Indeed, within high-secure psychiatric care, patients with an ASD (and therefore perhaps by definition high-risk individuals) were found to have lower PCL-R scores than other patient groups and that those PCL-R items that were present tended to be characterised by affective features including a lack of remorse or guilt, shallow affect, callousness/lack of empathy and a failure to accept responsibility for own actions (Murphy 2007b). Of clinical interest was the observation that only one individual with an ASD out of a sample of 20 was rated with a PCL-R score indicative of some psychopathic features, and this individual fell in a low violence history group. However, those individuals with an ASD rated with high violence histories had significantly higher social deviance and anti-social behaviour scores than the low violence history group. For all individuals, high PCL-R scores were associated with affective features such as displaying a lack of remorse and a failure to accept responsibility for actions. Of less importance appeared to be the interpersonal, lifestyle or anti-social features of psychopathy.

The independence of ASD and psychopathy has also been found among adolescent boys but with the idea of a 'double hit' for those who displayed an impairment of empathic responses to distress cues (e.g. Rogers et al. 2006). In a review of the violence characteristics of individuals with Asperger's syndrome who offend and those with psychopathy, Bjørkly (2009) highlighted some differences between these groups. Unlike those rated with psychopathy, those with Asperger's syndrome were rated as being more likely to present as naïve rather than manipulative, reactive rather than proactive in their behaviour and more likely to confess than deny their actions. Although the examination of psychopathy may be an important factor to include in any violence risk assessment of individuals with an ASD, the most sensible approach for the assessment would be to follow Hare's (2003) recommendation to 'exercise clinical judgement with the interpretation of psychopathic traits among individuals with unusual presentations'.

11.8 What Is the Experience of Individuals with an ASD Within Forensic Services?

A review by Robertson and McGillivray (2015) has highlighted that there has been limited research into this topic, with only three studies that have examined the prison experiences of individuals. Myers's (2004) examination of staff perceptions and experiences of individuals with an ASD within a range of forensic and non-forensic units in Scotland suggested that many individuals with a learning disability and/or ASD were 'multiply disadvantaged' in the context of prisons. Specifically, individuals with these conditions were considered at risk of being exploited, bullied and ostracised by other prisoners. Staff were also said to express the view that prisons were poorly equipped to meet the needs of individuals with an ASD.

Patterson's (2007) detailed description of two men with an ASD within prison environments suggested that whilst the offending, background circumstances, presenting difficulties associated with their ASD and relative co-morbid diagnosis differed, both were observed to have significant difficulties with prison life that could be attributed to the socio-communicative deficits and rigidity associated with having an ASD. Other authors, however, such as Allen et al. (2008) suggested following interviews with individuals with an ASD that they appear no more disadvantaged than individuals without an ASD within prisons and may benefit from the structured and routine nature of such environments, as well as the minimal social interference.

From their review, Robertson and McGillivray suggested four categories of difficulties that might be experienced by individuals with an ASD in prison environments. These included vulnerability to interpersonal difficulties, increased rates of isolation and seclusion, limited opportunity to engage in rehabilitation programmes and difficulties coping with the transition back to the community. Whilst all these difficulties may well be experienced by individuals with an ASD, personal experience suggests that the experiences of individuals with an ASD within the CJS can be varied. For example, a study of individuals with an ASD in one high secure psychiatric hospital (Murphy & Mullens, (n.d) accepted) suggested that whilst the group is small in number ($n = 7$), there was a diverse range of backgrounds; offending behaviours; experiences, as well as relative vulnerabilities; and objective measures of functioning (such as participation in occupational and therapeutic activities, number of problem incidents, periods in seclusion and views from staff). Although some individuals certainly expressed negative views and experiences of their care, as well as feeling that their difficulties were not understood by others, these were very much in the minority. Indeed, whilst most individuals described having negative experiences in custodial environments such as prisons, they were more positive about the forensic psychiatric system and valued the structure, predictability and routine of a hospital environment, as well as highly trained and sympathetic staff. Many individuals also described benefitting from the therapies they had participated in, as well as being actively involved in a range of occupational and educational activities. Most individuals also confirmed that their ASD had not been diagnosed until admission to high secure psychiatric care. Of interest were the views of two patients transferred from specialist ASD medium secure care and who both reported negative views of their care there and experiences with other ASD patients. Although it is not possible to generalise from these individuals, they do highlight the possibility that even within specialist ASD units, there can be negative experiences. Although the reasons for such different experiences need to be explored, impressions suggest some of those who do report negative experiences present with complex psychopathology including co-morbid mental illness and personality disorder. This in turn may have implications on how staff view and manage such individuals, as well as an individual's relative insight and presence of any other factors that may influence experiences such as paranoid ideation. Some objective measures of experience such as participation in activities, as well as any time spent in seclusion, appear unrelated to the views held.

Supporting the view of Robertson and McGillivray, whilst there is a need for more research in this area, there is also a need to recognise the varied backgrounds, the individual profiles of strengths and weaknesses and the presence of possible co-morbid conditions. It also remains to be established whether individuals with an ASD who become involved with forensic services have significantly different experiences compared to other vulnerable individuals such as those with a mental illness. With recent estimates suggesting that within the English prison system approximately 25 % of women and 15 % of men may have symptoms of a psychosis, 26 % of women and 16 % of men received mental health treatment before custody, and 46 % of women and 21 % of men have attempted suicide (Prison Reform Trust 2006), this is clearly an important area of research.

11.9 Criminal Responsibility, Litigation and Culpability

It has been suggested that the difficulties associated with having an ASD have the potential to impact on almost every aspect of the criminal justice process from interviews with the police, to the accused person's fitness to stand trial, a variety of defences to which an individual may be entitled, especially self-defence, mental impairment/insanity, provocation and diminished responsibility, as well as the sentencing process (Freckleton 2011). Of particular significance are the cognitive characteristics associated with having an ASD that may have a profound effect on an individual's decision-making, their capacity to retain or prioritise information as well as their memory for key information. An individual's communication, sensory and emotional regulation difficulties may also have implications on how they might present to the police during their initial contact (Debbaudt 2002) and subsequent interviews, as well as the impression they might give to a judge and jury.

A topic that has attracted some interest is whether individuals with an ASD are more vulnerable to suggestibility during interview (i.e. tendency towards being influenced by leading questions and ability to cope with 'interrogative' pressure). Studies to date, however, examining suggestibility within ASD have been limited to non-forensic and nonpsychiatric experimental samples who volunteered for research and who were paid for their time rather than clinical cases. Where adults with an ASD have been examined, no specific vulnerability towards being suggestible has been found in comparison to matched non-ASD controls (e.g. North et al. 2008 and Maras and Bowler 2012). However, North et al. (2008) found that individuals with an ASD were rated to be significantly more compliant than controls in terms of parental and self-report, as well as having higher scores in measures of depression, anxiety, fears of negative social evaluation and paranoia. Further comments were also made about individuals with an ASD appearing to be more reliant on questioning to facilitate recall, with some eagerness to please and/or avoid confrontation, as well as being more compliant to requests and demands.

The author's experience with victims of crime and offenders with an ASD is that whilst useful to assess (particularly where there may also be an intellectual disability), in line with the research findings, most individuals do not appear to have any specific vulnerability towards being suggestible to leading questions during interview. Indeed, many individuals are typically very specific about what was said to them and will clearly state if something was not said or if there was no information on which to make a decision or judgement. However, an area of potential cognitive dysfunction that may have some implication on interviewing individuals with an ASD and the reliability of the testimony is with autobiographical and episodic memory, i.e. the recall of personally experienced events and when these may have happened relative to other events or experiences (e.g. Maras and Bowler 2014). Such memory difficulties may have implications on how individuals with an ASD are formally interviewed or questioned regarding past events (e.g. Maras and Bowler 2010). To date, however, much of the research has been conducted with children and with 'experimental' non-forensic volunteers. There remain questions as to whether forensic cases display similar difficulties and whether additional co-morbid psychiatric diagnoses might complicate the assessment even more. There is also no research to date on assessing 'symptom validity' in any apparent memory dysfunction in ASD, i.e. where an individual might be deliberately exaggerating a memory problem in order for some perceived gain. Certainly clinical experience suggests individuals can vary enormously with regard to the reliability of their memory and that some caution is required as with all forensic assessments.

11.10 How Are Services Dealing with Individuals with an ASD Who Offend?

Many police forces within the UK provide autism awareness training, and qualitative reports suggest this has a positive impact on how police officers respond to individuals with an ASD. In addition, the National Autistic Society (NAS) within the UK has developed some guidelines for professionals working in the CJS on how best to respond to individuals with an ASD (National Autistic Society 2005), as has Debbaudt on his website (www.autismriskmanagement.com). The NAS also provides an autism alert card that individuals can wear and which can inform the police to their difficulties and who to contact in an emergency. Some specialist lawyers are also available to represent individuals with an ASD, and some encouraging research from the USA found that many judges considered that being aware of the potential implications that having an ASD might have for an individual offender may subsequently influence their sentencing recommendations (Berryessa 2014b).

Although it is difficult to assess the precise effect on service development, increased professional awareness of ASD over recent years seems to have been significantly influenced by the Adult Autism Strategy (2010) within England as directed by the Autism Act (2009). This initiative has placed ASD on the agenda of most government-run institutions and established a duty to provide appropriate ASD diagnostic assessments and staff training. Personal experience of the English prison system, however, suggests that whilst there has been an increased awareness by many staff groups including some prisons obtaining accreditation by the National Autistic Society (e.g. Lewis et al. 2013) of the specific difficulties and issues individuals with ASD can present with, there remains uncertainty with regard to how best address them. Within high-secure psychiatric care, it has been found that most staff who have direct patient contact recognised that patients with an ASD have difficulties and needs different from other patient groups. Of significance, however, most staff also felt they did not have adequate skills to work with ASD and would like to receive more training. Indeed, most staff expressed the view that such training should be mandatory (Murphy and McMorrow 2015). In addition to this general autism awareness training provided to staff, bespoke ward-based training has also made some positive impact on everyday management where particular emphasis is placed on the so-called NAS SPELL approach (i.e. placing emphasis on structure, a positive approach, empathy, low arousal and links with other professionals) that aims to reduce the likelihood of environmental triggers to problem behaviours. It might therefore be argued that for some individuals, the structure, routine and predictability of a prison environment or secure psychiatric care could suit them very well in the short term. However, this needs to be balanced against the negative consequences, such as sensory overload, further social exclusion and offending management programmes that may not be sensitive to the difficulties associated with ASD (Higgs and Carter 2015). It remains uncertain, though, whether it is less therapeutically useful or indeed potentially harmful to include individuals with an ASD in mainstream groups that address offending behaviours or whether to have ASD-only groups. Outside of specialist ASD medium- and low-security units, however, such ASD-only offending groups are unlikely to be possible. There may also be some argument for the view that all individuals, including those with an ASD, may benefit from participating in mixed groups by hearing different points of view and listening to other individuals' experiences. The qualitative reports by some individuals with an ASD seem to suggest that some group therapy experiences can indeed be useful, notably dialectical behaviour therapy that aims to promote positive coping and change unhelpful behaviours through recognising the cognitive and emotional triggers that increase stress.

Evidence for individual psychological work to address offending behaviours also remains at an early stage of evaluation. Whilst cognitive behaviour therapy (CBT) adapted for any cognitive and communication difficulties has been found to be a useful intervention with adults who have an ASD (e.g. Gaus 2007; Hare 2013), there has been limited exploration of how the approach can address offence-specific behaviours. Personal experience with several individuals has found that if a CBT approach is used to address risk or criminological issues among offenders with an ASD (such as improving victim empathy and an appreciation of consequences), there is a need to identify clear realistic goals and make specific further adaptations allowing for the presence of any cognitive, communication, sensory and emotional regulation difficulties, as well as any co-morbid psychiatric disorder (Murphy 2010). For many individuals, 'personalised' education about ASD can also be helpful as a way of improving an individual's understanding of his or her past and current difficulties. For example, one individual described to me being able to 'outthink' his ASD as a result of being aware of what his difficulties had been in the past.

However, whilst many individuals with an ASD do respond to individual psychological interventions (such as developing general problem-solving skills, working on basic social inference skills, encouraging appropriate assertiveness, reducing individual social anxieties, shifting preoccupations and obsessive thoughts, negative ruminations as well as developing perspective taking skills), it may be unrealistic to expect significant changes in cognitive style compared to other offenders who do not have an ASD. Engagement with those individuals who present with significant egocentricity, who take limited personal responsibility and reject their diagnosis, can be particularly problematic. Indeed, Hare (2013) has suggested that a primary goal in CBT with ASD is not to focus on cognitive changes but more to concentrate on behavioural changes which increase an individual's ability to function in everyday life, whilst being aware of difficulties in challenging dysfunctional cognitions and beliefs that may be present. For many individuals, there is also a role for pharmacological interventions that can assist with anxiety and co-morbid psychiatric disorder. Other activities including occupational therapy and further education can also have a very positive impact on social inclusion, self-esteem as well as opportunities to learn new skills.

As with all forensic patients, risk formulation and subsequent management are probably the most important aspect of care. For individuals with an ASD who offend, there is a strong argument that conventional risk assessment tools do not capture the difficulties associated with having an ASD and that may increase vulnerability towards offending. There may therefore be a need for good practice guidelines that clinicians can refer to when assessing and formulating risk for future reoffending within this group (Murphy 2013).

11.11 Summary

Whilst there is no robust evidence to suggest that individuals with an ASD are more likely to offend compared to other individuals in the general population or to commit particular crimes, there is a small but diverse group of vulnerable individuals who might engage in behaviours that can be at odds with social convention and which bring them into contact with the CJS. Experience suggests that although the relative seriousness of the offences committed by the majority of individuals is low, rather rare, unusual and extreme forms of offending can sometimes occur resulting in tragic consequences for all. It is these cases that attract media attention and which likely result in a stereotypical, distorted and confused misrepresentation of any link between ASD and crime. Research evidence and experience also suggest that the underlying precipitating factors for offending are typically due to a combination of cognitive, communication, sensory and emotional regulation difficulties (and sometimes preoccupations) that interact with a particular set of life circumstances. Understanding an individual's difficulties allows for more informed risk assessment and management interventions. However, an area of everyday functioning that would appear relevant in addressing some offending behaviour, but which is poorly understood in ASD, is how decisions are made and whether the same heuristics (the psychological processes that allow us to make choices and judgements) that influence non-ASD individuals apply. Some research has suggested that individuals with an ASD have difficulties making decisions (e.g. Luke et al. 2012), as well as making behavioural choices that are less influenced by information about reward contingencies (e.g. Damiano et al. 2012).

Whilst uncertainty with the exact number of individuals who have contact with the CJS makes commissioning of specialist forensic ASD services difficult, this does not make the position of those with an ASD who do present with difficulties that challenge mainstream services any less significant. It is also important to recognise that this group of individuals can be extremely diverse with regard to their circumstances and presenting difficulties, as well as an individual's position within the CJS not necessarily being fixed. For example, individuals can move between being supervised in the community by probation services and having a custodial sentence in prison or be detained in the different levels of the forensic psychiatric system. With reference to individuals with an ASD detained in high-secure psychiatric care or any secure forensic facility, whilst they may be considered at the higher end of the continuum of risk, they can enter via prison and leave through lower-security units to eventually community services. Future research should therefore be based on an individual's presenting difficulties rather than position within the CJS. Once within the CJS, the experiences of individuals can also vary. Whilst many individuals report positive environments and therapeutic interventions, some report negative experiences and services that fail to understand their difficulties. We need to learn from all these individuals to develop ASD-sensitive services and relevant interventions. Although the efficacy of most psychologically based interventions and programmes that address offending remains to be established for this population group, an effective and achievable way of making a real difference is greater ASD awareness among all professionals who might encounter individuals with an ASD.

Finally, whilst more collaborative multiservice research would be extremely informative in establishing numbers and identifying potential subgroups, it should also not be forgotten that because every individual with an ASD is unique, case analysis remains equally important. Much can be learnt from case studies on how to formulate individual difficulties, risks and needs, as well as provide guidance as to what has been or what might be therapeutically helpful. Ultimately our aim should be to identify and, where possible, to encourage, from a young age, key resilience or 'protective' factors that help an individual from offending or having contact with the CJS.

References

Allen D, Evans C, Hider A, Hawkins S, Peckett H, Morgan H (2008) Offending behaviour in adults with Asperger's syndrome. J Autism Dev Disord 38:748–758

Allely C, Minnis H, Thompson L, Wilson P, Gillberg C (2014) Neurodevelopmental and psychosocial factors in serial killers and mass murderers. Aggress Violent Behav 19:288–301

Barry-Walsh JB, Mullen P (2004) Forensic aspects of asperger's syndrome. J Forensic Psychiatry Psychol 15(1):96–107

Bjørkly S (2009) Risk and dynamics of violence in Asperger's syndrome: a systematic review of the literature. Aggress Violent Behav 14:306–312

Berryessa C (2014a) Judicial perceptions of media portrayals of offenders with high functioning autistic spectrum disorders. Int J Criminol Sociol 3:45–60

Berryessa C (2014b) Judiciary views on criminal behaviour and intention of offenders with high functioning autism. J Intellect Disabil Offending Behav 5(2):97–106

Berney T (2004) Asperger's syndrome from childhood into adulthood. Adv Psychiatr Treat 10:341–351

Chesterman L, Rutter S (1993) Case report: asperger's syndrome and sexual offending. J Forensic Psychiatry 4:555–562

Cooper S, Mohamed W, Collacott R (1993) Possible Asperger's syndrome in a mentally handicapped transvestite offender. J Intellect Disabil Res 37:189–194

Crocombe J, Mills R, Wing L (2006) Autism spectrum disorders amongst the female population of one special hospital. National Autistic Society, London

Damiano C, Aloi J, Treadway M, Bodfish J, Ditcher G (2012) Adults with autism disorders exhibit decreased sensitivity to reward parameters when making effort based decisions. J Neurodev Disord 4:13 Retrieved from www.jneurodevdisorders.com/content/4/1/1.

Debbaudt D (2002) Autism, advocates, and law enforcement professionals: recognising and reducing risk situations for people with autism spectrum disorders. Jessica Kingsley Publishers, London/Philadelphia

Dworzynsky K, Ronald A, Bolton P, Happé F (2012) How different are girls and boys above and below the diagnostic threshold for autism spectrum disorders? J Am Acad Child Adolesc Psychiatry 51(8):788–797

Fitzgerald M (2003) Callous/Unemotional traits and Asperger's syndrome? J Am Acad Child Adolesc Psychiatry 42(9):1011

Freckleton I (2011) Asperger's syndrome and criminal law. J Law Med 18:677–694

Frith U (1991) Autistic Psychopathy in childhood. In: Autism and Asperger syndrome . Cambridge University Press, Cambridge/New YorkChapter 2

Gaus V (2007) Cognitive behaviour therapy for adults with Asperger's syndrome. Guildford Press, New York/London

Ghaziuddin M, Tsai L, Ghaziuddin N (1991) Brief report: violence in Asperger's syndrome: a critique. J Autism Dev Disord 21:349–354

Gómez de la Cuesta G (2010) A selective review of offending behaviour in individuals with autism spectrum disorders. J Learn Disabil Offending Behav 1(2):47–58

Gould J, Ashton-Smith J (2011) Missed diagnosis or misdiagnosis? girls and women on the autism spectrum. Good Autism Pract 12(1):34–34

Hare D (2013) Developing psychotherapeutic interventions for people with autism spectrum disorders. In: Taylor JL, Lindsay WR, Hasting RP, Hatton C (eds) Psychological therapies for adults with intellectual disabilities. John Wiley & Sons, Chichester, pp 193–206

Hare D, Gould J, Mills R, Wing L (1999) A preliminary study of individuals with autistic spectrum disorders in three special hospitals in England. National Autistic Society, London

Hare R (1999) Psychopathy as a risk factor for violence. Psychiatry Q 70:181–197

Hare R (2003) Hare psychopathy checklist revised (PCL – R), 2 edn. MHS, North Tonawanda

Haskins B, Silva A (2006) Asperger's disorder and criminal behaviour: forensic psychiatric considerations. J Am Acad Psychiatry Law 34(3):374–384

Higgs T, Carter A (2015) Autism spectrum disorder and sexual offending: responsivity in forensic interventions. Aggress Violent Behav 22:112–119

Hipper K, Viding E, Klicpera C, Happé F (2009) Brief report: no increase in criminal convictions in Hans Asperger's original cohort. J Autism Dev Disord 40(6):774–780

Howlin P (1997) Autism: preparing for adulthood. Routledge, London

Huw J, Jones R (2010) Missing voices: representations of autism in British Newspapers, 1999-2008. Br J Learn Disabil 39:98. doi:10.1111/1468-3156.2010.00624

King C, Murphy G (2014) A systematic review of people with autism spectrum disorder and the criminal justice system. J Autism Dev Disord 44:2717–2733

Kohn Y, Fahum T, Ratzoni G, Apter A (1998) Aggression and sexual offending in Asperger's syndrome. Isr J Psychiatry Relat Sci 35(4):293–299

Kugmagami T, Matsuura N (2009) Prevalence of pervasive developmental disorder in juvenile court cases in Japan. J Forensic Psychiatry Psychol 20(6):974–987

Långstrom N, Grann M, Ruchkin V, Sjöstedt G, Fazel S (2009) Risk factors for violent offending in autism spectrum disorder: a national study of hospitalised individuals. J Interpers Violence 24:1358–1370

Lerner M, Haque O, Northrup E, Lawer L, Bursztajn H (2012) Emerging perspectives on adolescents and young adults with high functioning autism spectrum disorders, violence and criminal law. J Am Acad Psychiatry Law 40(2):177–189
Lewis A, Pritchet R, Hughes C, Turner K (2013) Development and implementation of autism standards for prisons. J Intellect Disabil Offending Behav 6(2):68–80
Luke L, Clare I, Ring H, Redley M, Watson P (2012) Decision making difficulties experienced by adults with autism spectrum conditions. Autism 16:612–621
Lyons A (2000) Examining media representations: benefits for health psychology. J Health Psychol 5:349–358
Maras K, Bowler D (2010) The cognitive interview for eyewitnesses with autism spectrum disorder. J Autism Dev Disord 40(11):1350–1360
Maras K, Bowler D (2012) Brief report: suggestibility, compliance and psychological traits in high functioning adults with autism spectrum disorder. Res Autism Spectr Disord 6(3): 1168–1175
Maras K, Bowler D (2014) Eyewitness testimony in autism spectrum disorders: a review. J Autism Dev Disord 44(1):2682–2692
Mawson D, Grounds A, Tantum D (1985) Violence and Asperger's syndrome: a case study. Br J Psychiatry 147:566–569
Milton J, Duggan C, Latham A, Egan V, Tantum D (2002) Case history of co-morbid Asperger's Syndrome and paraphilic behaviour. Med Sci Law 42(3):237–244
Mourisden S, Rich B, Torrben R, Nedergaard N (2008) Pervasive developmental disorders and criminal behaviour. Int J Offender Ther Comp Criminol 52(2):196–205
Mundy S & Murphy D (2003). Comparison of the cognitive, mentalisation and demographic profiles of a forensic and non-forensic sample of men with Asperger's syndrome. In partial fulfilment of an MSc in Forensic Psychology, University of Surrey
Murrie DC, Warren JI, Kristiansson M, Dietz PE (2002) Asperger's Syndrome in forensic settings. Int J Forensic Ment Health 1(1):59–70
Murphy D (2003) Admission and cognitive details of male patients diagnosed with Asperger's syndrome detained in a special hospital: comparison with a schizophrenia and personality disorder sample. J Forensic Psychiatry Psychol 14:506–524
Murphy D (2007a) Theory of mind and its relationship to clinical outcome, need and risk in mentally disordered offenders detained in high security psychiatric care. Crim Behav Ment Health 17:300–311
Murphy D (2007b) Hare PCL-R profiles of male patients with Asperger's Syndrome detained in high security psychiatric care. J Forensic Psychiatry Psychol 18(1):120–126
Murphy D (2010) Extreme violence in a man with an autistic spectrum disorder: assessment and treatment within high security psychiatric care. J Forensic Psychiatry Psychol 21(3): 462–477
Murphy D (2011). Computers and Autism - Computers; blessing or a curse? Research Autism Conference. Westminster, London, December, 2011
Murphy D (2013) Risk assessment of offenders with autism spectrum disorder. J Intellect Disabil Offending Behav 4(1/2):33
Murphy D (2014) Self-reported anger among individuals with an autism spectrum disorder detained in high security psychiatric care. J Forensic Psychiatry Psychol 25(1):100–112
Murphy D, McMorrow K (2015) Views of autism and training needs of staff working in high security psychiatric care. J Forensic Pract 17(3):231–240
Murphy D, Mullens H. (2017) Examining the experiences and quality of life of patients with an autism spectrum disorder in high secure psychiatric care. Advances in Autism 3(1):3–14
Myers F (2004) On the borderline? People with learning disabilities and or autistic spectrum disorders in secure, forensic and other specialist settings. Scottish Executive. Research Findings, Health and Community Care
National Autistic Society (2005) Autism: a guide for criminal justice professionals. National Autistic Society, London
Newman S, Ghaziuddin M (2008) Violent crime in Asperger's syndrome: the role of psychiatric co-morbidity. J Autism Dev Disord 38:1848–1852

North A, Russell A, Gudjonsson G (2008) High functioning autism spectrum disorders. An investigation of psychological vulnerabilities during interrogative interviews. J Forensic Psychol Psychiatry 19:323–334

Patterson P (2007) How well do young offenders with Asperger's syndrome cope in custody? Two prison case studies. Br J Learn Disabil 36:54–58

Palermo M (2004) Pervasive developmental disorders, psychiatric co morbidities and the law. Int J Offender Ther Comp Criminol 48:40–48

Philo G (1997) Changing media representations of mental health. Psychiatr Bull R Coll Psychiatry 21:171–172

Prison Reform Trust. (2006). Bromley briefings Prison fact file. Prison Reform Trust London. EC1V OJR.

Robertson C, McGillivray J (2015) Autism behind bars: a review of the research literature and discussion of key issues. J Forensic Psychiatry Psychol 26:719

Rogers J, Viding E, Blair J, Frith U, Happé F (2006) Autism spectrum disorder and psychopathy: shared cognitive underpinnings or double hit? Psychol Med 36:1789–1798

Scragg P, Shah A (1994) Prevalence of Asperger's syndrome in a secure hospital. Br J Psychiatry 165:679–682

Silva A, Ferrari M, Leong G (2004) The case of Jeffrey Dahmer: sexual serial homicide from a neuropsychiatric developmental perspective. J Forensic Sci 47:1347–1359

Siponmaa L, Kristianssson M, Jonson C, Nyden A, Gillberg C (2001) Juvenile and young adult mentally disordered offenders: the role of child neuropsychiatric disorders. J Am Acad Psychiatry Law 29(4):420–426

Tantum D (2012) Autism spectrum disorders through the lifespan. Jessica Kingsley Publishers, London/Philadelphia

Wahlund K, Kristiansson M (2006) Offender characteristics in lethal violence with special reference to anti-social and autistic personality traits. J Interpers Violence 21:115–130

Wing L (1981) Asperger's syndrome: a clinical account. Psychol Med 11:115–129

Wing L (1997) Asperger's syndrome: management requires diagnosis. J Forensic Psychiatry 2(8):253–257

Wolff S (1995) Loners: the life path of unusual children. Routledge, London

Wolff S, Chick J (1980) Schizoid personality in childhood: a controlled follow up study. Psychol Med 10:85–100

Wolff S, McGuire R (1995) Schizoid personality in girls: a follow up study – what are the links with Asperger's syndrome? J Child Psychol Psychiatry 36:793–817

Woodbury Smith M, Clare I, Holland A, Kearns A, Staufenberg E, Watson P (2005) A case control study of offenders with high functioning autistic spectrum disorders. J Forensic Psychiatry Psychol 16(4):747–763

Woodbury Smith M, Clare I, Holland A, Kearns A (2006) High functioning autistic spectrum disorders, offending and other law breaking: findings from a community sample. J Forensic Psychiatry Psychol 17(1):108–120

Woodbury Smith M, Clare I, Holland A, Watson P, Bambrick M, Kearns A, Staufenberg E (2010) Circumscribed interests and offenders with autism spectrum disorders: a case control study. J Forensic Psychiatry Psychol 21(3):366–377

Index

B. Barahona Corrêa, R.-J. van der Gaag (eds.), *Autism Spectrum Disorders in Adults*, DOI 10.1007/978-3-319-42713-3

MIX
Papier aus verantwortungsvollen Quellen
Paper from responsible sources
FSC® C105338

If you have any concerns about our products,
you can contact us on
ProductSafety@springernature.com

In case Publisher is established outside the EU,
the EU authorized representative is:
Springer Nature Customer Service Center GmbH
Europaplatz 3, 69115 Heidelberg, Germany

Printed by Libri Plureos GmbH
in Hamburg, Germany